THE
CEREBRAL
COMPUTER

An Introduction to the Computational Structure of the Human Brain

ROBERT J. BARON

The University of Iowa

 LAWRENCE ERLBAUM, ASSOCIATES, PUBLISHERS

1987   Hillsdale, New Jersey   London

Lawrence Erlbaum Associates, Inc., Publishers
365 Broadway
Hillsdale, New Jersey 07642

Library of Congress Cataloging in Publication Data

Baron, Robert J.
The cerebral computer.

Includes bibliographies and index.
1. Human information processing. I. Title. [DNLM:
1. Brain—physiology. WL 300 B265c]
QP398.B37 1987 612'.82 87-6738
ISBN 0-89859-824-9

Printed in the United States of America
10 9 8 7 6 5 4 3 2

For all students of brain function

CONTENTS

PREFACE

The human brain is the most complex and powerful computer known. It has been studied intensively for decades and has been the subject of thousands of books, tens of thousands of journal articles, hundreds of university courses, and even several television specials. Among the computational processes that have been investigated are memory, learning, language, visual and auditory perception and recognition, analogical reasoning, thought, attention, planning, and the control of movement. These studies have provided valuable insights into the computational nature of the brain.

However, even with all the advances in our understanding of human information processing, and even with our ever-increasing knowledge of computations in general, including the organization of knowledge, the nature of algorithmic processes and theoretical limits on computability, the human brain continues to elude our understanding. Among the reasons for this elusiveness are its incredible complexity, the redundancy of its circuitry and the variety of different ways that have evolved to reach the same computational goals. Because all of the computational processes which can be brought to bear on a particular problem seem to operate at the same time, the study of any one of them is difficult at best.

Recent investigations, particularly over the past three decades, have markedly increased our understanding of the human brain. Anatomical studies have given us detailed knowledge of the structure of various networks and the connections between them. Combined with clinical investigations, these studies have given major insights into the computations they perform. Clinical investigations, in particular, have characterized abnormalities resulting from localized brain damage. These abnormalities include deteriorated visual, auditory and tactile recognition, impaired language understanding and production, and abnormal planning and control of movement. Each syndrome gives considerable insight into the computational structure of the brain. Particularly with the advent of noninvasive techniques for determining the focus of damage, researchers are now able to determine the locations of the neural systems which are responsible for the underlying pathology. Neurobiological and neurophysiological investigations have also provided us with information regarding the computations of the various networks of the brain, and as a result, we are beginning to understand not only the biochemical mechanisms that underlie the computations but also details of the computations themselves.

The following excellent books have been written describing the human brain, its structure, its organization, and its function. I will therefore not introduce general topics which are so well presented elsewhere.

Nancy C. Andreasen (1984) *The broken brain.* **New York: Harper & Row.**
This book has an excellent introduction to the anatomy of the brain, and although its focus is on mental illness, the author describes recent techniques for the study of brain function.

Jack Fincher (1984) *The brain, mystery of matter and mind.* **New York: Torstar Books.**
This book has exceptionally nice illustrations of the anatomy of the brain but focuses mostly on topics of the mind: language, creativity, intelligence, feelings, and consciousness.

Dick Gilling and Robin Brightwell (1982) *The human brain.* **New York: Facts on File.**
This book is based on seven BBC-TV programs describing the human brain.

Bryan Kolb and Ian Q. Whishaw (1985) *Fundamentals of human neuropsychology* **(2nd ed.). New York: W. H. Freeman and Co.**
This excellent book presents both basic background information as well as clear, crisp, and thorough accounts of numerous clinical syndromes.

A. R. Luria (1973) *The working brain. An introduction to neuropsychology.* **New York: Basic Books.**
This book analyzes various clinical syndromes by showing how they result from damage to the underlying computational systems. Luria emphasizes the computational nature of the human brain.

Richard M. Restak (1984) *The brain.* **New York: Bantam Books.**
This book is based on the eight-part PBS television series "The Brain."

J. P. Schadé and Donald H. Ford (1965) *Basic neurology. An introduction to the structure and function of the nervous system.* **New York: Elsevier.**
This textbook presents excellent introductions to four significant areas: neuroanatomy, neurophysiology, neurochemistry, and neuropsychology.

Anthony Smith (1984) *The mind.* **New York: Viking Press.**
This book presents excellent introductions to the evolution, anatomy, and growth of the brain, in addition to overviews of consciousness, the senses, and ability.

The study of brain function is an interdisciplinary endeavor. My formal training was in mathematics, physics and computer science, but my goal, ever since I began to study the brain in 1966, was to understand how it represents and processes information. This endeavor has forced me to read the literature and talk to researchers in disciplines quite distant from my own. Breaking into an established discipline means learning a new vocabulary and new way of thinking. The process can be overwhelming. One goal, then, in writing this book is to summarize in one place the anatomical, physiological, and clinical facts which are essential for understanding the computational architecture of the brain. I hope to encourage new researchers to study the brain, particularly those individuals with strong mathematical and theoretical talents. Perhaps my effort will keep them from naïvely assuming properties of the brain which simply do not exist. For example, many theorists in the past have studied models of neural assemblies comprised of neurons which are connected together at random. Fortunately, the brain is not built that way, and we have come too far in understanding its structure to condone such naïve assumptions. Chapters in which I have presented fairly standard background material include Chapter 1 (neurons), Chapter 6 (memory), Chapter 7 (the visual system), Chapter 10 (the auditory system), Chapter 12 (the sensory-motor system), and the second half of Chapter 13 (the tactile and vestibular systems).

The principal goal of the book is to describe the computational structure and organization of the human brain. The theories presented here are, for the most part, mine although some have been improved by my students. Many of the ideas have been presented elsewhere as formal models, and several of them are included as appendixes to the appropriate chapters. Much of the material is new and under current investigation. For example, Scott Zimmerman and I are just now completing computer simulation studies of various parts of the movement control system discussed in Chapters 14 and 15, and Bryant Julstrom has just completed computer simulation studies of a model of parts of the spatial system, including spatial memory and the object buffers. We have not yet begun to simulate the body profile system described in Chapter 13, however.

The focus throughout this book is on information processing, but I will pay particular attention to information storage. Information storage is, after all, fundamental to virtually all intelligent activity. The first six chapters develop the theoretical framework needed for understanding the computational nature of the brain. Among the topics explored are the nature of information and the structures and functions of storage networks, information pathways, and information-encoding and transforming networks.

Chapter 1 describes the neuron, the basic computational element of the brain. Various properties of neurons are discussed, including the different logical operations they must perform and how they are organized into neural networks. The appendix to Chapter 1 presents a mathematical model for the neuron as a computational element.

Chapter 2 focuses on information and its characteristics. After all, neural networks store, transform, and transmit information, so an understanding of the nature of information is essential. Finally, several types of neural networks are introduced. These networks are components of many of the systems described later in the book.

Chapters 3 and 4 focus on information storage networks and their control. Chapter 3 describes the architecture of a typical associative storage network. It is described both in terms of its input, output and control functions and in terms of its internal organization: It is composed of numerous independent storage locations. The appendix to Chapter 3 presents a model for cortical storage.

Associative storage networks are crucial to brain function. Associative storage networks translate information from one representation to another. When we see a familiar object, we can name it. When we want to move a finger, we can move it. In the first case a visual representation is translated into a symbolic representation; in the second case a high-level intention is translated into a motor program. Both operations are performed by associative storage networks. Associative storage networks generate representations whose temporal characteristics are better suited to the next stage of processing than the previous representations. Phonemes vary rapidly as a function of time, words vary more slowly, ideas more slowly yet. Associative memory stores generate representations of phonemes from auditory patterns, representations of words from phoneme patterns, and representations of ideas from word patterns. While each representation varies more slowly than the previous one, it also lasts a lot longer. Each representation has vastly different temporal characteristics than the previous representation, which makes it more suitable for the next stage of processing. Chapter 5 lays the foundation for understanding these and other encoding and translating mechanisms.

Chapters 6 through 11 have a different flavor from the first five chapters. Whereas the first five chapters present issues of a conceptual or theoretical nature, Chapters 6 through 11 discuss particular sensory and storage systems and the representations they use.

Chapter 6 describes selected aspects of human memory and presents evidence that information is indeed stored by the human brain in storage systems of the type described in the previous chapters. It also shows that there are many different storage systems which differ from one another in structure, organization, function, trace permanence (immediate, temporary or permanent), trace time constants (rapidly varying to slowly varying) and pattern size (from a few elements to tens of millions of elements).

Chapters 7 through 9 focus on the visual system. Chapter 7 describes the low-level visual encodings and the networks which perform them. As you will see, the visual system extracts specific low-level features from the visual field and creates a set of storage representations which encode the world and objects in it. These storage representations use codes which enable the storage systems to locate related stored information. Chapters 8 and 9 describe high-level visual representations, including storage representations of visual experience, representations of mental images, and representations of the world and objects in it. Chapter 9 focuses on the permanent visual storage systems and describes how visual experiences can be recognized and how memories of visual experiences can be mentally scanned.

Chapter 10 describes the auditory system and draws parallels between auditory and visual processes. The nature of stored auditory experiences is explored.

Chapter 11 presents an introduction to understanding. We understand an utterance, gesture, or situation when we know how to respond to it. That is, we understand when we are able to control our mental and physical apparatus to process all appropriate information, both current and stored, and decide what to do. (Understanding does not mean that we will respond, however.) Mental procedures are one high-level encoding of knowledge and I show in Chapter 11 that understanding means we recall from memory or generate a mental procedure which, when executed, appropriately controls our response to the situation. A final section briefly suggests the minimum computational circuitry needed for a system to learn to use natural language.

Chapter 12, the first chapter that deals with the control of movement, describes muscle tissue and the anatomy of the sensory-motor system. This chapter lays the foundation for understanding how high-level intentions control actions.

Chapters 13 through 15 have a notably different flavor from previous chapters and describe a framework for understanding the control of movement. The ideas presented in these chapters are under current investigation and lack many details. Nonetheless, enough details are presented to show in principle how we control movements.

Chapter 16 describes the affect system and suggests how affects influence high-level decisions. The neural networks that process affects are only beginning to be understood so this chapter serves to introduce affects and their relationship to purposive behavior. The computations that underlie decision making differ from those which underlie sensory and motor processing, and this chapter illustrates the nature of the differences.

The final chapter attempts to organize the material presented in the previous 16 chapters. Networks introduced earlier in the book are grouped into the sensory, symbolic, and purposive systems according to the types of information they process. The spatial system deals with space, objects, the body, and physical interactions between them, and it maintains all the representations used for recognizing and manipulating objects, navigating, controlling locomotion, and so forth. The symbolic system creates and processes symbolic information and is responsible for natural language processing (recognition and production of speech, writing, reading, etc.), mathematical and logical thought, planning, and game-playing, to name a few. The purposive system makes all high-level decisions and ultimately controls itself and the spatial and symbolic systems. The purposive system includes the affect system which, when we are born, is controlled by innate (prewired) capabilities. All three systems work closely together for much of what we do, and some of the interactions between them are discussed. Finally, this chapter suggests how the brain learns to accept and process information. I conclude by reviewing Piaget's stages of cognitive development and relating them to the computational networks already described.

Although I have attempted to convey the computational nature of the human brain, in fact I have only laid the groundwork for that understanding. Almost nothing presented here is known for certain and our knowledge of the computational systems is just beginning to accumulate. When trying to understand how the brain works as a computer, and therefore how computations are implemented in neural circuitry, it is clear that we know very little. We know almost nothing about how the brain processes natural language, logical thought, musical thought, mathematical thought, concepts, or intuitions. We know almost nothing about how the brain encodes beliefs, dreams, hopes, desires, pleasure, pride, or self-esteem. We know almost nothing about how the brain generates plans. We know almost nothing about how the brain represents will, inclination, motive, purpose, or choice. Even with respect to sensory encoding, which is perhaps the best understood aspect of brain function, we are certain about almost nothing. We do not know how many different representations are generated and kept about the world or the objects in it. We do not know how physical properties of objects are represented. We do not know what types of coordinate systems the brain uses, nor do we know how it determines coordinates and uses them. We do not know how the brain translates between coordinate systems.

On the other hand, we are at least beginning to ask the right questions. We are beginning to understand how storage systems store, recognize, and recall information. We are beginning to understand the relationships between storage control, access control, and learning. We are beginning to understand how the low-level sensory networks create canonical representations for storage and what the organizations are within storage. We are beginning to understand the relationships between time and information encoding and modality. We are beginning to understand how recognition and perception occur. We will only understand human thought in general when we understand the underlying structures and representations used by the human brain, and this study is, I hope, a start in that direction.

Robert J. Baron

SUGGESTED READINGS

The following readings are of a general nature and are excellent sources for additional background information.

Clarke, E. & O'Malley, C. D. (1968). *The human brain and spinal cord. A historical study illustrated by writings from antiquity to the twentieth century.* Berkeley, CA: University of California Press.

Pribram, K. H. (1971). *Languages of the brain: Experimental paradoxes and principles in neuropsychology.* Englewood Cliffs, NJ: Prentice-Hall.

Restak, R. M. (1979). *The brain. The last frontier.* Garden City, NY: Doubleday.

Rock, I. (1984). *Perception.* New York: Scientific American Books, an imprint of W. H. Freeman and Co.

Russell, P. (1979). *The brain book.* New York: Hawthorne Books.

Scientific American (1979). *The brain. A Scientific American book.* San Francisco: W. H. Freeman and Co.

Wooldridge, D. E. (1963). *The machinery of the brain.* New York: McGraw-Hill.

ACKNOWLEDGMENTS

Many people have contributed to this book in one way or another. My uncle and dedicated teacher, Alexander Brodell, first stimulated my interest in science and art; his influence is immeasurable. My mentor, Henry David Block, a true educator and gentle man, introduced me to mathematical modeling and to the study of brain function. He, more than anyone else, showed me the importance of formal thinking in interdisciplinary research. This book is in memory of them both.

I am also greatly indebted to many individuals who helped me in the final preparation of the book. My son Robert and Heidi Fink did much of the original artwork, and the staff of Kinko's in Iowa City courteously helped me with the figures on a daily basis. My students Bryant Julstrom and Scott Zimmermann, and my friends Richard Fink and John Huntley gave me many valuable editorial suggestions. Harry Whitaker, David Waltz, Dana Ballard, Steven Kosslyn, and Tim Teyler reviewed the manuscript and made suggestions which greatly improved its quality. Thank you all very much. Finally, I am deeply grateful to all the authors and publishers who allowed me to reproduce their figures and illustrations. This book benefited greatly because of your generosity. I, alone, take credit for any errors or misinterpretations of the literature.

1

NEURONS:
THE COMPUTATIONAL
CELLS OF BRAINS

INTRODUCTION

The fundamental assumption that underlies this entire presentation is that the brain is a computer. It is comprised of some hundred billion computational cells called **nerve cells** or **neurons**, which interact in a variety of ways. This chapter will focus on neurons and how they interact with one another.

The brain is highly structured, with its major anatomical connections specified genetically. Some connections appear to be regulated by sensory stimulation early in life, but the extent to which the brain's architecture is determined by sensory stimulation is only beginning to be understood. In any event, once the physical connections between neurons have been established, they appear to remain fixed for the life of the system.

NEURAL NETWORKS AND THEIR ANALYSIS

Neurons are organized into well-defined and highly structured computational networks called **neural networks**. Neural networks are the principal computational systems of the brain and there are many types, including receptor networks, encoding and decoding networks, storage networks, and control networks. Many of them have been studied anatomically and have a well-known structure or **architecture**, and many also have a well-understood computational role. It is more often the case, however, that the brain's computational networks, which are sometimes called "nuclei," "centers," or "bodies" by anatomists, have been studied anatomically with their specific computational role not yet being understood. In many cases, certain computational networks are predicted but their anatomical location and structure are not known.

Each neural network receives inputs through specific input pathways, process

1

them in a well-defined way, and responds to them through specific output pathways in a manner that depends on current and past inputs. The ultimate goal of this research is to understand all computational activity of the brain in terms of these constituent networks, how they interact with one another, and for receptor networks, how they react to the environment. We are a long way from achieving this goal.

There are many facets to understanding the human brain and its computations. At the most elemental level we seek to understand the mechanisms of the nerve cell. In time, neural interactions will be understood in terms of cell structure, metabolic activity, transport mechanisms, and so forth, and this level of understanding should lead to descriptions of the networks in which both the statistical properties of the nerve cells (spike train statistics) and the electrical activity (presynaptic and postsynaptic potentials, refractory periods, synaptic delays, axonal conduction, etc.) will be quantitatively related to the activities of other neurons and nonneural elements (notably glial cells) that make inputs to the networks. This level of understanding will not be discussed at any depth here.

At a somewhat less elemental level we seek to understand the **logical** interconnections of small groups of cells. We seek to understand their input–output or **computational** behavior in terms of the activities of their cells. This is the black box level of modeling, and there are two different methodologies for studying neural networks at this level. One is to select a particular biological network to study, model the structure and interactions of its neurons, and determine by suitable mathematical analysis or computer simulation how the model network behaves. The validity of the model is then checked by comparing its computed properties with the corresponding properties of the biological system as determined experimentally. This methodology is generally adopted by the theoretical biologist when modeling networks such as the nervous system of the crayfish, the eye of the cat, the retina of the frog, the olfactory bulb, and the cerebellum. A second methodology is to define the desired input–output properties of a network and determine what types of neural interactions and structures are required to realize the desired behavior. Within this methodology, experimental and anatomical considerations are generally used to constrain the models. This is the approach I have adopted for studying information processing in the brain, including learning, visual and auditory recognition, information storage and memory, natural language processing, the control of movement, and the affect systems.

The most general level at which one can study brain function is in terms of its component information-processing networks and interactions between them. Thus one may consider a system that contains a receptor network (retina, cochlea, etc.), information-transforming networks, memory stores, adaptive control networks, and so on, without considering in detail the underlying neural activity. This is the system level of modeling. At this level of analysis one looks primarily at the psychological (behavioral) properties of the entire system in terms of its architecture—its functional components and their organization.

NEURONS

Since the primary concern throughout this book will be with the computational nature of the human brain, I will begin with an overview of the neuron and neural interactions. Two facts should temper this discussion. First, there is an enormous variety of neurons in the brain, with fundamental differences in morphology (structure), patterns of connections, and the way that neurons send and receive information. (See for example my discussions on the retina, the superior olive, and the cerebellum later in this book.) This discussion attempts to convey only those features that are common to most types of neurons—the average neuron, so to speak. Second, our current knowledge of neural interactions is limited in many respects, and although there is a large body of knowledge about certain aspects of neural interactions, other aspects are virtually unknown. This discussion describes only those aspects which are best understood.

A neuron consists of four parts essential to our understanding: the **cell body** or **soma**, **dendrites**, an **axon**, and **axon branches**, **collaterals**, or **terminal fibers**. See Figure 1.1. Dendrites are filamentous extensions of the soma which branch many times in the region surrounding the soma, forming the **dendrite tree**. The region in space occupied by the dendrite tree of a neuron is its **dendrite field**. The soma and dendrite tree are the receptors of signals from other neurons. A single axon originates at the soma, extends some distance, and divides often many times into a set of axon collaterals. The place on the soma where the axon originates is the **axon hillock**. Some axon collaterals progress to other parts of the brain where they divide even further before contacting other neurons. The regions in space occupied by the axon collaterals of a neuron are its **axon fields**. Each terminal fiber ends in a **synaptic button**, which almost contacts a dendrite branch or soma of another or the same neuron. Each such place of near-contact is called a **synapse**, and the space separating the two cells is called the **synaptic cleft**. See Figure 1.2. Synapses are essential for the information processing done by the neurons and will shortly be discussed in more detail.

A neuron normally maintains an ionic concentration gradient across its cell membrane, which produces an electric potential. When the membrane potential at the axon hillock is sufficiently disturbed, a self-sustaining **depolarization pulse** (sometimes called **impulse**, **pulse**, or **spike**) propagates along the axon and spreads throughout all axon collaterals. When the potential fluctuation caused by a depolarization pulse reaches a synapse, chemical transmitters are released. The chemical transmitters, which are ordinarily held in synaptic vesicles, are released and diffuse across the synaptic cleft to the cell membrane of the

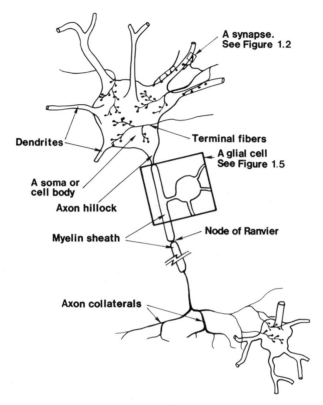

Figure 1.1   The structure of a typical neuron. Only a few of its synaptic contacts are shown.

postsynaptic neuron where they bind to receptor sites and may excite (tend to depolarize) or inhibit (tend to hyperpolarize) the postsynaptic cell. Within a short time after the chemical transmitters are released from the nerve endings, they are inactivated enzymatically, reabsorbed by the nerve terminals, or removed from the synaptic area by diffusion. The postsynaptic cell soon returns to its normal resting potential.

There are many different types of synapses as illustrated in Figure 1.3. Synapses of the type just described are axosomatic or axodendritic depending, on whether the contact is to a soma or dendrite. Axodendritic synapses may also terminate on specialized dendritic structures called dendritic spines, as illustrated at the top of the figure. Synapses between two axons are axoaxonic and those between two dendrites are dendrodendritic. Axosynaptic synapses, illustrated in the figure, are specialized structures often found in receptor networks; their intended computations are not yet understood. Finally, some synapses release chemical transmitters which control capillary constriction, muscle contraction (at structures called motor end plates) or in some unknown way the extracellular medium. The latter class of synapses are axoextracellular or free endings.

The influence that the presynaptic neuron has on the firing of a postsynaptic neuron is not exerted at one synapse alone but through many synaptic contacts that are distributed over parts or all of the soma or dendrite tree of the latter. The morphology of a neuron and the geometry and distribution of the contacts between itself and other neurons depends on the particular neuron and varies greatly between neurons in different parts of the brain. Figure 1.4 illustrates a few of the hundreds of varieties of neurons that can be found. Nonetheless, when a presynaptic neuron fires, the depolarization pulse causes the release of chemical transmitters at each of the synaptic contacts that it reaches. In this way one presynaptic cell may simultaneously influence thousands and perhaps tens of thousands of different postsynaptic cells, or in some cases only a single cell. The neurotransmitters that are released at a single synapse cause a slight fluctuation in the membrane potential of the postsynaptic cell in the region immediately surrounding the synapse, and these individual fluctuations spread from each focus of excitation. When a fluctuation arrives at the soma of the postsynaptic cell, its influence combines with all other influences that arrive at the same time from other focuses of excitation and may be of sufficient strength to initiate a pulse in the axon of the cell.

Although some neurons are contacted by a single presynaptic cell, most are contacted by many and often thousands of different presynaptic cells at thousands

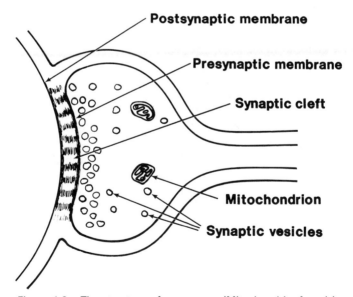

Figure 1.2.   The structure of a synapse. (Mitochondria, found in most cells, serve as the center of intracellular enzyme activity.)

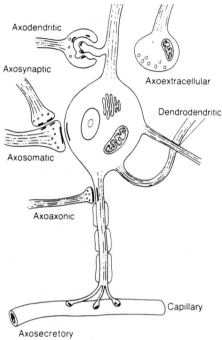

Axodendritic

Axosynaptic

Axoextracellular

Dendrodendritic

Axosomatic

Axoaxonic

Capillary

Axosecretory

Figure 1.3   Different types of synapses. (Reproduced, with permission, from B. Kolb & I. Q. Whishaw, *Fundamentals of Human Neuropsychology,* 2d ed. © 1985 by W. H. Freeman and Co.)

and perhaps tens of thousands of synapses. The fluctuations in the membrane potential at the soma, therefore, depend on the combined influence of all of the presynaptic cells. Furthermore, at a given synapse and at a particular moment of time, the effect of the neurotransmitters depends both on the quantity and type of neurotransmitter released. The magnitude of the resultant potential fluctuation in the postsynaptic cell also depends on the conductive properties of its dendrites, on the current state of the neuron's environment, on the current rate of cell metabolism, and on the presence of drugs, chemicals, and hormones which directly influence or regulate synaptic activity. At the present time there is not a single cell in a mammalian brain that is completely understood.

Although neurons are the logic elements of the brain, the brain consists of numerous other types of cells as well: blood vessels, connective and supporting tissue, and protective tissue. Within the brain, glial cells or glia occupy essentially all of the volume not occupied by neurons or blood vessels, and glia outnumber the nerve cells by an estimated 10 times. Glia provide both structural and metabolic support for the neurons and therefore directly influence neural activity. However, the way and the extent to which glia influence neural activity is not known in general.

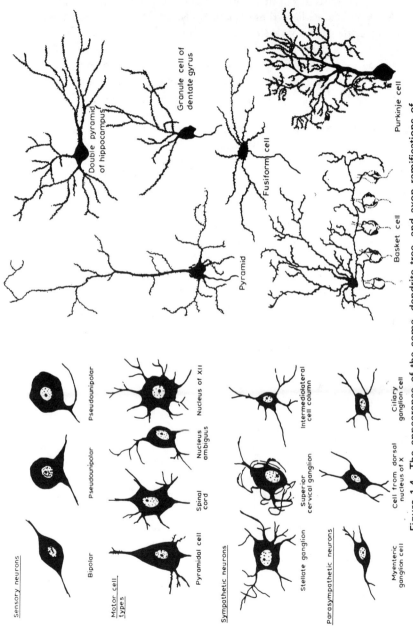

Figure 1.4 The appearance of the soma, dendrite tree, and axon ramifications of several types of neurons. (Reproduced, with permission, from J. P. Schadé & D.H. Ford, *Basic Neurology. An Introduction to the Structure and Function of the Nervous System.* © 1965 by Elsevier Biomedical Press.)

Double pyramid of hippocampus

Granule cell of dentate gyrus

Purkinje cell

Fusiform cell

Basket cell

Pyramid

Sensory neurons

Bipolar

Pseudounipolar

Pseudounipolar

Nucleus of XII

Nucleus ambiguus

Motor cell types

Pyramidal cell

Spinal cord

Intermediolateral cell column

Ciliary ganglion cell

Sympathetic neurons

Stellate ganglion

Superior cervical ganglion

Cell from dorsal nucleus of x

Parasympathetic neurons

Myenteric ganglion cell

Perhaps the oldest known and best-understood aspect of neural activity is the mechanism by which the cell membranes of neurons conduct potential fluctuations. As described earlier, these fluctuations, which result from synaptic activity, propagate away from each focus of excitation. Neural membranes are semipermeable to sodium and potassium ions and act as a pump, removing sodium ions from within the cell while pumping potassium ions into the cell. The cell membrane cannot be penetrated by most other components of intracellular fluids. The result of the pumping action is a potential gradient across the cell membrane of about 70 millivolts, negative inside the cell and positive outside. This is the cell's resting potential. A potential fluctuation at one region of the cell's membrane triggers a change in the conductance of neighboring regions to sodium and potassium ions. The stimulus trigger for the changing conductance is local current flow in the cell's membrane induced by the potential fluctuation. Sodium ions are first allowed to rush into the cell. This changes the membrane potential from approximately -70 millivolts to approximately $+40$ millivolts. A moment later potassium ions are allowed to rush out. The efflux of potassium ions restores the resting potential of the cell. After that, the cell membrane slowly expels the sodium ions and restores the potassium ions until the membrane once again reaches its resting potential.

For the axon of most neurons the situation is somewhat different. Most axons are surrounded by an insulating sheath of myelin, which is a sheet-like extension of one type of glial cell known as an oligodendrocyte. See Figure 1.5. The myelin sheath partly isolates the axon from the normal concentrations of ions found in most extracellular space and prevents the local currents from forming in the neural membrane. In fact, the potential fluctuation propagating into an axon would disappear entirely if it were not for one important fact. The myelin sheath is not continuous along the entire length of the axon but is interrupted every millimeter or so by a break called a node of Ranvier. The nodes of Ranvier are the gaps between myelin supplied by different glial cells. The only currents that can form pass through the nodes of Ranvier, and as a consequence, the potential fluctuations, the pulses, jump from node to node. Conduction in myelinated axons is called saltatory. A pulse entering one end of a myelinated axon essentially "jumps" from node to node until it reaches the other end of the axon, where the myelin sheath is no longer present. At that point the potential fluctuation is at its full strength. This accounts for the all-or-none conductive property of myelinated axons and enables one to characterize a nerve cell as "firing" or "conducting a pulse." The **rate of firing** of a cell is limited to about 1000 pulses per second because of the time constants of the underlying mechanism. Based on the all-or-none conductive property of axons, the firing rate of a neuron is taken to be the number of times its axon conducts a pulse per unit of time. Researchers often refer to spike train statistics when characterizing neural activity in this way.

In the peripheral nervous system, Schwann cells form the myelin sheaths around axons as shown in Figure 1.6.

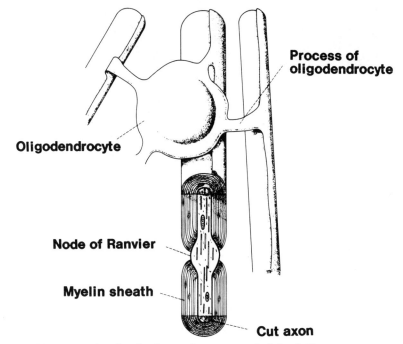

Process of oligodendrocyte

Oligodendrocyte

Node of Ranvier

Myelin sheath

Cut axon

Figure 1.5   An oligodendrocyte is one type of glial cell. The processes of the cell illustrated here form the myelin sheaths surrounding the axons of four different neurons of the central nervous system. The separations along an axon where two glial cells almost contact each other are the nodes of Ranvier. (Reproduced, with permission, from R. S. Snell, *Clinical Neuroanatomy for Medical Students.* © 1980 by Little, Brown, and Co.)

In summary, a neuron transmits information to other neurons along its axon in an all-or-none fashion. Depolarization pulses are generated at the soma, propagate along the axon and all collaterals, and release neurotransmitters which cause perturbations in the resting potentials of all postsynaptic cells. These cells integrate the effects of all arriving potential fluctuations and fire accordingly.

OTHER TYPES OF NEURAL ACTIVITY

Nonspiking Neurons

The "spiking" or "depolarization" of a neuron is generally associated with axonal conduction in myelinated axons. Keep in mind, however, the fact that the membrane potential of every neuron is in a constant state of fluctuation, and it is the fluctuation in membrane potential at a synapse, if sufficiently strong, that initiates the release of chemical transmitters. In line with this, some cells,

9

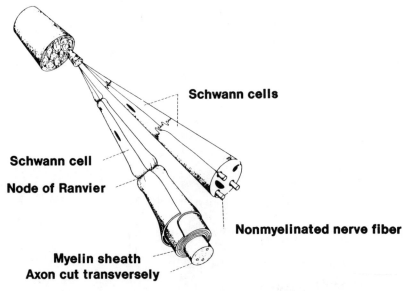

Schwann cells

Schwann cell

Node of Ranvier

Nonmyelinated nerve fiber

Myelin sheath
Axon cut transversely

Figure 1.6   Schwann cells form the myelin sheaths of axons of nerve cells in the peripheral nervous system. (Reproduced, with permission, from R. S. Snell, *Clinical Neuroanatomy for Medical Students.* © 1980 by Little, Brown, and Co.)

notably certain receptor cells, do not spike at all and in fact do not have axons. Information is conveyed from these nonspiking neurons to other cells through synaptic contacts that occur between cell bodies or cell body and dendrites. The fluctuations in a nonspiking cell cause corresponding fluctuations in the resting potential of the postsynaptic cell, which may in turn generate spikes in its axon. Nonspiking cells are highly specialized and have developed for specific information-processing tasks.

Chemoemissive Neurons

The synaptic contact, although by far the most prominent and best understood, is not the only type of information transfer between cells. Some neurons emit different types of molecules which affect the transmittive properties of all nearby cells. These nonspecific contacts have not been extensively studied, but the need for nonspecific information transfer, particularly to support various control processes, will become apparent in this and later chapters.

Logical Categories of Cells

For purposes of understanding the logic of neural networks it is convenient to define several logical categories of neurons. **Information input neurons** deliver information to a network for processing or analysis, and **information output**

neurons deliver processed information from a network to another. The output from one network is logically the input to another. For example, the optic nerve delivers the output from the retina and therefore consists of output cells. However, the optic nerve terminates in the lateral geniculate nuclei within the brain and therefore consists of input cells to those networks.

Control cells regulate the processing done by a network. The control inputs to one network may be the information outputs from another network.

A cell that is self-excitatory may be **bistable**. A cell is bistable if, when stimulated by other cells to an adequately high firing rate, its self-excitation will keep it firing indefinitely until turned off by an inhibitory input. If it is not firing, however, it remains off until it is stimulated by other cells. Such a cell is either **active** or **inactive**. The minimum firing rate that is required to activate an inactive bistable cell is its **threshold firing rate**. By analogy, an ordinary light switch can be lightly pushed without causing the switch to switch, but when pushed hard enough—beyond its threshold—it snaps and the light turns on or off. The switch is stable either in the "on" position or the "off" position; hence it is a bistable device.

When a single control cell is used to initiate activity in a network, that control cell is a **command cell**. If, for example, a single cell is used to initiate recall from a memory store, then that cell is a command cell. However, activity in a command cell may not be sufficient to initiate the action that it controls. Again by analogy, the playback button on an ordinary tape recorder is a command button. However, when the power is turned off or the batteries are removed, the playback button does not initiate playback.

Logical Categories of Neural Interactions

Different neurochemicals, such as neurotransmitters, peptides, enzymes, or pathological agents, influence neural transmission in a variety of ways. Inhibitors of biosynthesis prevent neurotransmitters from forming. Presynaptic blocking agents inhibit the release of transmitters at the presynaptic membrane. Presynaptic facilitators have the opposite effect. Postsynaptic blocking agents bind to receptor sites at the postsynaptic membrane preventing ordinary transmitters from doing so. This blocks their activity. Mimicking agents act as neurotransmitters, causing depolarization or hyperpolarization of the postsynaptic cell, depending on the type of mimicking agent. Some chemicals inhibit metabolic breakdown of the transmitters while others block their reuptake by the presynaptic cell. Still other chemicals alter the conductance of the cell membrane, thereby changing its transmission properties. Moreover, the affect that a particular chemical agent has depends on the normal neurotransmitter of the synapse. See, for example, Arnold (1984) for a detailed discussion and references to the literature.

Different neural networks perform markedly different information-processing

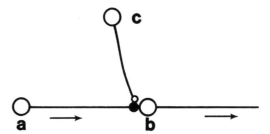

Figure 1.7 Two idealized neurons, a and b, which have uniform coupling regulated by
neuron c.

tasks, and the variety of requirements imposed on them accounts for the large
variety of mechanisms employed by the neurons themselves in their underlying
computations. Some networks simply route information from one place to
another. This implies a mechanism for blocking the transmission of all
information along a pathway. Networks which block transmission must act as
switches and have a very fast switching time. In contrast, some networks
transform information in a variety of subtle ways. Visual networks which
enhance the retinal image, for example, must transform their patterns in much
the same way that the contrast knob on a television set enhances the image.
Although we do not yet know what types of neural activity are used to
support any given information-processing task, and we are in fact only
beginning to understand the range of computational demands made on the
brain; still, the following sections suggest some of the expected types of
coupling needed by the brain to meet these demands. Only when researchers
specifically begin to look for these and other logical systems will we discover
which ones exist.

Regulatory Coupling. Neurons whose activity regulates the activity of other cells
are connected by **regulatory coupling**. Figures 1.7 and 1.8 each illustrate three
idealized cells, A, B, and C. In Figure 1.7, cells A and B have uniform coupling,
and cell C is a control cell with **negative regulatory coupling**. When control cell
C fires, the normal coupling between cells A and B, whether it be excitatory or
inhibitory, is reduced so that cell A makes a smaller contribution to the firing
rate of cell B. If cell C fires fast enough, then cell A makes no contribution to
the firing rate of cell B. When cell C does not fire, cell A is connected to cell
B as described earlier. Cell C **regulates** the coupling between cells A and B by
blocking their interaction and is said to have a **negative regulatory** effect.
Positive regulatory coupling is defined analogously and facilitates the inhibitory
and excitatory coupling between cells. In Figure 1.8, cells A and B have regional
coupling, and cell C is again a control cell having negative regulatory coupling.
When cell C fires, the coupling from cell A to cell B is reduced or blocked, but
only in that region influenced by cell C. Coupling elsewhere between cells A
and B is unmodified by the firing of cell C.

12

Transformational Coupling. In contrast to neurons which regulate the activity of other neurons, those which are connected together to process information use either **excitatory** or **inhibitory** coupling. Figure 1.9 shows a simple network having three sets of cells, I, C, and O. The collection named I is the input set, collection C is the control set, and collection O is the output set. A **neural network model** for the illustrated network consists of a complete and precise specification of the activity of each output cell when given the activity of each input and control cell for all time up to the present, and a complete specification of the state of each neuron's environment. For a biological network, a partial list of parameters needed for determining the firing rate of each output cell at time *t* is the following:

1. The structure of each output cell, including its size and the distribution of synaptic contacts from all presynaptic cells.

2. The rate of firing of each presynaptic cell.

3. The rate of release of neurotransmitters from each presynaptic cell as a function of its rate of firing, the current state of the neurons' environment, the effects of the control inputs on the release of neurotransmitters, and the history of all inputs to the network.

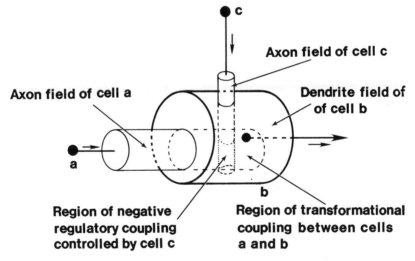

Figure 1.8 Two idealized neurons, a and b, whose coupling is regulated by neuron c. Transformational coupling occurs between neurons a and b within the volume enclosed by the larger intersecting cylinders. Control neuron c regulates the coupling between neurons a and b only within the volume enclosed by the smallest cylinder. Control neuron c also regulates the coupling between all other transformational neurons connected within that volume.

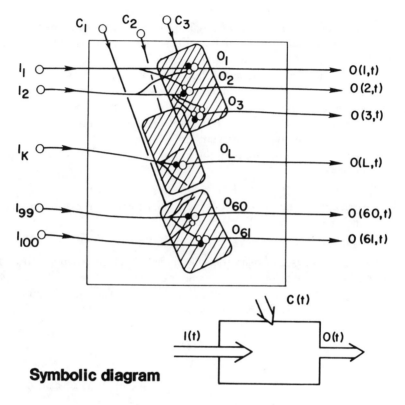

Symbolic diagram

Figure 1.9 A simple neural network composed of 100 input neurons, 3 control neurons and 61 output neurons.

4. The influence that the current state of each neuron's environment has on the movement of neurotransmitters from presynaptic to postsynaptic cells.

5. Any mutual influences that neurotransmitters released by different presynaptic cells have on one another.

6. The sensitivity at the current time of the postsynaptic cell toward depolarization (or hyperpolarization) due to the arrival of neurotransmitters, and any modification to that sensitivity due to the current state of its environment.

7. The influence that the current state of each neuron's environment has on its depolarization.

As the above list suggests, the influence that the presynaptic cells have on the firing rate of a postsynaptic cell is only one part of the interaction between cells. We call this component the **transformational coupling** between cells. In either

14

case, if one cell tends to cause another cell to discharge it is excitatory and if it tends to prevent another cell from discharging it is inhibitory. Transformational coupling determines the type of processing performed and is distinguished from control coupling, which regulates the transformation, and effectual coupling (to be described next) which initiates or effects a temporary or permanent change in coupling.

Effectual Coupling. The third and final type of neural coupling to be considered is effectual coupling. An input to a network is an **effectual input** and has **effectual coupling** in case its firing causes or initiates either temporary or permanent changes to take place in the transformational coupling characteristics of other cells. This differs from control coupling in that the changes do not directly affect neural transmission. Furthermore, the changes may persist after the effective neurotransmitters are no longer present. A neuron that initiates the consolidation process in a storage network makes an effectual input to that network. A neuron which makes an effectual input to one network may also make regulatory or transformational inputs to the same or other networks.

SUMMARY

The three types of coupling described here, regulatory, transformational, and effectual, are only beginning to be understood. From a logical point of view, all three types of coupling are necessary. However, the differences between control coupling and transformational coupling, for example, depend on the computational logic of networks, and the computational logic cannot be determined without knowing exactly what functional role the various neurons play in the computational process. Since computational roles are just beginning to be understood, these notions will become increasingly important as time passes. The relationship between cell morphology and its computational role will someday be understood, and when that happens, I expect researchers will find a direct relationship between cell morphology, coupling type, and coupling characteristics.

It should be clear that any attempt to formulate a complete and detailed model of the brain is, at the present time, impossible. We simply don't have enough quantitative information about the interactions between neurons to do so, and even if we did, the computational difficulties of specifying the activities of some hundred billion neurons with perhaps one hundred trillion synapses, their environment, and the entire history of inputs to the system is simply not computationally feasible. This, then, would be the end of this endeavor except for one very important fact. We know a lot about the computational processes of the brain. We know that representations of visual images are processed, that records are made of our experiences, that we manipulate mental models of the world, that we communicate with one another using natural language, that we can perform numerous types of logical computations, that we have emotional experiences, and that we control our own movements. Our way out of the dilemma of attempting to model the brain by studying its individual neurons, then, is to to build various computational networks which perform the same processes that occur in the brain, and use those neural network models as a guide to understanding the computational logic of the brain. The neural network models are constructed out of neuron-like elements called mathematical or abstract neurons, and by using our knowledge about the structure and function of the human brain we can build those models to resemble the networks of the brain closely. As our understanding of the brain increases, the models will be refined and approximate more closely the corresponding networks of the brain. This, then, will be the strategy followed throughout this endeavor.

SUGGESTED READINGS

The following excellent references are among many that present the biological ideas which motivated this chapter.

Arbib, M. A. (1972). *The metaphorical brain. An introduction to cybernetics as artificial intelligence and brain theory.* New York: John Wiley & Sons.
Arnold, M. B. (1984). *Memory and the brain.* Hillsdale, NJ: Lawrence Erlbaum Associates.
Kandel, E.R., & Schwartz, J. H. (1985). *Principles of neural science. (2d ed.).* New York: Elsevier.
MacGregor, R. J., & Lewis, E. R. (1977). *Neural modeling. Electrical signal processing in the nervous system.* New York: Plenum Press.
Morrell, P. & Norton, W. T. (1980). Myelin. *Scientific American, 242,* 88–118.
Ochs, S. (1965). *Elements of neurophysiology.* New York: John Wiley & Sons.
Schadé, J. P., & Ford, D. H. (1965). *Basic neurology. An Introduction to the structure and function of the nervous system.* New York: Elsevier.
Shepherd, G. M. (1974). *The synaptic organization of the brain. An introduction.* New York: Oxford University Press.
Snell, R. S. (1980). *Clinical neuroanatomy for medical students.* Boston: Little, Brown.
Stevens, C. F. (1979). The neuron. *Scientific American, 241,* 55–65.
Thompson, R. F. (1967). *Foundations of physiological psychology.* New York: Harper & Row.

APPENDIX 1
THE MATHEMATICS OF NEURAL INTERACTIONS[1]

This final section presents a formal model for neural interactions. The material is not essential to the remainder of the book and the reader may wish to proceed directly to Chapter 2.

---

[1]This material is reproduced, in part, from R. J. Baron (1970) A model for cortical memory, *Journal of Mathematical Psychology, 7,* 37–59.

As I suggested above, the model presented here describes the logical interactions between neurons and is an approximate description for the interactions between biological neurons. The model relates the output behavior of a network of abstract neurons to the behavior of the input and control neurons to that network. The model is linear and assumes statistical interactions between neurons.

When discussing different collections of neurons, either biological or mathematical, it is convenient to name them. For example, the retinal ganglion cells may be named RG whereas the cells of the olfactory bulb may be named OB. In order to distinguish one cell from another in a particular collection, we will enclose in parentheses a list of numbers which uniquely identify a particular cell in the collection. These are the **intrinsic coordinates** of the cell. If the collection is two-dimensional, then two number positions will be used, where the numbers in each position specify (in arbitrary units) the location of the cell in the collection. For example, the retinal ganglion cells may be designated RG(1,1), RG(1,2), RG(1,3) . . . RG(2,1), RG(2,2) . . . RG(M,1), RG(M,2) . . . RG(M,N), where M and N are the maximum number of cells in the two dimensions under consideration. If the collection is one-dimensional, then a single number position will be used, and if the collection is three-dimensional, then three number positions will be used. This notation clearly generalizes to any number of dimensions. When we wish to designate an entire collection only the name will be used and it will be set in boldface type.

If the coupling parameters between cells depend in a systematic way on the cell's intrinsic coordinates, then the network has **high neural specificity**. On the other hand, if the coupling parameters do not depend on intrinsic coordinates, the network has **low neural specificity**. The cells of a network having random coupling coefficients would have low specificity. If each cell on the retina is computationally distinguished by its position, then there would be a functional relationship between its cell number and its position on the retina and the retina would have high neural specificity. You will see that the human brain has high neural specificity. It is generally assumed that cell morphology and network architecture are genetically specified. Coupling parameters may not be genetically specified, depending on the specific network.

We define a **mathematical neuron** (hereafter called simply "neuron") as consisting of four parts: (1) a **soma**, (2) a **dendrite field**, (3) an **axon**, and (4) an **axon field**. The soma is a point whose geometric coordinates identify the neuron. The dendrite field is a three-dimensional volume containing the soma. The axon field is also a three-dimensional volume (not necessarily disjoint from the dendrite field), and the axon is a line connecting the soma with the axon field. See Figure 1.10.

When the axon field of one neuron, the **presynaptic neuron**, intersects the dendrite field of a second neuron, the **postsynaptic neuron**, the intersection is

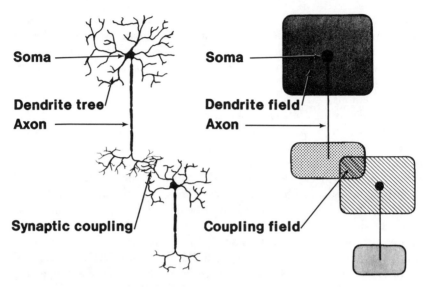

Figure 1.10 The relationship between biological neurons and mathematical neurons. (Adapted from R. J. Baron, A model for cortical memory. *Journal of Mathematical Psychology, 7,* 1970, 37–59.

called the **coupling field**. The coupling may be transformational, control, or effectual. Consider two neurons with nonempty coupling field. Neuron A, the **presynaptic neuron**, is said to **synapse on** neuron B, the **postsynaptic neuron**.

The **frequency** of a neuron is a nonnegative valued function of time, as illustrated in Figure 1.11. Let I be a collection of input neurons, O be a collection of output neurons, and C be a collection of control neurons as illustrated in Figure 1.9. Let I(J)(t) denote the frequency of cell I(J) at time t and similarly let O(K)(t) and C(M)(t) designate the frequencies of cells O(K) and C(M) at time t.

Finally, let E(x,y,z)(t) designate the **state** of the neural environment at time t and at geometric location (x,y,z). We say that the neural environment is in a **normal state** in case E(x,y,z)(t) has value 1.

When the neural environment is in the normal state and neuron I(J) fires at frequency I(J)(t), neuron I(J) releases **transmitter substance** to neuron O(K) throughout their coupling field at a rate density (quantity of transmitter substance per second per volume) given by

$$I(J)(t)c_{O(K)}^{I(J)}(x,y,z,C(t))$$

The parameters

$$c_{O(K)}^{I(J)}(x,y,z,C(t))$$

are called **coupling coefficients**, where the superscript identifies the presynaptic neuron and the subscript identifies the postsynaptic neuron. As indicated, the coupling depends on pre- and postsynaptic neurons and on the control input C(t) to the region of coupling (x,y,z). **Excitatory coupling** is represented by positive coupling coefficients, and **inhibitory coupling** is represented by negative coupling coefficients.

When the neural environment is not in the normal state it may influence the coupling between two neurons multiplicatively. Thus the rate of arrival of transmitter substance at O(K) from I(J) is given by

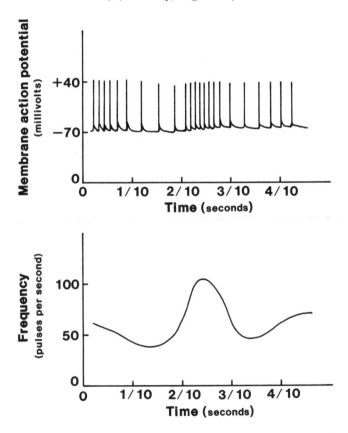

Figure 1.11   The relationship between the depolarization rate of a biological neuron and the frequency of a mathematical neuron. (Reproduced, with permission, from R. J. Baron, A model for cortical memory. *Journal of Mathematical Psychology*, 7, 1970, 37–59.)

$$I(J)(t)c_{O(K)}^{I(J)}(x,y,z,C(t))E(x,y,z)(t).$$

Since $E(x,y,z)(t)$ is 1 when the state of the neural environment is normal, this same expression is valid in general.

The axon and soma of our mathematical neuron do not play a central part in the model. Transmitter substance which arrives at the dendrite field of one neuron causes it to fire at a frequency given by integrating all contributions of transmitter substance which arrive throughout its dendrite field. However, the sensitivity of the postsynaptic cell to transmitter substances may not be uniform throughout its dendrite field. In any volume of the postsynaptic cell $O(K)$, the net rate density of arriving transmitter substance is given by

$$(\sum_{I(J)} I(J)(t)c_{O(K)}^{I(J)}(x,y,z,C(t)))\ E(x,y,z)(t)$$

where summation is over all neurons whose axon fields intersect the dendrite field of the postsynaptic neuron. The contribution toward depolarization of the postsynaptic cell may be modified by its **local sensitivity**, $k_{O(K)}(x,y,z)(t)$, at position (x,y,z). The contribution toward the frequency of the postsynaptic cell made by the arrival of transmitter substance at point (x,y,z) in its dendrite field is given by

$$k_{O(K)}(x,y,z)(t)\ (\sum_{I(J)} I(J)(t)c_{O(K)}^{I(J)}(x,y,z,C(t)))\ E(x,y,z)(t)$$

The frequency of neuron $O(M)$ is given by integrating all such contributions over its entire dendrite field. The final result is given by

$$O(M)(t) = POS(\int\int\int k_{O(K)}(x,y,z)(t)(\sum_{I(J)} I(J)(t)c_{O(K)}^{I(J)}(x,y,z,C(t)))$$
$$E(x,y,z)(t)dxdydz.$$

The function $POS(x)$ has value x if x is non-negative and zero otherwise. That is, cell $O(M)$ does not fire if the net effect of all arriving transmitter substance is negative.

DISCUSSION

The equation given above represents a mathematical model for the logical interactions between neurons in a neural network. In particular, it relates the output firing pattern $O(t)$ to the input pattern $I(t)$ and the control pattern $C(t)$. Once all parameters are specified, the frequency of each output cell can, in principle at least, be determined.

A few comments are in order. First, this model is statistical and does not take into account relative phases between spikes arriving from different presynaptic neurons. Second, the model is linear: All effects contribute linearly to the frequencies of the postsynaptic cells.

Perhaps more important are the biological counterparts of the various coupling contributions. Coupling contributions come from three places: presynaptic (the c's), interneuronal (the E's) and postsynaptic (the k's). The coupling coefficients (the c's) depend on the intrinsic coordinates of the pre- and postsynaptic cell, the position of contact, and any effects that the control patterns have on the coupling. This model therefore assumes that control inputs regulate the presynaptic release of transmitter substance rather than the interneuronal or postsynaptic parameters. The neural environment (the E's) contributes in a similar way to the coupling between all cells occupying the same volume of the network. Thus the environmental contribution is nonspecific. Finally, the postsynaptic neuron can also modify the coupling influence, and the postsynaptic cell's contribution (the k's) may vary as a function of position on the postsynaptic cell. When creating a specific neural network model, it is essential to assign values to the appropriate parameters in the equations, depending on the assumed origin of the contribution.

Notice that effective coupling has not been included in the equation. Effective coupling modifies coupling parameters and can be directly incorporated either in the definition of the coupling coefficients or the definition of the local sensitivity values, whichever is appropriate. For the storage model described in Appendix 2, the effective inputs determine when and where storage will take place and are the "store now" signals to the storage system. Storage in that model consists of establishing values for the local sensitivity values (the k's) of certain storage cells. In particular, the k's take on one set of values before storage and a different set of values after storage. The effective inputs to a storage location determine *when* the k's change values but have no other effect on the input–output relationships in the model.

REFERENCE

Baron, R. J. (1970). A model for cortical memory. *Journal of Mathematical Psychology*, 7, 37-59.

2

INFORMATION: ITS MOVEMENT AND TRANSFORMATION

INTRODUCTION

Many functions of the brain are similar to those of a modern digital computer. Both the brain and a computer accept information as input and produce information as output. Both encode and decode information. Both transform information in a variety of ways. Both store, search for and recall information. This chapter attempts to characterize information, how it is encoded, how it is transformed, and how it is transmitted from one place to another.

Information will be used here to mean two different things: (1) the pattern, arrangement, or configuration of constituent units that encode knowledge of form or event, and, (2) the signal impressed upon the input of a system and used to communicate knowledge of form or event. When used to encode knowledge, information is **static**; when used to communicate knowledge, it is **dynamic**. The terms static information pattern and dynamic information pattern, and static pattern and dynamic pattern will also be used.

STATIC AND DYNAMIC PATTERNS

Static patterns are the encoding of stored knowledge. The ink patterns on a page of text, the patterns of magnetic domains on a strip of recording tape, the grooves on phonograph records, the silver particles on a photograph, and the raised dots in braille are examples of static information patterns.

Dynamic patterns move or transmit knowledge from one place to another and interact with information-processing systems by supplying the energy needed to initiate information-processing operations. Light waves that convey printed information, electric signals generated by a playback head in a tape recorder, sound waves of speech, and firing patterns in collections of neurons are examples of dynamic information patterns.

Static patterns remain fixed in their supporting medium until modulated by an external activator; dynamic patterns, in contrast, are spatio-temporal patterns that exist because of a change in their supporting medium—an electric signal, a light wave, a mechanical movement. Static patterns are useless until converted into dynamic patterns: a book in the dark, a reel of magnetic tape with no tape deck, a phonograph record with no record player. The static patterns in these devices remains static, hence useless, without an appropriate playback mechanism. Once converted, however, static patterns are the source of all prior knowledge. When light shines on the printed page, when the magnetic tape is moved across a playback head, or when the grooves of a phonograph record move the stylus of a phonograph cartridge—these processes recreate the dynamic patterns that were originally present and stored when the static patterns were formed, and the recreated dynamic patterns once again become available for further processing and analysis.

For the printed page, the presence of a uniform external light source is necessary to convert from static to dynamic pattern; for a magnetic tape, the uniform movement of the tape across the playback head, and for the phonograph record the uniform movement of the record under the playback cartridge. Uniform light, uniform tape movement, and uniform record movement—these are the external modulators necessary for converting static patterns into dynamic information patterns.

Within the brain the dynamic patterns are the patterns of discharging neurons which convey signals from one network to another; the static patterns are the memory traces which are encoded as spatial patterns of biochemical markers. Chapter 3 will discuss information storage in detail, but for now let us take as self-evident the importance of static and dynamic patterns to brain function and continue to explore other facets of information.

CONTROL AND CONTENT PATTERNS

Information patterns can be loosely divided into two categories: **control patterns**, and **content patterns**. Consider a tape recorder that has three different recording channels. Two of the channels are used just as they are on any home stereo tape recorder: Each channel records a representation of the sound that arrives at a recording microphone in one part of the room. This tape recorder, however, has special circuitry that monitors the sound level in the room. If the sound level in the room increases during the recording session, the recording level of the two stereo channels is decreased. If the sound level decreases, the recording level is increased. (This optimizes the signal-to-noise ratio on the recording and enables a greater dynamic range without saturating the tape.) The third channel maintains a record of the recording level of the two stereo channels. If a tape consisting of just the two stereo channels is played back on an ordinary tape recorder, the average sound level during playback would remain constant even though the sound level during the recording session varied. However, on the special recorder being described, the information stored on the third channel is used in a special way during playback. If the recording level was reduced during the recording session, then the volume is increased during playback so the sound level in the room is the same as it was during recording. Similarly, if the recording level was increased during recording, then the sound level is decreased during playback. The information recorded on the third recording channel is **control information**, whereas the information recorded on the two stereo channels is **content information**. The control information is necessary for the proper operation of the tape recorder, whereas the content information plays no direct role in its operation. Control information relates to the circuitry—it controls a process; content information relates only to the quality of the information being processed.

Notice that from the point of view of the recording circuitry there is no difference between the content patterns and the control pattern. In fact, all three patterns are stored and played back in exactly the same way. The pattern stored by the third channel only becomes control information when used by the playback mechanism. *It is how information is used that distinguishes content from control information, not the format of the information itself.*

Notice also that information only becomes meaningful when it interacts with a system that can correctly interpret it. The control information stored on the third channel of the special tape recorder is only useful to that recorder. A book written in Chinese is only useful to a person who reads Chinese. *Information only has meaning to a system that is designed to interact with it properly.*

INFORMATION TRANSMISSION

There are many different ways that information can be transmitted. In computers, for example, numerical quantities are transmitted as electrical signals on collections of wires. For a given wire, a signal can either be present or absent. For a single wire at a given time, the presence or absence of a signal encodes either the value one (signal present) or the value zero (signal absent). Likewise, the presence or absence of signals on N wires can be used to encode up to 2^N difference values. For example, for two wires, if '00' indicates that neither wire has a signal, '10' indicates that wire 1 has a signal, '01' indicates that wire 2 has a signal, and '11' indicates that both wires have signals, then clearly all possibilities are exhausted. There are two wires and 2^2 or four different patterns. In each case, the pattern is dynamic since the electrical signals can directly interact with other computing devices which may be connected to the wires.

It is also possible to send time-varying dynamic patterns along wires. The electrical impulses along a telephone wire are one example. As a second example, consider the very simple case of one wire, and suppose that the presence or absence of an electrical signal is inspected every second. If we inspect the wire N times during a period of N seconds, then up to 2^N different sequences of on and off signals can be sent along the wire. In a collection of M wires, up to 2^{MN} different sequences of signals can be sent.

Within computers, information is transmitted from one component to another along **data buses**. Data buses are simply collections of independent wires, one for each component of the information being transmitted. When a signal is impressed on one end of a wire, it can be sensed almost immediately at the other. When one computer component is to transmit information to another component, it places signals on the wires of a data bus. In some cases a single signal is sent but in other cases a sequence of signals is sent and the receiving circuits must inspect the data bus at exactly the correct times to discover what the sequence is. In general, because of the critical timing involved, all components of a computer are controlled by a **master clock**, a circuit that periodically turns on and off a clock signal in a special control wire that goes to all components of the computer to coordinate their activity. The individual components use this clock signal to determine when to place data on the data bus and when to inspect the data bus.

INFORMATION ENCODING

In computers, static information patterns are encoded in many different formats but most often as the pattern of "on" and "off" **states** in sets of storage elements. The fundamental storage element of a modern computer is the **flip-flop**, an electronic switch that is either "set" (on) or "reset" (off). A **set** flip-flop holds the value '1' and a **reset** flip-flop holds the value '0.' This is analogous to a light switch which can either be on or off. Since a flip-flop can only hold two values, such a device is said to hold a binary digit or **bit**.

Although, like neurons, there are many different types of flip-flops, we will consider only one type here. Our flip-flop has one information input wire, one information output wire, and one control wire. See Figure 2.1a. When the control input is off, the state of the flip-flop remains unchanged, either set or reset, regardless of the value of the information input. The information output is on when the flip-flop is set, and off when it is reset. When the control input, called the **copy input**, is turned on, the flip-flop prepares to change state. The flip-flop does not change state, however, until the very instant the copy input turns off. At that instant, the flip-flop is set if the information input is on or reset if the information input is off. Thus the state of the flip-flop is determined by the input information (on sets it and off resets it) at the time specified by the control input. The output of the flip-flop subsequently reflects its new state. The

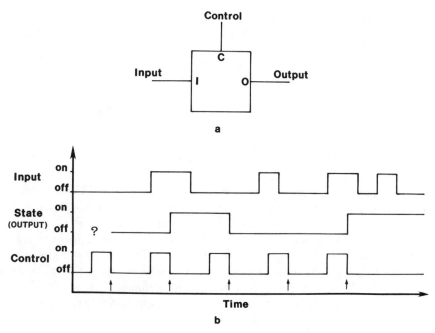

Figure 2.1. a) A flip-flop. b) A timing diagram showing the relationships between information inputs, control (or clock) inputs, and the state (hence output) of the flip-flop. For this flip-flop, a state change only occurs when the control input turns off (indicated by arrows). The new state is determined by the state of the input (on or off) at that instant. The question mark indicates that the initial state of the flip-flop is not known.

flip-flop then stays set or reset until the control input initiates another state change.

Flip-flops are generally grouped together into word-sized units which are controlled as a single device called a **register**. A register is a storage device that holds one word of information. See Figure 2.2. A four-bit register, for example, consists of four flip-flops and can therefore hold one four-bit word or one of 2^4 or 16 different patterns. An eight-bit register can hold one eight-bit word or one of 2^8 or 256 patterns. These patterns may represent numbers, characters, computer instructions, or some other set of logical quantities. The **copy input** to a register causes it to hold the value on the input lines just as the copy input to a single flip-flop caused that flip-flop to hold the last value on its input line. Table 2.1 shows several different four-bit information codes used today.

Registers are fundamental building blocks in computers. They are physically connected to other registers and other computer components (storage devices, processing units, and so forth) through data buses as described earlier. However, registers are not directly connected to data buses. They are connected to the

26

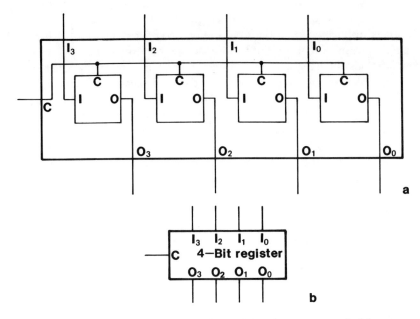

Figure 2.2. a) The circuit diagram for a 4-bit register composed of four flip-flops. b) The symbolic diagram of a 4-bit register.

TABLE 2.1
Common Four-bit Number Representations

Absolute Binary	Decimal	Sign Magnitude	One's Complement	Two's Complement	Excess 3	Binary Fraction
0000	0	0	0	0	−0	0
0001	1	1	1	1	−2	1/16
0010	2	2	2	2	−1	2/16
0011	3	3	3	3	0	3/16
0100	4	4	4	4	1	4/16
0101	5	5	5	5	2	5/16
0110	6	6	6	6	3	6/16
0111	7	7	7	7	4	7/16
0000	8	−0	−7	−8	5	8/16
1001	9	−1	−6	−7	6	9/16
1010	10	−2	−5	−6	7	10/16
1011	11	−3	−4	−5	8	11/16
1100	12	−4	−3	−4	9	12/16
1101	13	−5	−2	−3	10	13/16
1110	14	−6	−1	−2	11	14/16
1111	15	−7	−0	−1	12	15/16

buses through sets of switches, one switch for each bit in the register. This is illustrated in Figure 2.3. If the word size of a computer is four bits, then each register consists of four flip-flops and there are four switches that connect the four flip-flops of the register to the corresponding four wires in the data bus. The set of switches connecting a register to a data bus is called a **bus gate**, and in general the switches in a bus gate are all controlled by a single control signal which originates in the control unit of the computer. (Note that the control signal is such precisely because it is used as a control signal by the register.)

When the control signal opens the switches in a bus gate, the static pattern encoded by the register's flip-flops is impressed on the data bus. It is by this process that the static pattern in the register is converted into a dynamic pattern in the data bus that can be sensed by other components in the computer. Since the control unit generates the control signal that places data on the bus, it can at the same time signal other computer components to inspect the data bus and copy the information. It is by this very simple technique that information is transferred from one device to another during a computer's computations.

The brain is very different and vastly more complex than a digital computer. In the first place, neurons, which are the circuit components of the brain, are not simply on or off like flip-flops and wires. The information encoded in a collection of neurons is not represented by the states of the neurons at a particular time but by their rates of firing. Second, although information is conveyed from one part of the brain to another by the neurons themselves, the connections are not like the wires of a data bus that do not modify the signals they convey. Neurons *are* the computational elements of the brain, and computations often take place during information transfer. Finally, the number of neurons that encode patterns of information is significantly larger and the patterns themselves are markedly more complex than the patterns in a computer. The optic nerve, for example, which conveys the visual pattern from eye to brain, consists of more than a million elements; in a computer, a word size of 64 bits is considered very large!

NEURAL INFORMATION PATTERNS

Within a computer, the smallest indivisible unit of information is the bit, but the fundamental unit of dynamic information—the word—is the pattern of on-and-off signals in the wires of a data bus. Within the brain, the smallest indivisible unit of information is the rate of firing of an individual neuron but the fundamental unit of dynamic information is the **depolarization pattern**, the set of firing rates of the neurons in a specific collection of neurons.

The data buses of the brain are the **neural pathways** or **nerves**. Neural pathways are collections of myelinated axons of particular sets of cells. The information being transmitted by a particular neural pathway is the pattern generated by the neurons whose axons form the pathway. The transmitted pattern is the depolarization pattern sensed by the postsynaptic cells upon which the pathway terminates. The optic nerve is one example. It is comprised predominantly of the axons of retinal ganglion cells. The retinal ganglion cells perform the final stage of processing by the retina, so the optic nerve conveys the eye's representation of the ocular image to the brain. See Figure 2.4.

When describing neural information, one must always have in mind a specific collection of neurons, and the information pattern is specified by giving the rate of firing of each neuron in the collection, *not* by giving the state of each neuron at a particular time. For example, some of the axons in the optic nerve convey information from the brain to the eye. These efferent axons are not included in the pattern that describes the retinal output even though their activity may control the retinal output.

The **size** or **dimensionality** of a neural pattern is the number of axons conveying the pattern. Since there are approximately a million afferent axons (conducting information toward the brain) in the optic nerve, the afferent pattern conveyed by the optic nerve has size 1,000,000. In contrast, if it requires only three neurons to encode the color projected at a particular point on the retina, then the dimension of that subpattern is three.

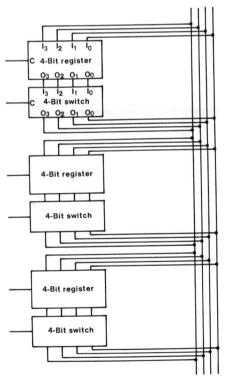

Figure 2.3. Three 4-bit registers connected to a 4-bit data bus using three 4-bit switches to regulate the connections. When the "C" input to a 4-bit switch is on, each input is connected to its output (I1 to O1, I2 to O2, etc. as labeled in the upper switch only), and hence all outputs of the register are connected to the data bus. When the "C" input is off, the register is disconnected from the data bus. Note that inputs to the registers are connected directly from the data bus. This is okay since a register does not change state except when its "C" input is turned off. Said another way, the register ignores its input unless it is clocked.

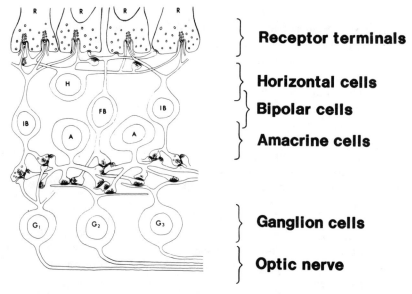

Receptor terminals

Horizontal cells

Bipolar cells

Amacrine cells

Ganglion cells

Optic nerve

Figure 2.4. The synaptic structure of the retina showing that axons of the ganglion cells form the final pathway of visual information. Note the specialized synaptic structures. Compare this figure with Figures 7.6 and 7.7. (Reproduced, with permission, from J. E. Dowling, Organization of Vertebrate Retinas. *Investigative Ophthalmology*, 9, 1970, 655-679.)

Neural information patterns in general are **spatial, time-varying patterns**. They vary both as a function of the particular neuron in the collection and as a function of time. Many information patterns are two-dimensional, where the two dimensions represent the geometric coordinates of the incoming sensory signals (e.g., position on the surface of the skin, position on the retina of the eye), or the geometric coordinates of the origin of the pattern within the brain (e.g., position on the cerebral cortex).

As stated earlier, the firing pattern in a collection of cells varies as a function of time. I will use the notation $S(N)(t)$ to designate the rate of firing of cell N in collection S at time t, and I will use $S(t)$ to designate the firing pattern in the entire collection at time t. If the retinal ganglion cells are named RG, for example, then $RG(t)$ designates the afferent information conveyed by the optic nerve to the brain at time t and $RG(3,6)(t)$ designates the rate of firing of retinal ganglion cell $RG(3,6)$ at time t. A similar notation was used in Chapter 1 to represent the frequency of a mathematical neuron.

This notion of neural information is based on the fundamental assumption that neural interactions are statistical and neural information is encoded in terms of the firing rates of cells. Pulse height and relative phases between spikes are assumed not to be of primary concern. However, for those brain systems where phase of depolarization is a critical parameter (for example, in the auditory system), this notion will need to be refined appropriately.

Describing Patterns in Neural Networks

The following descriptive mechanism is often convenient for describing the information in a particular collection of neurons. Imagine that each neuron in the collection can be connected to a small light bulb which glows with an intensity proportional to the rate of firing of the neuron. The light bulbs are then arranged in a geometric pattern determined by the intrinsic coordinates of the neurons in the collection. For example, light bulbs connected to retinal ganglion cells would be arranged in a pattern similar to the arrangement of the retinal ganglion cells themselves. An observer can now look at the light pattern just as he or she might look at a television screen and describe the neural activity as he or she would the picture on the screen. For example, he or she can describe the shape, size, position, and intensity of the activity within the collection.

Equality and Similarity of Information Patterns

The notion of equality of neural information patterns is fundamental and will be defined here. Two spatial neural patterns are **equal** in case two conditions hold: (1) There is a one-to-one correspondence between the cells in the two pathways that convey the patterns, and (2) The firing rates of each pair of cells under this correspondence are the same. Using the descriptive mechanism of the previous section, two patterns are equal if they look identical. Two spatial neural patterns are **similar** or **proportional** in case: (1) There is a one-to-one correspondence between the cells in the two collections, and (2) The ratios of the firing rates of each pair of cells under this correspondence is the same. For example, the firing patterns in two collections of cells are similar if the cells in the two collections correspond and the firing rate of each cell in the second collection is twice the firing rate of the corresponding cell in the first collection. Once again, using the descriptive mechanism of the previous section, two patterns are similar if they look the same only one is brighter than the other.

It is important to recognize that, according to this definition, two spatial neural patterns can be equal even if the corresponding neurons do not fire at corresponding times. It is only necessary that the **rates of firing** at corresponding times be equal.

I will now extend the notion of equality to spatial, time varying or **spatio-temporal** neural patterns. Two spatio-temporal neural patterns are **equal for T seconds** provided three conditions hold: (1) there is a one-to-one correspondence between the cells in the two pathways that convey the patterns, (2) there is a temporal correspondence between the onsets of the two depolarization patterns, and (3) the spatial neural patterns are equal at corresponding times. This can be stated mathematically as follows. If I and O are the pathways, cell I(M) corresponds to cell O(M), and t1 and t2 are the onset times of the two patterns, then $O(M)(t1 + t) = I(M)(t2 + t)$ for all t between 0 and T. Thus two spatio-temporal neural patterns are equal provided there is a spatial and temporal correspondence between the patterns.

Two spatio-temporal neural patterns are **similar** provided that (1) there is a one-to-one correspondence between the cells in the pathways that convey the patterns, (2) there is a temporal correspondence between the onset times of the two patterns, and (3) the spatial patterns are similar at similar times after pattern onset. Again, this can be stated mathematically as follows. Using our earlier notation, the patterns O(t2) and I(t1) are similar in case $O(M)(t1 + c1 \times t) = I(M)(t2 + t)$ for all t between 0 and T. Thus two spatio-temporal patterns are similar in case there is a spatial correspondence between them and one pattern either progresses faster or slower (or the same speed) than the other.

As an example, sentences read by the same person at different rates of speed are similar as are the images in a movie when played at normal speed or in slow motion.

Logical Categories of Patterns

Information input and output neurons were defined in Chapter 1 as were control and effector neurons. The patterns of information conveyed by these types of neurons are **input patterns**, **output patterns**, **control patterns**, and **effector patterns**. These are logical categories and depend not on the encoding of information in the pathways but on how the information is used.

SOME NEURAL NETWORKS

Having now built up a vocabulary for understanding the logical interactions between neurons, the final sections of this chapter will present several very simple neural network models for information transfer.

Transmission Lines

An **information pathway** consists of the set of myelinated axons of cells that transfer information from a **source** to a **destination**. The cells at the source whose axons form the pathway are **input cells**. They generate the **input pattern** that enters the pathway. The cells whose axons leave the pathway are **output cells**. They convey the **output pattern** from the pathway. The one requirement imposed on a pathway is that the input pattern equals the output pattern: The pathway must not modify the information.

The simplest realization of a pathway is when the input cells *are* the output cells so the pathway consists entirely of the axons of the input cells. In this case, the pathway is part of the source network. An alternate realization is that each input cell is either an output cell, or it connects to a single **intermediate** or **relay cell**. Each intermediate cell is either an output cell or it connects to another intermediate cell. Any number of intermediate cells may connect each input cell with one output cell, the connections all being sequential. When an input cell fires, the cell that it contacts fires, and so on until the output cell fires. Thus the output from a pathway is identical to the input except for a possible time delay in the pattern.

In the brain the most obvious candidates for pathways are the optic and auditory nerves. If, as in the auditory nerves, information is encoded in terms of the relative phases of depolarization between the cells, then the pathway must preserve the phase relationships or information would be lost or destroyed.

Switching Networks

A **switching network** is a network that has one or more collections of information input cells, one or more collections of information output cells, and one or more control inputs. The control inputs determine which information input cells will be connected to which information output cells. Three examples of switching networks and their graphic symbols are shown in Figures 2.5 through 2.7. The network in Figure 2.5 has one collection I of information input cells, two collections A and B of information output cells, and two control cells, C_1 and C_2, which have inhibitive regulatory coupling. When control cell C_2 fires, the coupling between the information input cells and the information output cells will be inhibited where shown. This means that the input cells are only connected to the output cells of collection A. Connections to the output cells in collection B are blocked. Similarly, when control cell C_1 fires, the connections to the output cells of collection A are blocked, and the inputs are connected to the outputs named B. If neither control cell fires, then both collections A and B will receive copies of the input pattern, and if both control cells fire, no information will be transmitted.

The network shown in Figure 2.6 has two collections I and J of input cells and one collection K of output cells. Both input sets I and J stimulate the output cells, which fire at the sum of rates of the corresponding input cells. However, if only one of the input sets I or J is active, then the output pattern is equal to that input pattern.

A third example of a switching network is a shift network. Figure 2.7 shows a shift network having one collection R of input cells, one collection S of output cells, and five control cells C_1 through C_5. When all five control cells fire, no information is transmitted from R to S. When control cell C_1 stops firing, the inputs are gated to output cells S_1, S_2, S_3, S_4, and S_5, respectively. When control

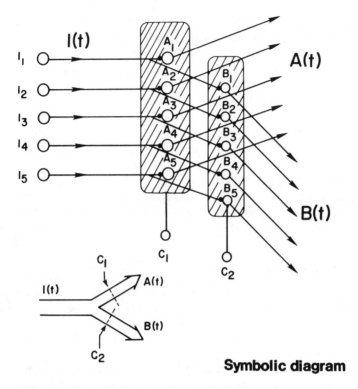

Symbolic diagram

Figure 2.5. One way to use negative regulatory coupling to control information transmission along two pathways.

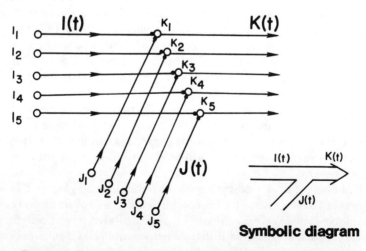

Symbolic diagram

Figure 2.6. The uncontrolled merging of two information pathways.

cell C_2 stops firing, the inputs are gated to output cells S_2, S_3, S_4, S_5, and S_6. When control input cell C_5 stops firing, the inputs are gated to output cells S_5, S_6, S_7, S_8, and S_9. The network shifts the input pattern in the output cells as determined by the control pattern C.

Masking Networks

The notion of switching can be generalized so that the information in one or more of the information input cells is *selectively* allowed to pass to the corresponding information output cell. Consider the network shown in Figure 2.8. Each information input cell is connected to a single information output cell, and each connection is regulated by a different inhibitive control cell. If a control cell fires, then information will be blocked between the corresponding information input and output cells. If a control cell does not fire, then information will be allowed to pass. By presenting a spatial pattern to the control cells, the corresponding pattern will be blocked by the network; it will be **masked**. Figure 2.9 shows the appearance of an input pattern, a control pattern or **mask** and the corresponding output pattern for the network. A graphic symbol for a masking network is also illustrated.

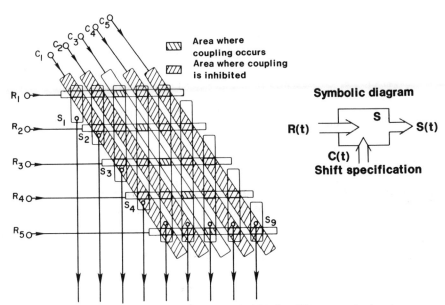

Figure 2.7. A shift network. Cells labeled R1 thru R5 convey the input pattern, cells labeled S1 thru S5 convey the shifted output pattern, and cells labeled C1 thru C5 control the amount of shift. The inset shows the symbolic notation for a shift network.

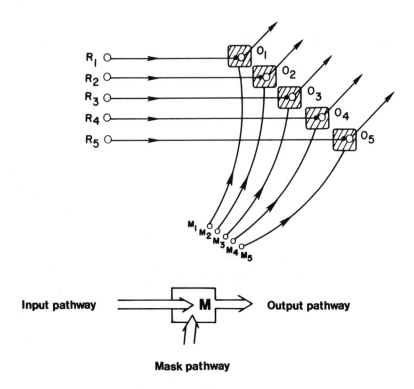

Symbolic diagram

Figure 2.8. A mask network. Cells labeled R1 thru R5 convey the input pattern, cells labeled O1 thru O5 convey the masked output pattern, and cells labeled M1 thru M5 convey the mask. The inset shows the symbolic notation for a mask network.

Receptor Networks

A **receptor network** is a collection of cells that converts nonneural information, a **stimulus pattern**, into neural information, a firing pattern called the **neural encoding of the stimulus pattern,** in a collection of cells making outputs from the network. Examples are the retina, which converts the light pattern projected on the rods and cones into the afferent pattern in the optic nerve, and the cochlea, which converts the sound pattern arriving at the ear into the afferent pattern in the auditory nerve. These receptors will be described in detail in later chapters.

There are three principal classes of receptor networks: passive, adaptive, and active or controlled. A receptor network is **passive** in case the same stimulus pattern always results in the same output pattern. A receptor network is **adaptive** in case is its only input is the sensory pattern and its output pattern depends on the history of sensory inputs. A receptor network is **active** or **controlled** in case it receives control inputs in addition to the sensory inputs, and the control inputs determine how the sensory patterns will be encoded as neural activity. The retina, for example, is adaptive since its output depends on previous inputs (bleaching of the rods and cones), and it also appears to be active since some of the axons in the optic nerve are efferent (sending information away from the brain). However, the effect of the efferent inputs on retinal encoding is not yet known.

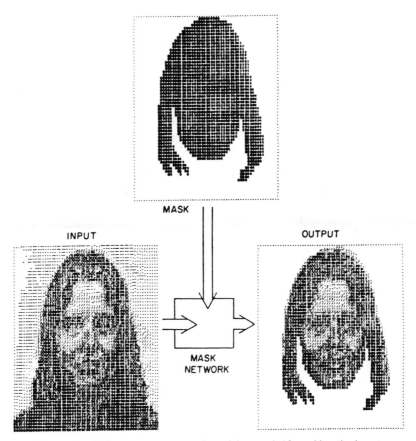

Figure 2.9. An input pattern, a mask, and the result of masking the input pattern with the illustrated mask. (Reproduced, with permission, from R. J. Baron, Mechanisms of human facial recognition. *International Journal of Man-Machine Studies*, 15, 1981, 137-178.)

CATEGORIES OF INFORMATION TRANSFORMATION NETWORKS

Just as with receptor networks, there are three basic classes of information-transforming networks: passive, adaptive, and active or controlled. An information transformation network is **passive** if its output depends only on its current input pattern. It is **adaptive** if the output pattern depends on the history of input patterns, and it is **active** or **controlled** if in addition to the input pattern, the network receives a **control pattern** that alters the transformation performed by the network. Examples of passive, adaptive, and controlled transformation networks are presented below.

Two examples of passive transformations that can be performed on a pattern are to compute its Laplacian and its x-gradient. The **Laplacian** of a pattern is a pattern which indicates how much faster or slower each cell fires than the average of its neighbors. Thus a network with symmetrical lateral inhibition can compute the Laplacian of its input pattern. The x-gradient of a pattern is a pattern that indicates how much faster or slower each cell fires than its horizontal neighbors, scanning from left to right across the input pattern. Suppose that an information pattern is generated at the retina in which the light intensities are encoded directly by the firing rates of the cells that receive the light from that position in the visual field. The Laplacian of this pattern represents places in the visual field where the light varies rapidly whereas the x-gradient represents places where the light increases when moving horizontally across the visual field. Figure 2.10 shows an input pattern, its Laplacian, and its x-gradient. Figure 2.11 shows a simple passive transformation for producing the Laplacian of an input pattern, and Figure 2.12 shows a simple passive transformation for producing the x-gradient. For each figure, the input and output cells are arranged on rectangular grids. For the Laplacian, each input cell connects to exactly five output cells. The coupling between an input cell and its corresponding output cell is excitatory with coupling coefficient $+4$, and the coupling coefficients between an input cell and its remaining four immediate neighbors is inhibitory with coupling coefficient -1 (lateral inhibition). For the x-gradient, each input cell connects to six out of nine of its adjacent and diagonal neighbors. The three cells on the right receive excitatory coupling with weight $+1$; the three cells on the left receive inhibitory coupling with weight -1. Try to distinguish between these two networks based only on their structure.

An example of an adaptive network and its graphic symbol are shown in Figure 2.13. The illustrated network is a **normalization network**. An information pattern is **normalized** in case the sum of squares of the firing rates of the cells conveying the output pattern is a specified constant, generally one. The input cells connect directly to the output cells in a one-to-one fashion but the coupling is regulated by a single control cell as shown. The output cells are monitored to determine the sum of squares of their firing rates. If the monitored rate exceeds one, the control cell fires at a faster rate. This uniformly decreases

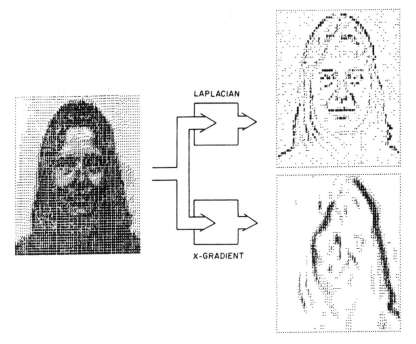

Figure 2.10. The Laplacian and X-gradient of an input pattern. (Reproduced, with permission, from R. J. Baron, Mechanisms of human facial recognition. *International Journal of Man-Machine Studies, 15,* 1981, 137–178.)

the connectivity between input and output cells. The result is that the sum of squares of the firing rates of the output cells is reduced while the ratios between firing rates of input to output cells remains constant. If the monitored rate of the output is less than one, the control cell slows down, resulting in a uniform increase in the coupling between input and output cells. The result is that the network produces a normalized output pattern that is similar (as defined earlier) to the original input pattern. The network is adaptive since the output pattern depends on the previous input pattern, and the adaptation is **bounded in time** since adaptation depends only on the most recent inputs. The masking network described earlier is also an active network.

SUMMARY

I have described the notions of information, information transmission, and information transformation. I have also described several fundamental types of

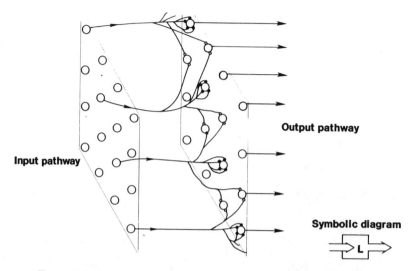

Input pathway

Output pathway

Symbolic diagram

Figure 2.11. A neural network for computing the Laplacian of an input pattern. Only a few connections are shown.

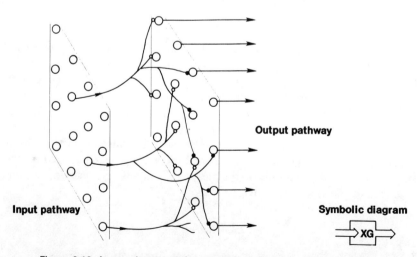

Input pathway

Output pathway

Symbolic diagram

Figure 2.12. A neural network for computing the X-gradient of an input pattern. Only a few connections are shown.

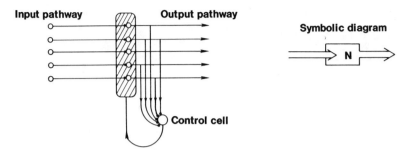

Figure 2.13. An adaptive network for normalizing an input pattern. The regulatory cell uniformly reduces the transformational coupling between information input cells and their corresponding information output cells when the average input value is too high, and increases the coupling when the average input value is too low.

neural networks for information transfer and transformation. The relevance of these and other networks to the brain will be the topic of later chapters in this book.

SUGGESTED READINGS

The following references describe neural networks and neural information processing in general and emphasize theoretical approaches to understanding brain function.

Baron, R.J. (1981). Mechanisms of human facial recognition. *International Journal of Man-Machine Studies*, 15, 137–138.

Caianiello, E.R. (Ed.). (1968). *Neural networks.* New York: Springer-Verlag.

Dowling, J.E. (1970). Organization of vertebrate retinas. *Investigative Ophthalmology*, 9, 655–679.

Grenander, U. (1976). *Pattern synthesis. Lectures in pattern theory.* (Vol. 1). New York: Springer-Verlag.

_____. (1978). *Pattern analysis. Lectures in pattern theory.* (Vol. 2). New York: Springer-Verlag.

Katchalsky, A. K., Rowland, V., & Blumenthal, R. (1974). *Dynamic patterns of brain cell assemblies.* Cambridge, MA: MIT Press.

Metzler, J. (Ed.). (1977). *Systems neuroscience.* New York: Academic Press.

Reichart, W. E., & Poggio, T. (Eds.). (1981). *Theoretical approaches in neurobiology.* Cambridge MA: MIT Press.

Sommerhoff, G. (1974). *Logic of the living brain.* New York: John Wiley & Sons.

Szentágothai, J., & Arbib, M. A. (1975). *Conceptual models of neural organization.* Cambridge, MA: MIT Press.

Wooldridge, D. E. (1979). *Sensory processing in the brain. An exercise in neuroconnective Modeling.* New York: John Wiley & Sons.

3
INFORMATION STORAGE

INTRODUCTION

I will begin this chapter with descriptions of two types of computer storage systems, addressed and associative, and I will discuss the hardware required for each of them. Since all of the storage techniques devised by computer architects while designing modern computers have occurred naturally during the evolution of man, a study of computer storage systems will serve as a gentle introduction into the mechanisms of information storage in the human brain. I will then describe neural storage networks and their computational and control structures. I will defer until Chapter 6 a discussion of human memory since an understanding of information storage in general must precede an understanding of the relationship between information storage and memory. The appendix of this chapter presents the details of one neural network model for cortical storage. The model emphasizes the control structures and mechanisms needed for converting dynamic patterns into static patterns and vice versa.

ADDRESSED COMPUTER STORAGE SYSTEMS

It is approximately correct to think of a computer storage system as a collection of registers together with their control circuitry. An N-word storage system, for example, consists of N register, together with the circuitry necessary for distributing information to them during storage and gathering information from them during recall. Historically, each register together with its control circuitry has been called a **memory location** and I will continue to follow that custom here.

Each register is connected to an **internal output bus** through a set of switches which are inside the register, and each register receives inputs from an **internal input bus**. Note that a correspondence is maintained between input bus wire and output bus wire throughout the system. Refer to Figure 3.1. One control input to each register, a **copy input** (labeled C in the figure), causes that register to store the value currently impressed on the internal input bus. However, unless the copy input is turned on, the register ignores the value on the internal input bus. A second control input to each register (labeled En in the figure), an **enable output** input, connects the register to the internal output bus. The value held by a register is only impressed on the internal output bus when the enable output signal is turned on. The control circuits of the computer generate the copy and enable output signals. The control circuits also guarantee that only one register is ever connected to the output bus at a time.

An **addressed memory system** generally has two distinguished registers that do not store information but are used as part of its control circuitry. A **memory buffer register** is used to temporarily hold and make available for output the information that has just been recalled from a memory location. A **memory address register** is used to hold the number or index of the memory location that is storing or recalling information. The number or index of a memory location is its **address**, which can range from 0 to N − 1 in an N word storage system. If the the memory address register has K bits, then the storage system can hold at most 2^K words.

Figure 3.2 illustrates the major components of an addressed storage system. The wires numbered C1 through C8 are control wires that receive signals directly from the computer's control unit. Their use, summarized below, will be described shortly.

C1   gate the contents of a memory location onto the internal output bus
C2   gate the memory input onto the internal input bus
C3   gate the contents of the memory buffer register as an output from the storage system
C4   gate an address value into the memory address register
C5   enable an output from the address decoder
C6   store a value in a memory location
C7   store a value in the memory buffer register
C8   store a value in the memory address register

The **address decoder** shown in Figure 3.2 accepts both information and control inputs. Its information input is the value held in the memory address register. The control input is an **enable** input (control wire C5 in Figure 3.2). The enable input causes the address decoder to generate exactly one output. The output from the address decoder is a signal on a single output wire that corresponds to the address currently held in the memory address register. If the memory address register holds the value 1, then output wire number 1 is turned on; if the memory address register holds the value 2, then output wire 2 is turned on, and so forth. *In summary, the address decoder generates a signal on one and only one of its output wires.*

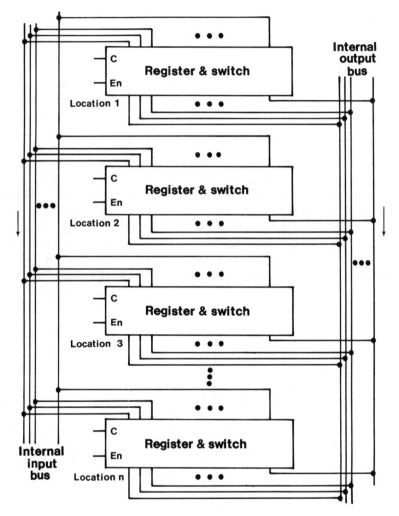

Figure 3.1. The registers and pathways that comprise a computer's memory store.

As shown in Figure 3.2, each output wire from the address decoder goes to a different memory location. The output wire labeled 2, for example, goes to memory location number 2. Each control wire divides and goes to two switches at its target memory location. Switches appear as semicircles in the figure, with inputs on the left and a single output on the right. The output is on only if both inputs are on. The lower of the two switches enables the register to place its value on the internal output bus. A memory location will place its value on the internal output bus only when both the memory address register holds its address, and hence the control wire to that memory location is active, and when control wire C1 is turned on (by the control unit of the computer). The other switch is connected to the copy input of the register. The register will store the value from the internal input bus only when the memory address register holds its address and when control input C6 is turned on (by the control unit of the computer). When a value is stored, it is always the value impressed on the internal input bus, which is also the input value to the storage system.

I will now describe exactly how an addressed storage system works. Suppose the goal is to store the value 123 in memory location 3. The control circuitry of the computer first sends the value 3 to the memory address register of the storage

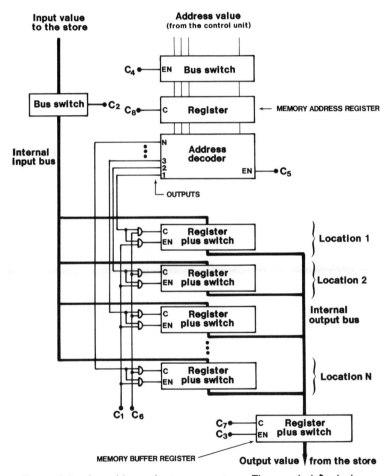

Figure 3.2. An addressed storage system. The symbol ⊃ designates a switch. Both inputs (arriving at the left) must be on for the output (exiting on the right) to be on. Individual wires of the data busses are not shown. The control inputs, C_1 through C_8, are described in the text.

system. At the same time it sends control signals along control wires C4 and C8. Control signal C4 gates the value 3 into the memory address register and control signal C8 causes the memory address register to store this value. Thus the memory address register stores the address of the desired memory location. Next, the control circuitry of the computer sends the value 123 to the storage system and sends signals along control wires C2, C5, and C6. Control wire C2 gates the value 123 into the internal input bus which distributes it to all memory locations. Since the memory address register is holding the value 3, a signal on control wire C5 causes the address decoder to place a signal on its output wire numbered 3 which goes to the two switches at memory location 3. The signal along control wire C6, the "store now" signal, arrives at the switch in location 3. Since both inputs are turned on, the switch sends a signal to the copy input of the register in memory location 3. Memory location 3 therefore stores the current value on the internal input bus, 123, exactly as desired.

The sequence of control signals C4-C8, C2-C5-C6 will always cause a value to be stored in a memory location and is called a **microprogram**. The value stored is the input value to the store when C2-C5-C6 occurs and the memory location that stores the value is the one whose address is input when C4-C8 occurs.

A similar process is used for recalling a value from memory. First the address of the desired location is input to the store and signals are sent along control wires C4 and C8. This stores the address of the desired memory location in the memory address register in preparation for the read operation. Next, signals are sent along control wires C1, C5, and C7. Control signals C1 and C5 open the bus gate from the location whose address is in the memory address register to the internal output bus, and control wire C7 causes the memory buffer register to store the value on the internal output bus. Finally control wire C3 is turned on. Control wire C3 gates the recalled value, the value now in the memory buffer register, as an output from the storage system.

The microprogram C4-C8, C1-C5-C7, C3 always causes a value to be recalled from memory, and the selected location is the one whose address is input when control signals C4 and C8 occur.

It should be clear for a storage system that some information is content information (the information being stored and recalled) and some information is control information (the control signals C1 through C8 and the control signals generated by the address decoder). But what about the addresses themselves? There is no definitive answer. They can be thought of either as content or control patterns depending on one's point of view.

The main points to keep in mind are:

1. The memory locations themselves are all identical; only their contents may differ.
2. Control signals determine when and where information is to be stored.

3. Control signals determine when and from where information is to be recalled.

4. The information pattern that is last stored in a memory location is the only information that can subsequently be recalled from that memory location.

5. Storage is the conversion of the dynamic pattern on the internal input bus into a static pattern in a register in the storage system.

6. Storage occurs when the "store now" signal is turned on.

7. Recall is the synthesis of a dynamic copy of a static stored pattern.

ASSOCIATIVE COMPUTER STORAGE SYSTEMS

An associative storage system, like an addressed storage system, consists of one register for each word of storage together with the necessary control circuitry to store, search for, and recall information. An associative storage system generally has four distinguished registers that do not store information but are used by the control circuitry for holding temporary values during storage, search, and recall. A **memory buffer register** holds the value just recalled from a memory location. An **argument register** holds a value to be searched for, and a **mask register** holds a pattern that indicates which bits in the argument register hold the sought after value. A **match register** indicates which storage locations contain the sought after information. Finally, a single **match signal** indicates if any of the bits in the match register are set. The argument and mask registers are the same size as the words in the memory locations, whereas the match register has one bit for each word in the storage system. See Figure 3.3.

In an addressed storage system, the memory address register holds the address of the word that will participate in a storage or recall operation. In an associative storage system, the match register is used for that purpose. The words may be thought of as ordered from top to bottom. The word that can be accessed, if any, is the highest word whose match bit is set. The problem that the control circuits of an associative storage system must solve is how to set the proper bits of the match register so the desired words can be accessed.

In an associative storage system, the idea is to access information not by address but by the values in some of the bits of the words in storage. For example, the desired word may contain the pattern '10110' in its first five bits. The mask register is used to indicate exactly which bits of the words will be compared. If a mask register bit is set (value 1), the corresponding bit is "masked out" and does not participate in the search. If the mask register bit is reset (value 0), that bit does participate. Thus if the words are eight bits long and we are looking for a word with '10110' in bits 1 through 5, then the mask register would be set to '00000111' and the argument register bits would be set to '10110???',

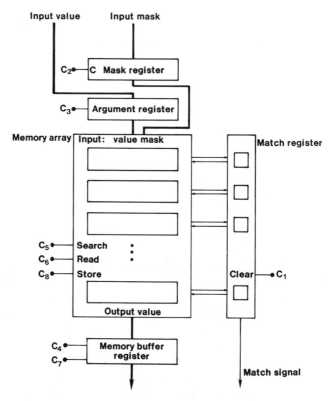

Figure 3.3. The major components of a computer associative memory. Comparison logic and storage circuitry within the memory array and match register array are not shown.

where question marks are "don't care" bits since they do not participate in the match. They are masked out. The mask register bits indicate that the first five bits of the argument register wil be compared and the last three bits will be ignored while the argument register's first five bits are '10110', which is the desired subpattern.

Figure 3.3 does not show the comparison circuitry of the memory locations but it does show the eight control wires that cause the storage system to operate. The control wire functions are:

C1   clear the match register
C2   store a value in the mask register
C3   store a value in the argument register
C4   store a value in the memory buffer register
C5   search memory
C6   read memory and reset the match bit of the selected word

48

C7   output the value in the memory buffer register
C8   store a value in memory and reset the match bit of the selected word

Control wire C1 resets all bits in the match register and therefore blocks access to all words of storage. Control wire C2 sets the mask register value to the input value, control wire C3 sets the argument register to the input value, and control wire C4 sets the memory buffer register to the value on the internal output bus. Control wire C5 causes memory to be searched. The value in every word is simultaneously compared with the value in the argument register, but only the bits corresponding to '0' bits in the mask register are actually compared. If all unmasked bits in a word of storage are identical to the corresponding bits in the argument register, that word's match bit is set. Otherwise that word's match bit in not changed. Control wire C6 causes the highest word in memory whose match bit is set to be read; its value is placed on the internal output bus and copied into the memory buffer register. At the same time the match bit of that memory location is reset. Control wire C7 causes the value in the memory buffer register to be sent as an output from the storage system, and control wire C8 causes the input value to the storage system to be stored in the highest word in memory whose match bit is set. At the same time the match bit is reset.

Here is how the associative store operates. First the mask and argument registers are set to the desired values. This is done by inputting the mask and placing a signal on control wire C2 and inputting the argument and placing a signal on control wire C3. Next control wire C1 is turned on to clear the match register in preparation of the search. Next control wire C5 is turned on. This causes the search to occur: the match bits of words in memory having the desired property are set. The values of words whose match bits are set can now be read. The memory locations are **activated**. In order to read a value, control wire C6 is turned on. This copies the value in the first activated memory location into the memory buffer register, and control wire C7 outputs this value so it can be inspected by the computer. As the word in memory is read, its match bit is reset. Thus a subsequent read operation will read the next word whose match bit is set (i.e., the next activated word). To read the next word, the computer again sends the control signals C6 and C7 in sequence and inspects the memory output. This can be done any number of times. When no more words can be accessed the match bit shows value '0' and the process is terminated.

In order to store a word in memory, the match bit of the desired word must be set, the value to be stored must be input to the storage system, and control wire C7 must be turned on. The problem is how to set the correct bit in the match register. If the current contents of the word to be changed are known, the mask bit can be set just as for a read operation. Otherwise all match register bits can be set (by performing a search with a mask register containing all '1' bits), and the match register bits above the desired word can be reset by sequential read operations. When the match bit of the desired word is the highest bit set, the storage signal (control wire C7) can be turned on. This will cause the input value to be stored in the desired memory location.

This method of storing a word in an associative memory is very slow and therefore not very satisfactory. An alternative solution is to give the storage system a memory address register and add circuitry, which sets the match register bits according to the value in the memory address register. Such a storage system is both addressed and associative and has the advantages of both systems.[1]

STORAGE IN NEURAL NETWORKS

Neural networks for storing, analyzing, and retrieving information are fundamental to brain function. Let me begin this discussion with the notion of **neural information storage**. Consider the situation depicted in Figure 3.4. A neural pathway is shown having one **sensory microelectrode** implanted in each axon. A sensory microelectrode is an electrical probe which senses the state of the neuron. The signal derived from each sensory microelectrode is sent to a separate channel on a multichannel tape recorder where the individual signals are amplified and stored on magnetic tape. When the RECORD button is depressed, recording starts and continues until the tape runs out or until the RECORD button is released. As soon as the RECORD button is released, the tape is automatically rewound. After the tape is rewound, the PLAYBACK button can be depressed. When the PLAYBACK button is depressed, the recorder begins to play back the information stored on the tape. Each output from the recorder connects to a **stimulating microelectrode** that stimulates the same pathway element that the corresponding sensory microelectrode was probing. Thus there is a one-to-one correspondence between the input cells from which the recording was derived and the output cells that are stimulated during playback. If, during playback, each output cell is stimulated to fire each time the recording indicates that the corresponding cell fired previously, then the output pattern synthesized during playback is equal to the input pattern that arrived during storage. We say that the depolarization pattern was **stored** by the recorder and later **recalled** by the recorder during playback.

An analogous neural **netlet** for storing and recalling information is shown in Figure 3.5. A netlet is a small, functionally distinct collection of cells within a larger network, and in this diagram a netlet corresponds to a single memory location in a neural storage system. The **input pathway** corresponds to the pathway originating at the sensory microelectrodes in the previous system, the cells labeled "to output pathway" correspond to the outputs connected to the

---

[1]Associative stores are not common today because of their slow speed and the cost of the circuitry to perform the associative search. This discussion gives the features of an associative store without facing the technical problems of actually building one.

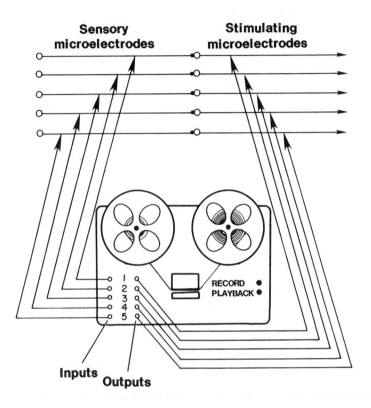

Figure 3.4. The tape-recorder analog of a memory location.

stimulating microelectrodes, the **initiate storage input cell** is an effectual input that corresponds to the RECORD button, the **initiate recall input cell** is a command input that corresponds to the PLAYBACK button, and the cells shown inside the netlet correspond to the magnetic tape and the tape-recording hardware. Also analogous to the previous system is the fact that there is a one-to-one correspondence between the information input cells and information output cells in the netlet.

A detailed model of a storage network comprised of netlets of this type will be deferred until the appendix of this chapter. Fortunately, the internal details need not be specified in order to understand its behavior and control functions. In particular, we may assume that this netlet behaves essentially like the recorder just described. In particular, time-varying neural patterns can be stored and recalled.

51

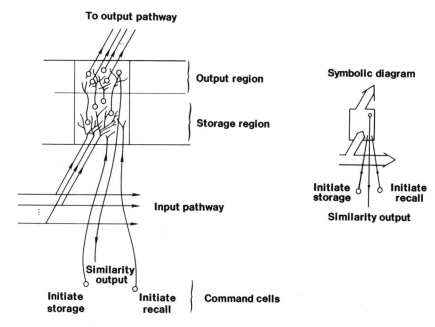

Figure 3.5. The components of one storage location.

I will now describe the behavior of one storage netlet. When the initiate storage cell fires, the netlet begins to record the activity present in the information input neurons. Storage occurs in real time, and the network stores the spatial, time-varying firing pattern arriving along the input neurons. The entire process is called **storage**. **Consolidation** is the internal process of modifying the coupling parameters that effect storage. Storage terminates either when the initiate storage input stops firing or when the memory location, because of physical limitations, can hold no more information. When the initiate recall input fires, the netlet synthesizes a copy of the information that was stored during the storage process. **Recall** is the synthesis of a copy of the stored pattern and its transmission to the output pathway of the storage system. The recalled pattern varies in time exactly as the stored pattern did during storage, and the recalled pattern equals the stored pattern under the correspondence between input and output cells.[2]

A **memory store** is a storage network that receives inputs through a collection of information input cells and delivers recalled information through information output cells. A **memory system** is a memory store together with the networks

---

[2] Storage in this network differs from storage by the tape recorder in that during recall, the axons do not necessarily depolarize at corresponding times but only at corresponding rates. This is because of the statistical nature of the neurons and the complementary notion of equality of information.

that control its activity. See Figure 3.6. The information input cells to a memory store distribute the input pattern to all memory locations in the memory store and the information output cells gather together the recalled information from each storage netlet. There is a one-to-one correspondence between information input cells and information output cells. Two command inputs to each memory location regulate storage and recall. An **initiate storage** input to a memory location is an effectual input that causes the storage process to begin, and storage continues either until no more information can be accepted or until the initiate storage signal ceases. An **initiate recall** input is a command input that causes recall to begin. Recall continues until there is no more information to recall or until the initiate recall cell stops firing.

Hereafter, unless explicitly stated to the contrary, I will use these notions of information storage and recall and have in mind a storage network having the characteristics described herein. The relationships between storage networks and well-known psychological topics such as learning, remembering, forgetting, adaptation, and so forth, will be explored in depth in later chapters.

Types of Memory Stores

Within a memory store, those physical coupling parameters of the storage cells that are established during consolidation are **memory traces** or **memory engrams**. A memory store which can recall information without changing its memory engrams has **non-destructive recall**. A memory store whose memory traces are destroyed during recall has **destructive recall**. A memory store whose memory engrams once made are never changed is a **permanent memory store with non-degrading memory traces**. A memory store whose memory engrams are changed continuously to reflect the current input is an **immediate memory store** or **memory buffer**. A memory store whose memory engrams slowly degrade over a long period of time is a **permanent memory store with degrading memory**

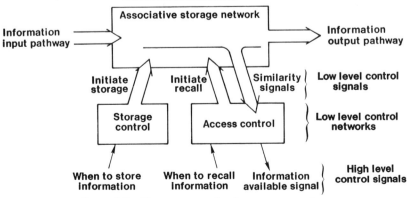

Figure 3.6. The components of a memory system.

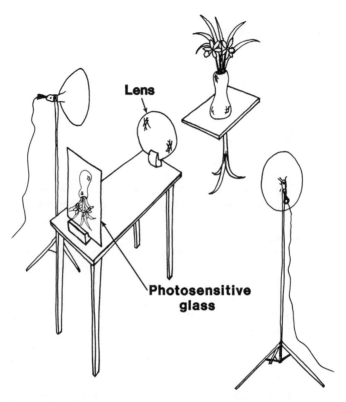

Lens

Photosensitive glass

Figure 3.7. A piece of photosensitive glass can be used as a storage medium in a continuously adaptive optical storage system.

traces. A memory store whose memory engrams can be modified during repeated presentations of input information has **adaptive memory traces**. Finally, a memory store which can delete one memory trace and replace it with a new one is a **temporary memory store**.

As an example, a home tape recorder is a temporary memory store with nondegrading memory traces and nondestructive recall. The magnetic domain patterns on the tape are the memory engrams, the electrical signals which are sent to the recording amplifiers during storage comprise the input patterns and the electrical signals produced by the playback amplifiers during playback comprise the recalled pattern. The physical process of modifying the magnetic domains on the tape during a recording session is consolidation.

As a second example, consider the situation depicted in Figure 3.7. A lens is shown that focuses an image of a scene on a piece of photosensitive glass. After a few seconds, the glass turns dark wherever the focused light is bright and remains clear where the focused light is dim. When the light is turned off, the photosensitive glass retains an image of the scene, but the image fades away after a short time. The glass together with the lens and light source are a storage system having continuously adaptive memory traces and destructive recall.

A **memory location** is one independently controlled storage unit within a memory store. A memory store consisting of 10 netlets of the type illustrated in Figure 3.5 would have 10 memory locations. Each netlet is one memory location. Such a network is illustrated in Figure 3.8. However, it is not always true that the memory locations are functionally or spatially distinct. The cells of the network might appear as shown in Figures 3.9 and 3.10. Figure 3.9 shows a memory store with **locally distributed memory traces** and Figure 3.10 shows a memory store with **totally distributed memory traces**. By definition, individual memory locations are controlled by independent command cells, and this situation pertains in all the networks illustrated. The command cells always determine which memory location will participate in storage or recall at any given time. The command cells are an **index** into the memory store and the memory store is **indexed**. In an indexed memory store, a specific piece of information can be recalled by initiating recall from the appropriate memory location, say location number 1, location number 2, and so forth. The **address** of a memory location is its number in the memory store. For memory stores having independent or locally distributed memory traces, the physical position of a memory location is equivalent to its index and therefore its geometric position relative to a two-dimensional coordinate system suitably imposed on

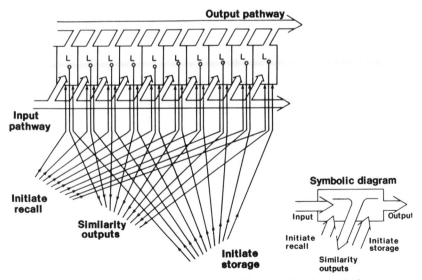

Figure 3.8.   The internal organization of storage locations within an associative memory store. (Reproduced, with permission, from R. J. Baron, Mechanisms of human facial recognition. *International Journal of Man-Machine Studies*, **15**, 1981, 137-178.)

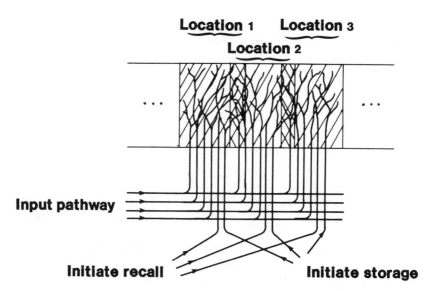

Figure 3.9. A memory store with locally-distributed memory traces.

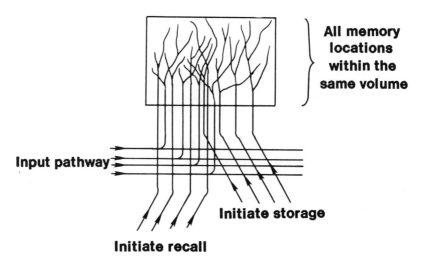

Figure 3.10. A memory store with totally-distributed memory traces.

the memory store is also equivalent to its index. In general, the intrinsic coordinates of control neurons are an index into a biological memory store.

An **associative memory store**, also known as a **content addressable memory store**, is a memory store in which the location or address of a piece of stored information can be determined *by the memory store* by presenting to it an information input pattern that is similar to the desired stored pattern. An associative memory store may also be indexed. Each memory location in an associative memory store is a computational netlet that determines for each input pattern the similarity between it and the information stored in that memory location. Each memory location delivers similarity information, a **similarity coefficient**, as an output through a **similarity output cell**. The **similarity pattern** from an associative memory store is the firing pattern in the set of similarity output cells. This is illustrated in Figure 3.11. The similarity coefficients evaluated by the memory locations can be used by the control networks of the storage system to determine which memory locations to recall information from. This will be discussed further in Chapter 4.

An associative memory store operates as follows. Inputs to the memory store are delivered through information input cells. Whenever an initiate storage cell is activated, the corresponding memory location stores the current input pattern. Several memory locations may concurrently store the input pattern. Simultaneously, each similarity output cell fires at a rate which indicates the similarity between the current input pattern and the pattern stored in that memory location. When an input pattern is not being sent to the memory store, recall can be initiated. The memory location that receives an initiate recall signal recalls its stored information and the recalled information is delivered as an information output pattern from the memory store.

The only essential difference between an associative memory store and an indexed memory store is the existence of the similarity outputs. However, this

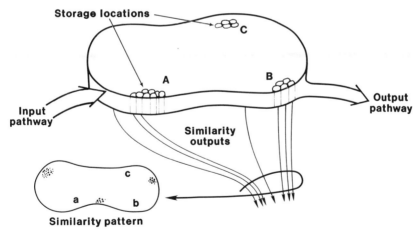

Figure 3.11. The similarity pattern is the pattern of activity in the similarity output pathway of an associative memory store. Strong activity at position "a" in the similarity pattern means that memory locations in corresponding position "A" within the store measure high similarity with the input pattern. The same is true at "b" and "B" and "c" and "C." Thus the similarity pattern is an index to regions of the store holding similar stored patterns.

difference has major significance. An associative memory store does more to the input patterns than just store them: It **analyzes** them. Whenever an input pattern arrives at an associative memory store, the similarity outputs indicate *if* any stored patterns are similar to the current pattern, *how similar* they are, and *where* in the memory store they are located. An associative memory store is an **analyzer network** (Luria, 1966) that continually monitors the input pattern and determines if there is similar stored information and where it is located.

Time and the Memory Trace

An information pattern is a **dynamic pattern**, which is an active encoding of information. In contrast, a memory trace is a **static pattern**, which is a passive encoding of information. Memory traces are encoded in terms of neural coupling parameters within a memory store, and storage entails the conversion of a dynamic pattern into a static pattern. Recall, in contrast, entails the conversion of a static pattern back into a dynamic pattern.

In a tape recorder, time is encoded into position on the moving magnetic tape. As the tape advances across the tape head during storage, the magnetic fields produced by the recording head cause magnetic domains to be formed along the tape. Movement of the tape during storage enables the conversion of the dynamic, time-varying, input pattern into a static pattern on the tape. During playback the tape again moves. This time, the magnetic fields produced by the magnetic domains on the tape moving across the tape head are detected by the tape head, which in turn produces electrical signals, depending on the direction of magnetization. When amplified, the signals are identical to the ones sent to the tape head during recording. Movement of the tape during playback enables the conversion of the static pattern on the tape back into a dynamic pattern.

There are several possible mechanisms within a neural storage network for converting between time of input and position. First, time can be divided into discrete intervals, for example, one-tenth of a second long, and the input pattern that arrives during each interval can be stored in a different storage location. The stored pattern in one location could be the average pattern that arrived during the corresponding time interval or it could be a sample of the input. During recall, the output firing rate of a given cell would either be the average firing rate of the corresponding input cell during the interval of storage or the sampled rate. A storage network of this type requires that distinct locations be given the initiate storage signals in sequence, both during storage and during recall. Either the memory store itself or external control networks would determine the sequence of memory locations to be used and therefore control the way in which dynamic patterns are converted into static patterns and vice versa. A memory location in such a memory store consists of all netlets controlled by a single initiate storage and initiate recall cell. See Figure 3.12.

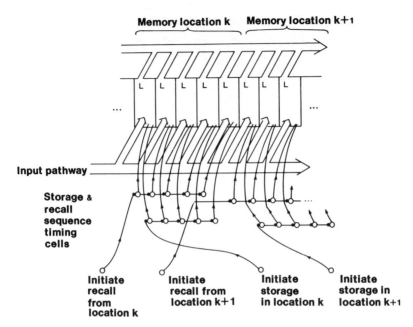

Figure 3.12. A storage system whose time of input is distributed among independent storage netlets within each memory location.

An alternative mechanism for converting between time of input and position in the memory store is to control the region of coupling between cells of each netlet. Consider the netlet shown in Figure 3.13. This netlet represents the same storage location illustrated in Figure 3.5 with one difference: 5 **timing control cells** C_1 through C_5 have been added. These timing control cells have negative regulatory coupling: Each timing control cell blocks the release of transmitter substance by the input cells. During storage and recall, all timing control cells fire except one. When control cell C_1 stops firing, the coupling between other cells of the netlet is restricted to the domain bounded by its axon field. Similarly, when control cell C_2 stops firing, the coupling is restricted to the domain bounded by its axon field. During storage, the timing control cells are stopped in sequence, first control cell C_1, then control cell C_2, and so forth. Likewise during recall, the timing control cells are stopped in sequence, first cell C_1, then cell C_2, and so forth. The control cells partition the coupling fields of the cells in the storage netlet into spatial regions where time of input is converted into position. Each "slice" of a netlet, determined by the geometry of the timing control cells, can store a different input pattern. One netlet of this type can hold the same information that five netlets of the previous type can hold. And with more elaborate timing control cells, the storage density can be further increased.

If the storage netlet is associative, the differences between the previous two

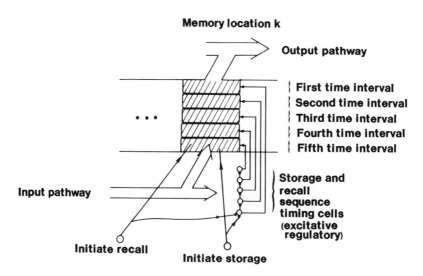

Figure 3.13. A storage system where time of input is converted into position of storage within one memory location using regulatory cells for sequencing.

networks are significant. In the first storage system (Figure 3.12), the current input pattern would be independently correlated against the stored pattern in each memory location. In order to determine whether or not the entire input pattern is similar to the stored pattern, the similarity signals from each storage netlet would have to be checked in sequence. The similarity signal produced at the first memory netlet would have to be high during the first time interval, the similarity signal produced by the second netlet would have to be high during the second time interval, and so forth. In the second storage system (Figure 3.13), all timing control cells except cell 1 would be firing. As soon as a memory location gives a high similarity signal, the remaining timing control cells would be stopped in sequence, beginning with timing control cell 2. This would restrict the network so that only those stored patterns having times corresponding to the time of the current input pattern would be correlated. If the similarity signal is high during the entire presentation of the input pattern, then the input pattern and the stored pattern are similar; otherwise they are not.

There is a third possibility for a mechanism for converting time of input into position in a storage network. The nonneural environment might provide the same type of timing mechanism that the control cells do in the previous system. Such a mechanism would completely relieve the neural circuitry from the responsibility of generating the appropriate timing signals, which is a very practical advantage. The storage system described in the appendix to this chapter is a system of this type.

The existence of a mechanism for converting between time of input and position in a storage network, and vice versa, is of central importance to understanding brain function. Such a mechanism organizes the information that is stored in the storage network into accessible **packets**. Take for example, our ability to recite the months of the year. This is an easy task. The fact that it is difficult to recite them backwards suggests that the information is organized into packets that can only be recalled in forward sequence. Our ability to read is an example of the reverse process, where time of input is critical to recognition. A sentence makes no sense at all if its words are jumbled up. (Example a supporting this is sentence.) But put the words in the correct sequence, and the sentence can easily be read and understood. (This sentence is a supporting example.) Similarly, a sentence is difficult to read if it does not have timing markers to indicate the onset of the words. (Thissentenceisacaseinpoint.) But insert the timing markers and the sentence is easy to understand. (This sentence is a case in point.)

Temporal order and external timing signals are essential for recognition of time-varying patterns.

I will assume hereafter that the memory timing mechanism is controlled automatically for storage, recognition, and recall. This assumption is independent of the type of timing mechanism: location sequencing, timing cells within locations, or nonneuronal timing. It is also independent of the type of storage network: temporary or permanent.

The Making of Memories and Their Recall

Memory traces can be made in two very different ways. At one extreme, information enters the storage network once and the memory traces are made during or immediately following that single presentation. This corresponds to the way a tape recorder makes a tape. At the other extreme, memory traces may be made slowly during repeated presentations of the same or very similar information patterns. For such a network, the memory traces would have to be adaptive.

Both types of memory trace appear to be used by human memory stores. Memories of experience appear to be made as the experiences are lived. They appear to be laid down much as a tape recorder records the input signals that it receives. In contrast, people appear to learn skills only after long hours of practice, repeating time after time the same motions, slowly improving them, until they are perfect. Once learned, such motor skills can be used without conscious thought, as if the motor patterns are simply recalled in sequence from a memory store and played back through the appropriate muscles. This is only partly correct as you will see later.

There is an important difference between the stored encodings of experience and the stored patterns that control our motor skills. Experiences which arise from the outside world are not under the control of the brain and occur just once. In contrast, motor skills are the result of motor patterns that are generated by the brain during practice. The onset of a motor pattern is determined by the brain, and as a result the timing signals are present that are required for synchronizing the input pattern with the memory timing mechanism. This is necessary for a storage system that has adaptive memory traces.

Information can be recalled in two very different ways. At one extreme, the speed at which recall proceeds may be fixed by the neural tissue: The recalled pattern progresses in time only at the speed that the initial pattern did during input. At the other extreme, the speed of recall may be variable, regulated by control inputs arriving at the memory store. This seems to be the case for the execution of motor skills, which can be performed at a variety of speeds. In either case (depending on the timing mechanism), it might be possible to suspend recall and at a later time resume recall from the point of suspension.

Similarity Measures for Neural Patterns

The ability of an associative memory store to locate stored information by association depends both on the type of information to be located and on how the similarity signals are generated. The similarity signals determine a **measure of similarity** between information patterns, one being the dynamic input pattern and the other being the static stored pattern. In a computer, information is encoded as states in registers, and when a computer uses an associative memory store, a memory location is identified provided that the input pattern exactly matches the corresponding stored pattern (subject to the masking out of certain bits). The result of the similarity computation is simply a "yes" or a "no" response in the match register. In a neural network there is no such simple criterion that can be used to identify a memory location. The firing rate of a similarity output cell depends on the mathematical computation performed by the memory location, and the criterion for choosing one memory location over another one is not clear.

There are two aspects to similarity that are relevant to neural systems. First, two patterns must be **spatially similar**. That is, the firing rate in each input cell must be similar to the firing rate that occurred in the same cell during storage. If a network holds visual encodings, the input pattern and the stored pattern must "look" the same.

The second aspect of similarity concerns the temporal characteristics of the two patterns. Two patterns are **temporally similar** only if they are spatially similar for a long enough long interval of time. The time interval required for agreement, however, need not be the entire interval for which a stored pattern is defined. Suppose that an associative memory store holds in one memory location the entire verbal encoding of the words of a poem. It may be that only the first few words of the poem are needed in order to generate an adequate similarity signal to identify and enable access to the remainder of the poem.

(Jack and Jill went . . .) Regardless of the type of encoding, there must be some mechanism for synchronizing the input pattern with the stored pattern during the similarity computation. As indicated earlier, a high initial similarity signal may be used to initiate the timing mechanism for subsequent similarity tests within in that memory location. Another possibility is that the onset of an input pattern is used to start the timing mechanism concurrently for all memory locations in the memory store. This would enable synchronization between the input pattern and all stored patterns.

The time interval of agreement need not be the starting interval for the stored information. Consider the following: ". . . that I have but one life. . . ." The given words are generally adequate to enable recall of information about the quotation. However, recognizing a sentence when given a few central words appears to be a much more complex task than recognizing a sentence when given its first few words. Recognition when given a few central words is often done during rehearsal or upon a second or third presentation of the given pattern—for example, while rereading the sentence. During such a repeated presentation, the brain has control of the onset of the input pattern and therefore control of the timing signals necessary for its recognition. This internal control process appears to be necessary for synchronizing the input pattern with the memory timing mechanism during this type of associative search.

MIXED MODALITY MEMORY STORES

Figures 3.14 and 3.15 show two different storage networks for concurrently storing more than one information pattern. The network shown in Figure 3.15 is identical to the network in Figure 3.14 except that the cells of the various memory locations have been physically merged in the same volume, and the two networks share the same control inputs. Both networks are **mixed modality memory stores**. A mixed modality memory store is a memory store having more than one collection of information input and output cells, and each memory location can simultaneously store and recall more than one pattern. Because of the one-to-one correspondence between input and output cells, information that arrives through one set of inputs will always be correlated against patterns that arrived through that same set of inputs and they will always be recalled through the corresponding set of outputs. Information from the two modalities remains independent. For the associative mixed modality memory stores shown in Figures 3.14 and 3.15, the similarity signal could be the sum of the similarity signals generated by either of the modalities independently, it could be the maximum of the two values, or it could be some other combination of them. (Note that a mixed modality memory store can associate two different patterns of the same modality if both sets of inputs [and therefore outputs] deliver information of the same modality.)

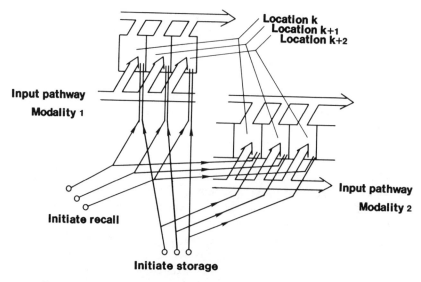

Figure 3.14. A mixed modality memory store with physically separate memory traces for each modalaity.

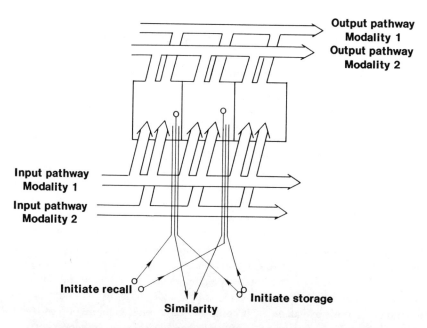

Figure 3.15. A mixed modality memory store where the memory traces from different modalities are stored within the same physical location.

The behavior of a mixed modality memory store is as follows. Whenever the initiate storage signal is active, the network begins to store information. If information arrives through input cells of both modalities, then input patterns of both modalities are independently stored. If only one of the input modalities is active, then only that one pattern is stored. A null pattern would be stored in the other modality corresponding to the input neurons not firing. Similarly, when the initiate recall signal is active, independent patterns are recalled, each recalled pattern being delivered from the storage network through the information output cells of that modality. If only one pattern was stored, then only that pattern would be generated; the outputs of the other modality would deliver a null pattern, as the output cells would not fire.

Associated Information

There are two different ways that information patterns can become **directly associated** by an associative memory store. Two patterns of different modalities become directly associated if they simultaneously arrive at a mixed modality store and are stored in the same memory location. (Two storage netlets that are controlled by the same control cells are a single memory location.) When this happens, input information in either modality may be used to locate stored information, and recall of the stored information gives rise to two different associated patterns, one in each of the modalities. If two patterns are of the same modality, they may become directly associated if they arrive at a memory store close together in time so they are stored in the same information packet. When this happens, recall of information generates an entire sequence of stored patterns. All patterns in such a sequence are directly associated. These two types of association are illustrated in Figure 3.16.

Two patterns P and Q are **associatively linked** or **associated** if there is a sequence of patterns $P_1, P_2, \ldots, P_K$, where $P = P_1$, $Q = P_K$, and P_i is directly associated to P_{i+1} in the sequence. An associative memory store has **associatively linked information** if the last pattern stored in each information packet is also the first information pattern stored in a subsequent information packet. Associative linking sequentializes data over a long period of time just as the memory timing mechanism sequentializes information over a short period of time. The parameters of the memory stores determine whether a memory timing mechanism or associative linking can be used to sequentialize particular information patterns.

Association Stores

The most common type of storage network to have been modeled and hence the best understood theoretically is the **association store**, a network which differs considerably from the storage networks described so far in this chapter. The differences will be described below.

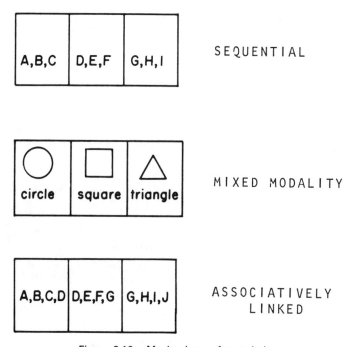

Figure 3.16. Mechanisms of association.

Consider the two associative memory stores shown in Figure 3.17. Each memory location is controlled by an initiate storage command cell and an initiate recall command cell, and each memory location makes a similarity output. As illustrated in Figure 3.17, a single external input initiates storage in one memory location of each of the memory stores; thus both networks store information concurrently. Also implied by Figure 3.17 is the fact that the similarity output from one memory location is the recall input to the corresponding memory location in the second storage network, and vice versa. If an initiate storage signal is externally generated, memory locations in both memory stores will store their respective input patterns. Two patterns stored in corresponding memory locations become **associated** by virtue of the hardware of the storage system. All incoming patterns that arrive at the storage system are compared with all patterns already stored there. If a similarity output from one memory location is high, recall is automatically initiated from the corresponding memory location in the other memory store. Recall occurs without intervening control of any kind. The arrival of information to one memory store initiates recall of associated information from the other, which is why networks of this type are called association stores. If two or more memory locations in one of the memory stores contain similar information, recall from both of the corresponding memory locations in the other memory store will be initiated and the output pattern will be a combination of the two recalled patterns. (If the statistical neuron described in Chapter 1 is used, the firing rate in each output cell would be the sum of firing rates of the corresponding output cells.) If the associated patterns are very different, the recalled output pattern may not resemble either of the associated patterns. If, however, they are similar, then the recalled output pattern will resemble them both.

In summary, an association store is a storage network from which information is recalled automatically, without intervening control, whenever an input pattern is presented. It is important to note that two associative memory stores with suitable control functions may operate as an association store. You will see in later chapters that the memory stores which control skilled behavior initially operate as associative stores but later operate as association stores when appropriate motor programs are stored. It is not generally the case that association stores can operate as associative stores.

Association stores having a much simpler architecture are well known. Perhaps the oldest and most thoroughly understood association store is the perceptron (Minsky & Papert, 1969; Rosenblatt, 1962). See Figure 3.18. The perceptron is a three-layered adaptive neural network which operates as follows. Two patterns arrive at the network simultaneously: the **input** or **stimulus**

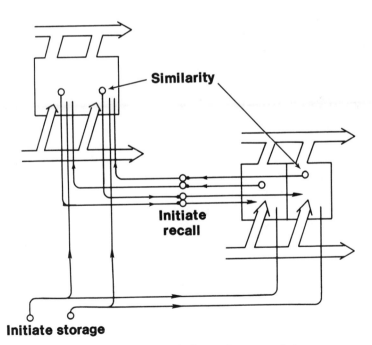

Initiate storage

Figure 3.17.   An association store built out of two associative memory stores.

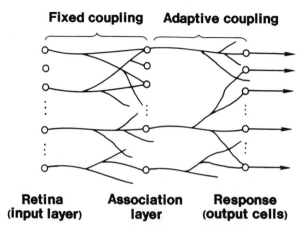

Fixed coupling   **Adaptive coupling**

Retina   **Association**   **Response**
(input layer)   **layer**   **(output cells)**

Figure 3.18.   The structure of a perceptron.

pattern, and the **desired response pattern**.[3] The desired response pattern is an effectual input to the perceptron. Upon presentation of a stimulus pattern, if the desired response pattern is elicited by the network, no changes are made. However, if the desired response is not elicited, coupling parameters between the association layer and response layer of cells in the perceptron are systematically modified until the correct output is derived. The procedure for modifying cellular parameters is **adaptation**. After the perceptron is modified to respond correctly for the first stimulus and desired response pattern pair, a second stimulus and desired response pattern pair are presented and the same adaptation procedure followed. When the perceptron responds correctly to the second stimulus pattern, the first stimulus and desired response pattern pair are again presented and the adaptation procedure once again carried out. Each time a new stimulus and desired response pattern pair are presented, the adaptation procedure is followed. Afterwards, all previous stimulus and desired response pattern pairs are again presented and the adaptation procedure followed for them. This process of presenting a new stimulus and desired response pattern pair, modifying the system, and then repeating for all prior stimulus and desired response pattern pairs is called **training**. Rosenblatt and his colleagues proved that if there is any set of coupling parameters that will enable the network to respond correctly for all stimulus patterns, then his adaptation and training procedures guarantee that such a set of coupling parameters will be found.

Within a network of this type, the memory traces do not resemble the stimulus or response patterns and there is no way of recalling a previous stimulus

---

[3]In the usual presentation of a perceptron, the desired response pattern is an implicit rather than explicit input pattern and is only used for changing the coupling parameters of the perceptron. Neurons conveying the desired response pattern are generally not described.

pattern unless the response pattern is also the stimulus pattern. This is in principle very different from the mixed modality memory stores described earlier which enable recall of either or both of the input patterns. (In the perceptron, the desired response pattern is an input pattern, so that at least one of the input patterns is recalled.) The concepts of memory locations, similarity signals, and so forth have no meaning for perceptrons. Finally, the internal structure of a perceptron is much simpler than the internal structure of the associative memory stores described earlier.

SUMMARY

The notion of information storage is fundamental to all information processing systems. At the neural level several parameters of a storage system must be considered:

Permanence of the memory trace
• Permanent
• Temporary
• Degrading

Mechanism of trace consolidation
• Continuously adaptive
• Made during a single presentation of the input pattern
• Adaptive—made during multiple presentations of the input pattern

Duration of the input pattern
• Short (less than .1 second) such as for phonemes of speech or the letters of words during reading
• Medium (about 1 second) such as the words during speech or reading
• Long (greater than 1 second) such as the sentences during spoken language or the images formed during an analysis of a visual scene

Dimensionality of the input pattern

Number of memory locations in the store

Number of input modalities to the store
• Single modality
• Mixed modality

The first and second of these parameters are determined by the biochemical properties of the storage networks themselves. The third parameter is determined by the wiring diagram of the networks using the memory store but is highly dependent on the first and second parameters. The final two parameters are relatively independent of the first parameters but depend on the architecture of the neural network and how it is used. Other storage properties will be discussed as necessary later in this book.

Association stores and associative memory stores differ markedly in their behavioral characteristics and both are likely to be found in the brain. However, in any attempt at understanding brain function, it is imperative that the various properties of the storage networks be understood and made explicit. In this way a critical evaluation of their properties for brain function is possible.

REFERENCES

Luria, A. R. (1966). *Higher cortical functions in man.* New York: Basic Books.
Luria, A. R. (1980). *Higher cortical functions in man. (2d ed.).* New York: Basic Books.
Minsky, M., & Papert, S. (1969). *Perceptrons. An introduction to computational geometry.* Cambridge, MA: MIT Press.
Rosenblatt, F. (1962). *Principles of neurodynamics.* Washington, DC: Spartan Books.

SUGGESTED READINGS

The following references, which describe information storage in general, information storage in neural networks, and models for human memory, supplement the material presented in this chapter.

Hinton, G. E., & Anderson, J. A. (1981). *Parallel models of associative memory.* Hillsdale, NJ: Lawrence Erlbaum Associates.
Jacks, E. L. (1971). *Associative information techniques.* New York: American Elsevier.
von Neumann, J. (1958). *The computer and the brain.* New Haven: Yale University Press.
Norman, D. A. (Ed.). (1970). *Models of human memory.* New York: Academic Press.

APPENDIX 2: A MODEL FOR CORTICAL MEMORY[4]

The model presented here, called a **memory block**, suggests a possible structure for one distinct memory store of the human brain. Understanding this material is not essential to understanding the remainder of this book. A memory block may represent either a temporary or permanent memory store depending on the parameters, and the memory traces may either be temporary, permanent, or degrading in time. Outputs from a memory block will be formulated in terms of all current and prior inputs.

A **memory block** is a collection of interconnected neurons together with the medium surrounding them. See Figure 3.19. It is divided into **memory locations** which can store the incoming pattern that arrives during a particular interval of time. A **memory timing mechanism** is introduced for converting dynamic input

---

[4]This appendix is reproduced, in part, from R. J. Baron, A model for cortical memory, *Journal of Mathematical Psychology,* 7, 37–59. © 1970 by Academic Press, New York. The discussion comes, in part, from R. J. Baron, In search of the memory trace. *SISTM Quarterly/Brain Theory Newsletter* II, 1979, 16–19.

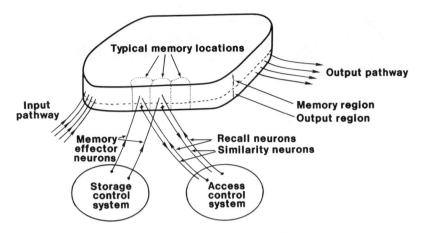

Figure 3.19. The structure of a memory block. Memory neurons are not shown. (Redrawn from R. J. Baron, A model for cortical memory. *Journal of Mathematical Psychology*, 7, 1970, 37-59.)

patterns into static stored patterns, and vice versa. This mechanism is a wave of activity which moves vertically upward at a velocity v through the nonneuronal medium. During storage, each level z in the active memory location receives transmitter substance for one instant of time only. The local sensitivity value at a dendritic position on one of the **memory neurons** is set proportional to the net amount of transmitter substance that arrived at that point during storage. In this way, time of input is encoded into vertical position within a given memory location. During recall the memory timing mechanism is again used, this time to convert the static stored pattern into a dynamic output pattern. The recalled pattern is an exact copy of the stored pattern and varies in time exactly as the incoming pattern did during storage.

When a memory location is neither executing storage nor recalling information, the memory timing mechanism does not function. However, each memory location automatically correlates the incoming pattern with its stored pattern. The resulting **similarity signal** is high only when the stored information is similar to the incoming information. This enables the memory block to be searched associatively. Recall is then immediately possible.

Properties of the memory block model are:

1. Information patterns to be stored arrive at the memory block through a specific collection of input neurons.
2. These **input patterns** are stored continuously in time.
3. Recall is a nondestructive process.
4. The recalled patterns are exact copies of the patterns which were stored; they vary in time exactly as the input pattern did during storage.

5. The memory block is associative. It is able to locate any stored information which is similar to the input information.

6. Changes which support consolidation are changes in the properties of the neurons themselves, not changes in the structure of the memory block.

External to the memory block are two control systems which regulate the flow of information to and from the memory block. The first control system is a **storage control system**. It signals the individual storage locations to initiate storage. The second control system is an **access control system**. It signals the individual storage locations to initiate recall. The memory block model specifies how signals from these control systems regulate its behavior but not how they work. They are not part of the memory block model. The following are assumed functional properties of the control systems:

1. All input patterns which are delivered to the memory block for storage are normalized:

$$\Sigma \ (P(j, \ k)(t))^2 = 1$$

Summation is over all neurons in the input pathway.

2. When an input pattern is delivered to the memory block, the access control system will not initiate recall from any memory locations.

3. When an input pattern is delivered to the memory block, the storage control system will signal the appropriate memory location or locations to initiate storage.

4. When a memory location is filled, the storage control system will signal the next storage location or locations to initiate storage. (A memory location is filled once the memory timing mechanism passes entirely through the memory location.)

THE MODEL

Before defining the structure of the memory block, some insight into its operation may be helpful. Input information that arrives through the input pathway is distributed to every location in the memory block. Each memory location operates independently under the control of its **memory effector neuron** and **recall neuron**. Information which arrives at each memory location is transformed into a new pattern of activity in the memory neurons. Similarly, the pattern of activity in the memory neurons is transformed into a pattern of activity in the output pathway. The specific transformation is determined by the coupling coefficients, local sensitivity values, and geometry of the memory block, which will be presented below.

The coefficients given below make each storage location store information in much the same way that a Fourier hologram stores optical information. (See Pribram, Nuwer & Baron, 1974, for a further discussion of the holographic hypothesis of memory structure.) The input layer of each storage location Fourier-transforms the input pattern. If the local sensitivity values of all the memory neurons were unity, the firing pattern in the memory neurons of each memory location would represent the Fourier transform of the input pattern. In actuality, the firing pattern for the memory neurons in a given memory location represents the product of the Fourier transform of the input pattern with the spatial pattern of local sensitivity values of the memory neurons in that memory location. If a pattern was already stored there, these local sensitivity values represent the complex conjugate of the Fourier transform of the stored pattern. Hence the memory location computes the product of two patterns: the Fourier transform of the input pattern and the complex conjugate of the Fourier transform of the stored pattern. The product pattern is represented as the dynamic pattern in the memory neurons of the given memory location and is evaluated in real time. The memory engram in this system is, in a sense, a hologram of the input firing pattern. Compare this method of information storage with the methods proposed by Beurle (1956, 1959), Kabrisky (1966), and van Heerden (1968). Keep in mind the fact that because of the coupling coefficients, the net amount of transmitter substance which arrives during storage at any point of a memory neuron is exactly proportional to the Fourier transform of the input pattern to the memory block. Consolidation takes place when the local sensitivity values at each point are set proportional to this amount.

After consolidation, the pattern of activity of the memory neurons in each memory location represents the product of Fourier transforms as just described. Therefore, the output pattern of each memory location is the crosscorrelation of the input pattern with the stored pattern. This is an immediate consequence of the convolution theorem. (For mathematical details, see Stroke, 1966.) The output generated by each storage location, therefore, is a measure of the similarity between input and stored patterns. When only the recall neuron to a memory location fires, uniform transmitter substance arrives at each memory neuron. The firing pattern of the memory neurons, under this circumstance, equals the complex conjugate of the Fourier transform of the stored pattern. When this pattern is transformed for output, the output pattern is a synthesized copy of the pattern which was originally stored.

The Fourier transform of a positive-valued pattern may be both negative and complex. In order to maintain the assumption that neurons fire at positive frequencies only, and in order not to introduce negative local sensitivity values during storage, multiple-neuron encodings are used in the memory block. Four neurons are used to represent each value: one represents the positive real component, one represents the negative real component, one represents the positive complex component, and one represents the negative complex component. Within the equations presented herein, r corresponds to the positive complex components of the Fourier transform pattern and the variable s distinguishes between positive and negative frequencies and positive and negative local sensitivity values.

The structure of the memory block will now be presented. Proofs that the memory block operates as I just described appear in Baron (1970) and will not be reproduced here. There are six types of neurons within the memory block: **input neurons, output neurons, memory neurons, memory effector neurons, recognition neurons**, and **recall neurons**. Input neurons comprise the input pathway to the memory block. Output neurons convey the recalled patterns from the memory block. Memory neurons are the neurons within the memory locations whose local sensitivity values effect storage. Memory effector neurons are effectual inputs which signal the memory neurons to consolidate information. Recall neurons initiate recall from the memory locations, and similarity neurons evaluate the similarity between input and stored patterns. Similarity neurons deliver their evaluations as outputs from the memory locations.

Only those parts of the neurons which are contained in the memory block itself will be described. In particular, only the axon fields of the input neurons, memory effector neurons, and recall neurons will be described, and only the dendrite fields of the output neurons and similarity neurons will be described. The dendrite fields and somas of the input, memory effector, and recall neurons, and the axon fields of the similarity and output neurons are outside the memory block and will not be considered.

Figures 3.20 and 3.21 show the cross section of a memory block and define its neurons. A memory block is a three-dimensional structure having an upper or memory region and a lower or output region. Each memory location is a vertical column extending from the top to the bottom of the memory block. There are B memory locations in the memory block, each having an equal cross sectional area. The memory locations are indexed by the integer variable b, b ranging from 1 to B.

There are JK different input neurons to the memory block. An input neuron will be labeled (j,k) and its frequency at time t will be denoted $P(j,k)(t)$. The variables j and k are integer variables, j ranging from 1 to J and k ranging from 1 to K. These are the intrinsic coordinates of the input neurons. The axon field of each input neuron is the entire memory region of the memory block, and the soma and dendrite field of each input neuron is outside the memory block and will not be considered. Refer to Figure 3.20.

There are JK different output neurons. An output neuron will be labeled $[j,k]$ and its frequency at time t will be denoted $O[j,k](t)$. See Figure 3.20. (For convenience, square brackets denote neurons which make outputs from the memory block while round brackets denote neurons which make inputs or are within the memory block.) The soma of an output neuron lies within the

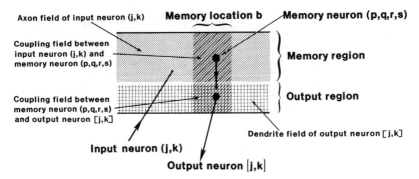

Figure 3.20. The cross section of a memory block showing how the axon fields of input neurons are distributed, how memory the dendrite and axon fields of memory neurons are distributed, and showing how the dendrite fields of output neurons are distributed. (Redrawn from R. J. Baron, A model for cortical memory. *Journal of Mathematical Psychology*, 7, 1970, 37-59.)

memory region of its memory location, and the dendrite field of each output neuron is the entire output region of the memory block. The axon fields of the output neurons are outside the memory block and will not be discussed.

There are 8JK different types of memory neurons. A memory neuron will be labeled (p,q,r,s) and its frequency at time t will be denoted P(p,q,r,s)(t). The variables p, q, r, and s are integer variables, p ranging from 1 to J, q ranging from 1 to K, r being either $+1$ or -1, and s being either 1, 2, 3, or 4. The variables p, q, r, and s are the intrinsic labels of the memory neurons. See Figure 3.20. The memory region of each memory location contains the soma of one of each different type of memory neuron. Therefore, there are 8BJK memory neurons in the memory block. The dendrite field of a memory neuron is the memory region of the memory location containing its soma, and the axon field of a memory neuron is the output region of its memory location.

Each memory location contains the axon field of one recall neuron. See Figure 3.21. The recall neuron whose axon field is in memory location b will be denoted (b) and its frequency at time t will be denoted Rcl(b)(t). The axon field of recall neuron (b) is the output region of memory location b.

Each memory location contains one similarity neuron. See Figure 3.21. The similarity neuron whose soma is in memory location b will be labeled [b] and its frequency at time t will be denoted Rgn[b](t). (Rgn stands for "recognition," which is what similarity signals are used for.) The dendrite field of similarity neuron [b] is the output region of memory location b. The axon field of similarity neuron [b] is outside the memory block and will not be considered.

Each memory location contains the axon field of one memory effector neuron. Memory effector neurons are effectual inputs and do not alter the

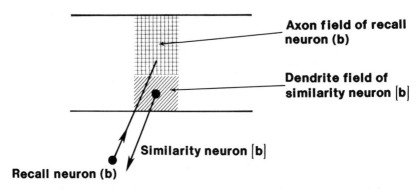

Axon field of recall neuron (b)

Dendrite field of similarity neuron |b|

Similarity neuron |b|

Recall neuron (b)

Figure 3.21. The cross section of a memory block showing how the dendrite fields of recall and similarity neurons are distributed. (Redrawn from R. J. Baron, A model for cortical memory. *Journal of Mathematical Psychology*, 7, 1970, 37-59.)

frequencies of other neurons in the system, but inputs from the memory effector neurons signal the memory neurons to execute storage.

The coupling coefficients between neurons will be denoted as follows:

1. c_{pqrs}^{jk} between input neuron (j,k) and memory neuron (p,q,r,s)
2. c_{jk}^{pqrs} between memory neuron (p,q,r,s) and output neuron [j,k]
3. c_{pqrs}^{b} between recall neuron (b) and memory neuron (p,q,r,s)
4. c_{b}^{pqrs} between memory neuron (p,q,r,s) and recognition neuron [b]

For all neurons other than memory neurons, the local sensitivity values will remain fixed. Therefore, for simplicity, I will assume they all have constant value 1.

Although a memory block is formally defined and highly structured, such a carefully defined structure is not necessary. Computer simulations have shown that the presence of noise such as the spurious firing of neurons, death of neurons, overlapping coupling fields among neighboring memory locations, and so forth, does not severely hinder the operation of the memory block. With 30% noise, the fidelity of the recalled image is only slightly reduced while the similarity signals remain fairly acute.

The **memory timing mechanism**, a nonneural property of the memory block, is a wave of activity that inactivates all but a thin horizontal layer of the memory block. Consider memory location b and fix a coordinate system whose X-Y plane is the interface between the memory and output regions and Z is measured positive upward (into the memory region). Let t_b be the time when either the memory effector neuron or the recall neuron to memory location b began firing. Then $E(x,y,z)(t) = \delta(z/v - (t - t_b))$, where δ designates the Dirac delta function, v is the velocity of the timing wave, and z is assumed greater than or equal to zero. Once the control neuron (either the memory effector neuron or the recall neuron) stops firing, the memory timing mechanism resets; that is, the nonneural medium returns to the normal state. (The particular linear form of the timing wave was chosen primarily for mathematical simplicity. Cylindrical, spherical, or spiraling waves of activity would work equally well.)

Consolidation consists of "setting" the local sensitivity values in the memory neurons. When the memory effector neuron to memory location b fires, the local sensitivity values for the memory neurons in that memory location are set proportional to the net amount of transmitter substance present during the storage process. Let (x,y,z) be a point in the dendrite field of memory neuron (p,q,r,s) and let t_{b_0} be the time when the memory effector neuron to memory location b began to fire. Then for $t_{b_f} = t_{b_0} + z/v$, the local sensitivity values at point (x,y,z) will be set to an initial value given by

$$k_{pqrs}(x,y,z)(t_{b_f}) = POS\left(\pm \sum_k P(j,k)(z/v + t_{b_0})\, c_{pqrs}^{jk}\right),$$

where the positive sign is chosen if $s = 1$ or 2, and the negative sign is chosen if $s = 3$ or 4. For a permanent memory store, the local sensitivity values, once set, remain fixed for the life of the system. For a temporary memory store, the local sensitivity values can be reset at a later time.

The coupling coefficients given below guarantee that the memory block behaves as I described above. Proofs that the similarity signals measure the crosscorrelation of the input with stored patterns and that the recall neuron causes a copy of the stored pattern to be synthesized as an output from the memory block are presented in Baron (1970).

$$c_{pqr1}^{jk} = c_{pqr3}^{jk} = -c_{pqr2}^{jk} = -c_{pqr4}^{jk} = \frac{1}{\sqrt{JK}}\cos\left(\frac{pj}{J} + \frac{qr}{K} + \frac{r}{8}\right)2\pi$$

$$c_{jk}^{pqr1} = c_{jk}^{pqr2} = -c_{jk}^{pqr3} = -c_{jk}^{pqr4} = \frac{1}{\sqrt{JK}}\cos\left(\frac{pj}{J} + \frac{qk}{K} + \frac{r}{8}\right)2\pi$$

$$c_{b}^{pqr1} = c_{b}^{pqr2} = -c_{b}^{pqr3} = -c_{b}^{pqr4} = c_{00}^{pqr1}$$

$$c_{pqr1}^{b} = c_{pqr3}^{b} = -c_{pqr2}^{b} = -c_{pqr4}^{b} = c_{pqr1}^{00}$$

DISCUSSION

There is uniform agreement among scientists that permanent memories are encoded as coupling parameters between brain cells. What are the coupling parameters and how do they support storage? How are they established and modified, and when?

The theory presented here suggests that the memory engrams are encoded as local sensitivity values in the dendrites of special memory cells within the storage system. Moreover, the theory suggests that the local sensitivity values are set proportional to the net amount (excitatory less inhibitory) of transmitter substance arriving there during storage.

In order to convert a dynamic input pattern into a static pattern of local sensitivity values, a memory timing mechanism is introduced. The timing mechanism, a structural property of the neural system, generates a wave of activity which prevents the release of transmitters from the input cells in all but a thin region of the storage network. The timing wave may either block the release of transmitters or prevent depolarization pulses from reaching the synaptic terminals. In either case, the timing wave moves through the storage medium and its movement, like the movement of a magnetic tape across the head of a tape recorder, converts the dynamic input pattern into a static pattern of neural transmitters in the storage system. The memory effector signal, an effectual input, signals the memory neurons to consolidate that pattern—by changing local sensitivity values—as structural changes in their dendrites. How this might be done is an open question (but see Walker & Hild, 1969).

Any theory of human information storage must account for the tremendous capacity for information storage as well as our ability to access stored information rapidly, by association. Evidence abounds that our streams of conscious experience are stored throughout our lifetimes. If it were not for an inhibitory mechanism that prevents us from accessing all our experiences, we should, in theory, be able to recall in detail anything that occupied our focus of attention. Some of the evidence will be presented in Chapter 6 of this book. If a person is awake for 11 hours per day for a lifetime of 80 years, he or she lives about 10^9 seconds. There are roughly 10^{11} neurons in the brain, so that if experiences are stored throughout a person's lifetime, then there are available for storage only 100 neurons per second. If only one-tenth of all neurons are memory neurons, then the available number is reduced to about ten neurons per second. If we further assume that the patterns that make up our experiences have dimensionality 300, which I will later show to be reasonable, and if a neuron is the fundamental storage unit, then only one neural pattern can be stored every 30 seconds. This is clearly inconsistent with our common experience. One must conclude that the neuron is not the fundamental level at which experiential information is stored.

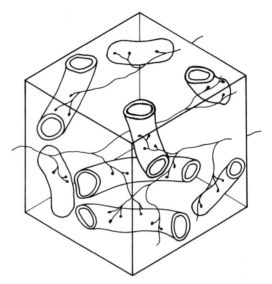

Figure 3.22. A cortical micro-volume showing a few of the many axonal and dendritic branches and contacts between them. (Redrawn from R. J. Baron, In search of the memory trace. *SISTM Quarterly*, 2, 1979, 16-19.)

Each cortical neuron receives several thousand synaptic contacts and its axon branches contact several hundred postsynaptic cells at several thousand contact points. Each of these contact points is a potential site of information storage in the same way that most current theories propose that the net coupling between neurons is responsible for storage. However, if all synaptic contacts function alike, then why have the contacts distributed throughout the brain tissue? Why have the duplication when there is not enough storage capacity without duplication?

For purposes of exploration, suppose that memory is at the synaptic level rather than the neural level. This leads to another very natural question: If storage is at the synaptic level, then what is the mechanism that distinguishes between the local sites of storage—between the synapses? How, in essence, are some of the synaptic contacts utilized at one time while others are not?

From a theoretical point of view, in order to transform the incoming information patterns into static patterns so that both storage and association can take place, it is necessary to gather information from all cells that comprise the input pattern. This implies that each cortical volume having representative inputs from all input cells is potentially capable of information storage. This quantity of cortical tissue, a **microvolume,** is illustrated in Figure 3.22. In particular, a microvolume may be much smaller than the extent (axon or dendrite trees) of a given cell, but it must be large enough to contain representative parts of all pre- and postsynaptic cells involved in the storage process. Such a microvolume may be a solid volume, a spherical shell, a cylindrical shell, or some other cortical volume.

Now suppose that microvolumes within one cortical region can be activated sequentially with a memory timing wave. Then each collection of cells in the cortex that is capable of information storage becomes capable of storing incoming information patterns for several seconds or longer, continuously in time, rather than being limited to a single "snapshot." This assumes that the speed of propagation of the timing wave is sufficiently slow. If a timing mechanism is present, there would be sufficient storage capacity (theoretically) in the brain to store the information that enters the stream of consciousness for an entire human lifetime, and this suggests that perhaps such a mechanism exists but has not yet been discovered experimentally.

Hereafter I will use the term "memory timing mechanism" to denote the biological activity that supports memory timing and the term "memory timing wave" to denote the corresponding wave of inactivity. The following questions are among many that come to mind:

1. What is the underlying biology of the memory timing mechanism?
2. What is the geometry of the timing wave?
3. How is a timing wave initiated?
4. What are the parameters of the timing wave?

These remain open questions for the neurobiologist. (For an excellent up-to-date presentation of memory research, see Arnold, 1984.)

There are two other questions that the neurobiologist must someday address. What is the nature of the memory engram? How is trace consolidation initiated?

The theory suggests that memory engrams are encoded as local sensitivity values in the dendrites of memory neurons. However, because each part of a dendrite can represent part of a memory engram, in order to measure the structural changes, one must restrict one's measurements to a small portion of the dendritic membrane. At present, there is no way to make such measurements in a laboratory, and even if there were, we do not know which neurons are memory neurons and where in the cortex they are located. Thus the problems associated with experimentally verifying the theory are presently unsolved.

As far as the signal which initiates storage, one would expect a system whose neurons release a special chemical transmitter which is interpreted by the memory neurons as a "store now" signal. What the chemical is, how it signals the memory neurons to initiate consolidation, how they interpret the signals (on the one hand) and how they inform the dendrites to modify sensitivity values (on the other hand) are simply unknown. All of these questions await development of more sophisticated experimental techniques and appropriate research.

REFERENCES

Arnold, M. B. (1984). *Memory and the brain*. Hillsdale, NJ: Lawrence Erlbaum Associates.

Baron, R. J. (1970). A model for cortical memory. *Journal of Mathematical Psychology, 7*, 37-59.

_____ (1979). In search of the memory trace. *SISTM Quarterly/Brain Theory Newsletter* (Vol. 2), 16-19.

Beurle, R.L. (1956). Properties of a mass of cells capable of regenerating pulses. *Philosophical Transactions of the Royal Society of London (B), 240*, 75-82.

_____ (1959). Storage and manipulation of information in the brain. *Journal of the Institute of Electrical Engineers, 5*, 75-82.

Kabrisky, M. (1966). *A proposed model for visual information processing in the human brain*. Urbana, IL: University of Illinois Press.

Pribram, K. H., Nuwer, M. & Baron, R. J. (1974). The holographic hypothesis of memory structure in brain function and perception. In D. H. Krantz, et al. (Eds.), *Contemporary developments in mathematical psychology* (Vol. 2), 416-457.

Stroke, G. W. (1966). *An introduction to coherent optics and holography*. New York: Academic Press.

van Heerden, P. J. (1968). *The foundation of empirical knowledge*. Wassenaar, the Netherlands: N.V. Uitgeverij Wistik.

Walker, F. D. & Hild, W. J. (1969). Neuroglia electrically coupled to neurons. *Science, 165*, 602-603.

4
THE CONTROL OF ASSOCIATIVE STORAGE SYSTEMS

INTRODUCTION

In order to understand human memory one must not only know what is stored and how but also how the storage networks are controlled. The previous chapter described how information might be stored, and coming chapters will describe what is stored. This chapter will focus on storage control networks and how they might control the organization of stored information and access to it. The material presented here is theoretical. No one knows, for the present, either where the control networks may be found or how they are implemented in neural circuitry. Nonetheless, networks which perform these functions must be present, and this chapter suggests their nature.

Storage control networks determine where information will be stored and therefore how stored information is organized. **Access control networks** determine what information can be accessed and therefore both what will be remembered and what will be forgotten. Both organization and access of information are fundamental to learning and will be major topics of this chapter.

In this chapter I will describe a very simple neural network for controlling access to an associative memory store. I will show that the storage access system is crucial to the behavior of the storage system. I will also describe several different storage policies and show that the organization of stored information as determined by the storage control system is also crucial to the behavior of the storage system.

CONTROL OF A MEMORY STORE

There are two primary **control functions** for each memory store: **initiate storage**, and **initiate recall**. Associated with each of these control functions are two **decision functions**: **when** should information be stored, and **where** (in which memory location); and **when** should information be recalled, and **from where** (from which memory location). For a given memory store, the decision functions may be "wired in" as an **innate** part of the store, or they may be determined externally by control networks that can use different decision policies under different circumstances. Both types of control networks appear to be present in the human brain.

As an example of storage and recall decision functions, consider an indexed associative memory system. All memory locations in the memory store are ordered, from location 1 to location N, where N is the total number of memory locations. Every input pattern that arrives is to be stored. (This specifies **when** to store information.) The input pattern will be stored in the next sequential memory location under the given ordering. (This specifies **where** to store the information.) In this store, information is organized according to its time of arrival. Using such a memory system, the following recall decision functions may be used to control recall of information. Whenever information is delivered to the storage system, the similarity signals are monitored. The access system assigns to each memory location a **match threshold**. If the value of the similarity signal from that memory location exceeds its match threshold, then recall from that memory location will be allowed. The memory location is said to be **activated**. When no patterns are being presented to the memory store, recall of information will occur. This specifies **when** to recall information. Recall will be initiated from the first activated memory location in the specified ordering. This specifies **where** to recall information from. (Compare this control strategy with the one used by the computer associative memory described in the previous chapter.) Among all memory locations whose similarity signals exceeded their thresholds of recall, the memory location is selected for recall that most recently stored information. This is a consequence of the chosen storage policy. (Part of one decision network for this recall policy is presented later in this chapter.)

One consequence of a sequential storage policy is that by presenting a piece of information to the network and analyzing the similarity signals, it is possible to determine when similar information was previously stored. The memory store is a **temporal analyzer**. Our own ability to determine when it was that we saw, heard, or did something strongly suggests that the records of our experience are stored sequentially. Our ability to recall specific events in sequence suggests that those records are also associatively linked.

As a second example, consider the following. Information is to be stored only when the storage system receives an external signal specifying that it should store the input information. (The **when** decision is external to the network.) During input, the similarity signals will be monitored. The input pattern will be simultaneously stored in one or more memory locations. If no high similarity signals are produced, the input pattern will be stored in one randomly selected memory location. (This specifies where to store the information.) However, if high similarity signals are produced, a copy of the input pattern will be stored in each neighborhood of the store that generates a high similarity signal. (This also specifies where to store the information.) Multiple copies of the input pattern may therefore be made in different parts of the memory store.

Using this storage policy, information will no longer be organized according to its time of input. Instead, it will be organized according to how similar[1] stored patterns are to one another. Initially, different information patterns will be stored at random. However, after a while, a pattern will be presented that is similar to one that is already stored. The new pattern will be stored near the old one. As the process continues, clusters will form according to the similarity of the input patterns. Patterns that correlate highly will be localized, whereas patterns that differ will likewise be distributed throughout the memory network in a random way. If, for example, the network stores encodings of visual images, if the encodings are iconic, and if the storage network correlates these encodings according to pictorial similarity, then the information in the memory system will be organized according to pictorial similarity: things that look the same will be stored nearby and things that appear to be different will be stored apart from one another.[2] If the network stores auditory encodings of words, then words that sound the same will be stored in nearby memory locations. The memory store is a **conceptual analyzer**, where concepts are defined in terms of similarity as measured by the storage network.

AN ACCESS CONTROL NETWORK

In the associative memory stores described earlier, the recall decision function associated with selecting a memory location for recall was assumed to be external to the memory store. In this section a **decision network** is described for selecting a particular memory location for recall. This decision network corresponds to the match register of the the computer associative memory store described in Chapter 3, but it is different in two fundamental respects. First, the values of the similarity signals sufficient to enable access to store information are variable parameters of the system. As a result, access to a storage location at one time does not guarantee access to the same storage location at another time. Second, the control mechanism in the computer storage system that enables access to the highest activated storage location is not implemented in this network. (Control networks for sequential access to activated memory locations will be discussed later in this chapter.) Using this

---

[1]Similarity is measured by the storage locations and depends on how they compare patterns as well as on how information is encoded for storage.

[2]This is actually an oversimplification of what probably occurs. I will show later that the encodings of visual images are substantially more complex than this, and the formation of natural conceptual groups by this mechanism occurs for several different visual attributes.

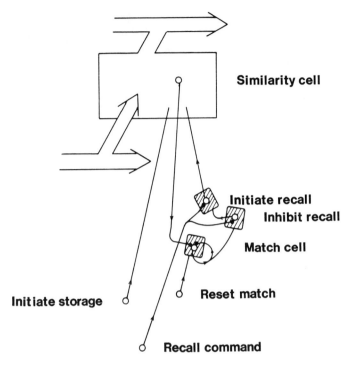

Figure 4.1. A recall decision network for a memory location in an associative memory store.

decision network, the memory store begins to display properties that we call learning and forgetting. Human learning and forgetting, however, are considerably more complex than this, as you will see.

Figure 4.1 shows one memory location in an associative memory store and part of a recall decision network for that memory location. For this memory store, each memory location receives three external control inputs: an **initiate storage** command input, a **recall command input**, and a **reset match** command input. The initiate storage input is an effectual input that initiates the consolidation process. The decision network contains the **initiate recall cell**, a **match cell** which is bistable, and an **inhibit recall cell**. The match cell receives inputs from itself (it is self-excitatory), from the similarity output of the memory location, and from the external reset match command input. The match cell makes three outputs: itself, the inhibit recall cell (as a negative regulatory input), and the external networks.

The match cell is stimulated by the similarity cell. If the resulting firing rate of the match cell exceeds its match threshold, it becomes active and the memory location is said to be **activated**. The **match threshold** of a memory location is the minimum firing rate necessary for the similarity cell to activate the match cell.

The match cell continues to fire until it is turned off by the reset match command input, which is a negative regulatory input to the match cell. Once the match cell is turned off, it remains off until it is turned on by the similarity cell at a later time.

Because of the match cells, the decision network is a temporary memory store, a temporary memory store without any memory traces! The temporary records are maintained by the activity of the bistable match cells. Once the match cells are turned off, the temporary records are lost. In this network, the temporary records are **active**: They are maintained by neural discharges. This is in contrast to static memory traces which are maintained by changes in neural coupling parameters (either temporary or permanent).

The **inhibit recall cell** is stimulated by the recall command cell but it is inhibited by the match cell. If the match cell is active, then the inhibit recall cell stays off even if the recall command cell is firing. The inhibit recall cell makes a negative regulatory input to the connection between the recall command cell and the initiate recall cell. If the inhibit recall cell fires, then the recall command cell can not stimulate the initiate recall cell and recall of stored information can not occur: Recall is **blocked**.

The **recall command cell** now replaces the initiate recall cell as an external input to this system. The coupling between the recall command cell and the initiate recall cell is determined indirectly by the match cell. If the match cell is firing, then the recall command cell can stimulate the initiate recall cell. However, if the match cell is not firing, then the recall command cell also stimulates the inhibit recall cell, which inhibits the connections between recall command cell and initiate recall cell. This blocks recall of the desired information.

The general behavior of a memory store using this control network is as follows. Input patterns are delivered to the memory store through the information inputs and may be stored just as in any storage network. The input patterns are correlated against the stored patterns just as they are in any associative memory store. The similarity cells therefore indicate how similar the input pattern is to the stored patterns. If the similarity signal exceeds the match threshold for a particular memory location, then the match cell for that memory location is turned on and remains active. That memory location is activated and **matches** the input pattern. If no patterns are being input to the memory store, recall may be initiated. If a recall command signal is generated (externally), and if that signal goes to a memory location that is activated, then the initiate recall cell fires and the information is recalled exactly as it was in the previous system. If a recall command signal arrives at a memory location that is not active, however, then nothing happens. The network cannot recall the stored data. The match cells "remember" when similarity signals exceed the match thresholds for memory locations, and they enable recall from those memory locations. The match cells can be turned off by the external networks at any desired time, and once turned off, they remain off until they are associatively turned on by the similarity cells.

AN ASSOCIATIVE STORE WITH ADAPTIVE ACCESS

Using the access control network just described, an input pattern is **associated** with all stored patterns that are activated by that input pattern. If one or more memory locations are activated by an input pattern, the input pattern is **recognized** or **matched** by the memory store. If no memory locations are activated, the input pattern is not recognized. The match thresholds now play a fundamental role in the ability of this storage system to recall stored information. If the match thresholds are all set at zero, then the memory store is simply an addressed memory store. The match cells will always be on and any attempt to recall information will succeed. If the match thresholds are all set too high so that a match can never occur even if the input pattern is identical to a stored pattern, then recall can never occur. The similarity information is still available but the stored information can not be recalled. It is the situation between these two extremes that is most interesting. If the similarity thresholds are sufficiently high so that most input patterns do not cause matches, but matches do occur when an input pattern is very similar to a stored pattern, then the decision network is a **discrimination network** that allows restricted access to stored information. Those memory locations that contain information that is very similar to recently presented patterns will be activated; others will not.

If the match thresholds for an associative memory store are fixed, then the same memory locations will always match the same input patterns. However, if the match thresholds are adaptive, then a given memory location may match different input patterns at different times and is said to have **adaptive access** to stored information. Patterns that are at one time associated may at a later time not be associated, and vice versa. As a result, adaptive match thresholds are crucial to understanding learning and forgetting.

FORGETTING CAUSED BY ADAPTIVE ACCESS

As a specific example of an adaptive control system, suppose that the match threshold of each memory location is initially set at a low value, so that many patterns enable recall from that memory location, and suppose also that the match threshold changes as follows: If information is successfully recalled from a memory location, then its match threshold is slightly decreased. The match threshold is slightly increased for each day that the match cell does not fire. Now, if the memory location does not match any input patterns for a long, long time, then the match threshold will increase and fewer and fewer patterns will be matched by that memory location. Ultimately, it will never match any input patterns. All information in that memory location will be inaccessible or "forgotten."[3] In contrast, if a memory location matches information and the associated information is subsequently recalled, then the match threshold will be reduced. That memory location will be more likely to match other new (different) inputs and therefore more likely to be used for subsequent recalls. The memory store, by virtue of this adaptation procedure, "learns" to associate new patterns with old.

Using this adaptation procedure, the system's performance changes even though the memory traces do not change. Learning and forgetting (in the restricted sense used here) depend on the access to stored information and not on the stored information itself. The memory system is adaptive (by virtue of the match thresholds) even though the memory traces are permanent and do not change.

One final thing to notice about this system is that two new types of "memory" have been introduced. The match cells, while active, keep track of the fact that recent input information was similar to the corresponding stored information. The memory store "remembers" when input information is matched to stored information. This match information is temporary. Once the match cells are turned off, the information is lost. But as long as the match cells are on, all associated information is available for recall. By this mechanism, the system can, at very little cost, keep track of a large amount of associated information.

Second, the match thresholds "remember" which information is to be readily accessible and which is not. Changes to the match thresholds change the behavior of the system and can account for many interesting properties of the storage system. These changes, then, are themselves "memories" of a sort, even though no sensory information is stored.

ACCESS TO INDIVIDUAL ITEMS OF INFORMATION

The preceding sections discussed access parameters to individual memory locations. An equally important question is the mechanism by which one storage location is selected for recall from among all activated memory locations. One suggestion made earlier is that the active memory location selected is the

---

[3]In this discussion, no commitment is yet made as to what information is being stored. The goal here is to give a rather detailed characterization of an adaptive access associative storage network, and begin to study its formal properties. Once we have established an adequate definitional framework for discussion, we can then explore the relationship of these networks to brain function, the encodings of stored information, and the psychological implications of the models. Until that time, however, the use of such terms as "learning" and "forgetting" should only be understood in the restricted sense defined here.

one that most recently stored information, but this policy is quite restrictive. In general, the mechanism of access to memory locations will depend very strongly on the organization of information within the store and therefore also on the networks that control storage.

As a particular example of a network that implements sequential access to stored information, consider an associative storage network with the storage policy that new information is stored in consecutive memory locations. If similar patterns arrive at random, they will be distributed randomly throughout the memory store. Now imagine that the memory locations are distributed across a two-dimensional network, and consider the resulting pattern of activated memory locations when a given input pattern is presented for association. High similarity signals will be distributed throughout the store. The question, then, is: What mechanism should be used to select one activated memory location over all others for recall? If a most recently stored policy is adopted, then the access control network must scan all memory locations, starting with the most recently used for storage, for the first one which is activated.

One access control network for activating memory locations in such a memory store was presented earlier in Figure 4.1, but no mechanism was proposed to enable access to a single memory location. If that access control network is modified as shown in Figure 4.2, then sequential access can easily be performed. The newly added cells form a transmission line that has one input as shown on the left of the figure. The transmission line consists of a sequence of cells which can propagate a signal from one to the next unless inhibited by one of the negative regulatory inputs shown. The negative regulatory inputs come from the match cells of the various memory locations. If none of the match cells are active, then the recall input propagates along the entire transmission line and attempts to initiate recall from every memory location in the store. However, since none of the match cells are active, recall will not occur. Now suppose that one or more of the match cells are active. Then the match cell from the memory location which most recently stored information will prevent the recall input from propagating any further along the transmission line, and recall will be attempted (and successful) from the active location which most recently stored its information. Note that I have assumed that the storage policy is consistent with the order that the locations are "wired together" by the transmission line. This shows how close the relationship must be between the storage and access control networks.

In order to enable sequential access to all active memory locations, it is only necessary to deactivate a memory location that has just executed recall. Deactivation will occur if the recall input from the transmission line makes a negative regulatory input to the match cell. However, deactivation must take a sufficient length of time to enable all stored information to be recalled, and this can be accomplished by selecting appropriate coupling parameters for the cells under consideration.

The access control network just described has the advantage that only a

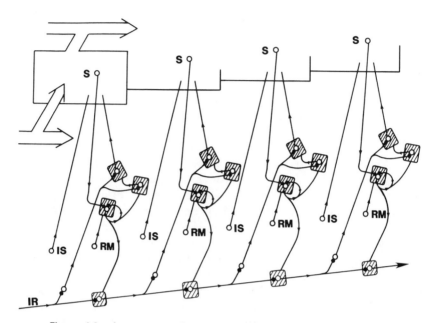

Figure 4.2. A sequence of memory locations controlled by a single initiate recall command signal. The initiate recall command signal can only propagate to the first activated memory location. Key: S, a similarity cell; IS, an initiate storage cell; IR, the initiate recall signal; RM, a reset match cell.

single external control input is required to initiate recall from many active memory locations. However, it has two distinct disadvantages. First, recall is strictly sequential among all active memory locations, so that access to a particular piece of information is likely to take a long time. Besides, the network is highly susceptible to trauma: If the transmission line is damaged, then access to all memory locations beyond the damage will be impossible. It is therefore unlikely that such a network is used in the brain.

However, a realistic alternative is that the memory locations in the store are grouped together, and these groups are controlled by a sequential access policy. The global control networks would then have immediate access to one of the patterns in a group, and sequential access would be possible within the groups. One advantage is the immediate access to information which was stored at markedly different times although sequential access would still be necessary if similar items are stored at nearby times.[4] Finally, such a network would be much less sensitive to traumatic damage.

---

[4]Note that sequential access as described here is over and above the memory timing mechanism assumed present within the individual memory locations. Thus there are at least two different forms of sequentialization inherent in networks of this type.

As a second example of a recall control network, consider a conceptual analyzer, which is an associative memory store with the storage policy that similar patterns are stored in nearby memory locations. For such a network, an input pattern would most likely activate many locations in one local region of the store. If the goal is to recall information from one active memory location, the problem for the access control network is to enable access to the most appropriate memory location within a conceptual group. But which one is most appropriate? One possibility is to enable recall from the memory location that generates the strongest similarity signal for the activating input pattern. But this information is lost by the networks described earlier: The match cells are either active or they are not. The question becomes, how can the control network be modified so that only one memory location within a given region is activated, and that memory location is the one whose similarity signal is strongest? This can be done as shown in Figure 4.3, which is the same network as shown in Figure 4.1 with a minor modification: The similarity signals from each memory location make inhibitory inputs to the match cells of neighboring memory locations. By this mechanism, local memory locations compete with one another to become active. Networks of this type have **competitive inhibition** and have been studied in detail by several researchers. For a network of this type, the one memory location having the strongest similarity signal tends to

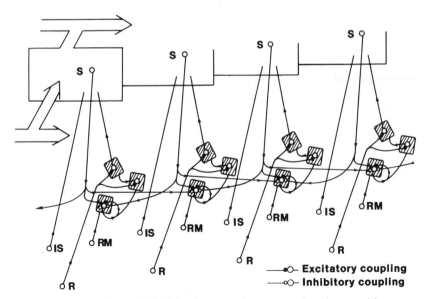

Figure 4.3.   Lateral inhibition from nearby memory locations enables only the memory location with the strongest similarity signals to become activated. Key: S, a similarity cell; IS, an initiate storage cell; IR, the initiate recall signal; RM, a reset match cell.

inhibit the activation of its neighbors—it "wins out," so to speak. Recall, therefore, is enabled from at most one memory location in a given group. Since conceptual groups form in local areas (by assumption that the storage network uses the conceptual storage policy described earlier), this mechanism guarantees access to at most one memory location in each conceptual group.

There are numerous types of access control networks for memory stores and two types have been described here: sequential access and access by competitive inhibition. These access networks illustrate the general problems that must be considered and show that a necessary part of the description of a storage system is a careful and precise description of the storage and access policies for the network. Without these, the behavioral properties of the storage system cannot be determined.

LEVELS OF ACCESS CONTROL

The principle of grouping together small numbers of memory locations for access control can be applied on many levels, forming a hierarchical access structure. For example, consider an associative memory store having a million memory locations, and suppose such a store has access groups consisting of one hundred memory locations controlled directly by networks as illustrated in Figures 4.2 or 4.3. At the next higher level in the control hierarchy, one hundred groups can be controlled by a similar access control network. For this network, the low-level groups can send signals which indicate how many active memory locations are present, and these signals replace the similarity outputs generated by the memory locations themselves. That is, the signals that indicate the count of active memory locations determine which groups of memory locations are to be activated at the next higher level in the control hierarchy. Either a competitive inhibition policy or a sequential access policy could be used at any level of control in the hierarchy.

Using the same hierarchical structure once again, the second level of the hierarchy can be controlled by yet another access control network of the same type. For a store having a million memory locations and a grouping factor of one hundred as described, this third level in the hierarchy would be the highest level, and at this level only two external control signals would be necessary: a recall command input, and a reset match cell command input. The entire responsibility of selecting a specific item of information for recall would be assumed by the control hierarchy, and at the highest level the entire control function would be reduced to a "recall now" input and a "reset match cell" input. The reset match cell input would inactivate all memory locations in preparation for the next associative search.

It should be clear that any imaginable hierarchy of control structures can be proposed and implemented in neural circuitry. My goal here was to separate the storage functions from the functions of associative search, memory location activation, and recall selection. As I will show, it appears that different human memory stores use different storage and access policies, and each store must be studied with the particular goal in mind of understanding its own particular access policy.

It should also be clear, even to the most naïve student of brain function, that there can be many different neural realizations for the same access function. At the present time there is no reason, based solely on anatomical considerations, to choose one realization over another. Thus it must be emphasized that the particular neural networks proposed in this chapter do not have any special significance. Rather, they illustrate with suitable detail some of the various possible access mechanisms and how the storage networks will differ in behavior when different access mechanisms are selected. Whenever a particular network model of a brain function is proposed, the relationships between the various encoding and access policies must be made clear to the experimentalist in search of data which can be used to select one model over another.

SUMMARY

There are three fundamental aspects of storage systems that must be studied and understood: the decision functions relating to placement of information within the storage system, the access mechanism that enables or restricts access to stored information, and the encoding of the stored information itself. Each aspect must be understood before one can gain a thorough understanding of the many psychological properties of memory, such as learning, remembering, and forgetting.

SUGGESTED READING

The following rather specialized reference describes a variety of neural networks and approaches to understanding them. The papers dealing with competition in neural networks may be insightful in understanding storage control systems.

Amari, S., & Arbib, M. A. (Eds.). (1982). *Competition and cooperation in neural nets.* Lecture Notes in Biomathematics, Vol. 45. New York: Springer-Verlag.

5
INFORMATION ENCODING AND MODALITY

INTRODUCTION

In the previous four chapters I discussed neurons, neural information, information transmission and transformation, information storage, and finally the organization and access of stored information. In this chapter I will discuss the encoding of information in neural networks. In particular, I will focus on information modality, tagged encodings, and techniques for converting between different representations of information.

POSITIVE AND NEGATIVE VALUES IN NEURAL NETWORKS

Many external signals can be characterized by their degree of presence. For example, the intensity of a particular color of light reflected by the surface of an object can range from zero (absent) to some maximum value which can be detected by the eyes without damaging them. The intensity of sound at a particular frequency can range from zero (none) to some maximum value which will not damage the ears. In the neural domain, if these sensory properties are converted by the eyes and ears into firing patterns in receptor cells, a firing rate of zero may represent the absence of the external signal while the maximum firing rate of the receptor cell may represent the maximum detectable value of the signals. Intermediate firing rates would then represent the presence of intermediate amounts of the sensory signals.

The receptor organs for every sensory modality encode information in such a way that the magnitude of the resulting sensation is logarithmically proportional to the intensity of the stimulus. For example, the eyes encode the intensity of the reflected light so that doubling the intensity increases the perceived brightness by a constant amount. This is the famous Weber-Fechner law, which suggests that the firing rates of sensory cells are logarithmically proportional to the sensory stimulus they measure. Logarithmic encodings enable a wide range of sensory signals to be encoded, often as many as 10 orders of magnitude, between the minimum and maximum detectable signals.

For information such as brightness and loudness, non-negative firing rates are adequate to convey the desired information. However, for many sensory attributes, both positive and negative values must be used. This happens, for example, when the sensory organ is encoding the change in a sensory signal. Consider the change in reflected light as one looks from left to right across the surface of an object. If the object is dark on the left and light on the right, the change in brightness is a positive quantity. However, if the object is light on the left and dark on the right, the change in brightness is a negative quantity (see Figure 2.10). Thus the eyes need a way of encoding both positive and negative values.

First, what is the significance of a negative value? In mathematics the significance is clear: Positive values add while negative values subtract. In the neural realm, the significance should be that a neuron contacting a postsynaptic cell with positive coupling and firing at a positive rate should tend to depolarize its postsynaptic cell, whereas if firing at a negative rate it should tend to hyperpolarize its postsynaptic cell. The opposite would be true for a neuron with inhibitory coupling. That means the type of neurotransmitters released at a given synaptic contact would have to change from excitatory to inhibitory when the firing rate changes from positive to negative, and that simply does not make good biological sense. The assumption that neurons can fire at negative firing rates is simply not realistic.

How then can negative values be encoded in the nervous system? Two possibilities immediately come to mind. First, a neuron firing at some intermediate or background rate represents the value zero. The same neuron firing at a slower rate represents a negative value while the same neuron firing at a faster rate represents a positive value. This is called a **biased encoding**. The second possibility is that two different neurons encode a single numeric value. If neither cell fires, the value zero is represented. The firing of one cell represents a positive value whose magnitude is proportional to that cell's firing rate; if the other cell fires, the value is negative with magnitude proportional to its firing rate. This is a **two-cell encoding**. Both of these encodings appear to be present in the human brain as you will see.

There is considerable evidence that vector quantities are also encoded in the nervous system, quantities that represent both a direction and a magnitude. Vector quantities that the brain encodes include velocity, acceleration, and surface orientation of visually perceived objects. Since the world is three-dimensional, these vectors each have three distinct components whose values may be positive or negative.

One way the brain might represent a three-dimensional vector is with 6 neurons which are logically grouped into three pairs, each pair representing one component of the vector. There are, of course, other ways of representing vector quantities, but the differences are not of central concern for this discussion.

In mathematical systems, numbers are not only positive and negative but also real and complex. A complex number may be thought of as a pair of real numbers, where one of the real numbers is the real component of the complex number and the other is its imaginary component. Equally important is the fact that specific mathematical operations are defined for complex numbers, which is where their significance arises. In a neural system complex numbers can also be represented. They can be represented as a pair of real numbers and hence either by two cells if a biased encoding is used or by four cells if a two-cell encoding is used for each real number. Furthermore, the mathematical operations for complex numbers can easily be implemented by the appropriate choice of coupling parameters. The memory block model presented in the appendix to Chapter 3 illustrated a multiple cell encoding for complex numbers. In either case, we can and will assume that positive and negative values as well as real and complex values can be represented.

TAGGED INFORMATION

The notion of information in computers was introduced in Chapter 2. In this section I will introduce the notion of tagged information and indicate its relevance for neural systems.

Most computers are capable of performing arithmetic on several different types of numbers. Among the better-known number representations are absolute binary integers, sign-magnitude integers, and floating-point numbers. For an absolute binary integer, the right-most bit denotes the value 1, the next bit from the right denotes the value 2, the next bit 4, the next bit 8, and so forth, with the Nth bit denoting $2.^{1-N}$ Table 2.1 (page 27) showed several numbers and their absolute binary encoding. For sign-magnitude integers, the leftmost bit designates the sign, and the remaining bits are the magnitude encoded in absolute binary. A sign bit of '0' generally indicates a positive number while a sign bit of '1' indicates a negative number.

There are many different representations for floating-point numbers. In general, a floating-point number consists of a mantissa and an exponent. The exponent base is assumed. In scientific notation, for example, 432×10^4 designates the decimal integer 4320000 and 432×10^{-4} designates .0432. The value 432 is the mantissa, the values 4 and -4 are the exponents, and 10 is the assumed exponent base. For computers that use floating-point numbers, several leftmost bits of a word are generally used to encode the exponent; the remaining rightmost bits encode the mantissa. The exponent base is understood and depends on the particular computer. As a specific example, consider an eight-bit floating point number, where the left four bits encode the exponent in sign-magnitude notation, the rightmost 4 bits encode the mantissa in sign-magnitude notation, and an exponent base of two is assumed. Several numbers and their floating-point encoding are listed below:

$$01110111 = 7 \times 2^7 = 896$$
$$00000111 = 7 \times 2^0 = 7$$
$$00000001 = 1 \times 2^0 = 1$$
$$00000000 = 0 \times 2^0 = 0$$
$$00001001 = -1 \times 2^0 = -1$$
$$00001111 = -7 \times 2^0 = -7$$
$$01111111 = -7 \times 2^7 = -896$$
$$10010001 = 1 \times 2^{-1} = 1/2$$
$$10011001 = -1 \times 2^{-1} = -1/2$$
$$11110001 = 1 \times 2^{-7} = 1/128$$
$$11111001 = -1 \times 2^{-7} = -1/128$$

Any eight-bit register can hold any of these numbers as well as any other eight-bit encoded value, including all those listed in Table 2.1.

Suppose that a computer is instructed to add two numbers which are held in memory. If only one kind of numeric encoding is used, then the values must be represented in that encoding and the adder circuitry simply adds the numbers. If the computer allows two different numeric encodings such as sign-magnitude and floating-point numbers, and the computer has hardware for adding numbers in each encoding, then the question is, which adder should be used when adding two values that are stored in memory?

Two different solutions have been used for this problem. For some computers, different instructions are used, depending on the type of stored data. One instruction is an integer add instruction: Its two operands must be sign-magnitude integers. A second instruction is a floating-point add instruction: Its two operands must be floating-point numbers. It is the responsibility of the programmer to guarantee that the values stored in memory are the correct types for the add instruction being executed. For other computers an entirely different solution has been adopted. All data are stored with a "tag" which indicates the type encoding of the stored data. Whatever numeric encodings are used, the word size is generally a few bits larger, and the value in these extra bits indicates the type of the stored data. The hardware automatically inspects the tags and uses the correct arithmetic circuitry for the stored data. As a result, a single add instruction is all that is necessary.

As a specific example, assume that the computer uses eight-bit sign-magnitude integers and eight-bit floating-point numbers as described earlier, and further suppose that the computer has a word size of 10 bits. The left two bits will be a tag field. If the value in the tag field is '00', the number is sign-magnitude. If the value in the tag field is '01', the number is floating-point. If the value is either '10' or '11' then the data are neither sign-magnitude nor

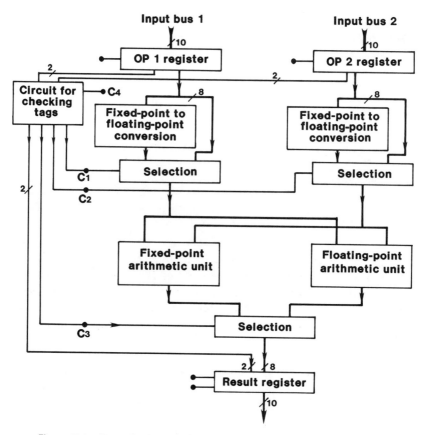

Figure 5.1. Part of the arithmetic circuitry of a computer that uses tagged data. See text for explanation.

floating-point and hence cannot be added. We will not consider this case further.

Figure 5.1 shows part of the arithmetic circuitry for this machine. Two input buses carry the two operands to registers where they are held prior to an arithmetic operation. The outputs from the two operand registers are divided into their tag and arithmetic parts. The left-most two bits from each register go to circuitry, which checks the tags and determines what type of arithmetic to perform. In the figure, a slash through a data bus and an adjacent integer indicates the number of bits in the data bus. The right-most eight bits from each register go to two places: (1) circuitry for converting fixed-point values into their equivalent floating-point values, and (2) selection networks, which receive the converted representations as well as the unconverted representations. Each selection network selects one of its input representations and delivers it as an output. For example, if the left-most selection network receives a signal on control line C1, it selects its second input, which is the unconverted value in operand register one. Otherwise it selects its first input, the floating-point equivalent of the value in operand register one. The same is true for the right-most selection network and the control signal C2.

The circuit for checking tags generates control signals C1, C2, and C3, depending on the tag values it receives. If both tags indicate fixed-point numbers, it generates signals on control lines C1 and C2, but not on control line C3. Both upper selection networks choose the unconverted values held by the two operand registers, and because the lower selection network receives no control signal, it selects its first input which is the value determined by the fixed-point arithmetic unit. In this case, both operands are fixed-point numbers and the result is a fixed-point number. If both tags indicate floating-point numbers, the circuitry for checking tags generates signals on control lines C1, C2, and C3. Once again, the upper selection networks choose the unconverted numbers, which are floating-point numbers, and the lower selection network selects the result computed by the floating-point arithmetic unit. In this case, both operands and the result are floating-point numbers. However, if one of the tags indicates a fixed-point number and the other tag indicates a floating-point number, then the circuitry for checking tags generates C3 (to select the floating-point result) and the proper signal, C1 or C2, to select the floating-point equivalent for the operand that is fixed-point. As a result, both operands received by the arithmetic units are floating-point, and the floating-point result is selected.

A control output labeled C4 is generated by the circuit for checking tags in case one or both of the tags indicates a representation which is neither fixed-point nor floating-point. The signal C4 goes to the control unit of the computer and is used to interrupt the computation: In this case an error condition is detected.

For a computer that does not used tagged numbers, special instructions are provided for converting numbers from one representation to another. For example, if an integer is to be added to a floating-point number, the integer must first be converted into a floating-point number. After conversion, the floating-point adder is used. The availability of the tags in the second computer enable the hardware to take the responsibility of checking the types of data to be processed, thereby relieving the programmer of that responsibility. However, there are nontrivial costs: the word size of the computer must be large enough to incorporate the tags and the circuitry that inspects the tags and performs the proper data-type conversions is more costly.

When viewed using the terminology of Chapter 2, the information in the tag field is control information, whereas the information in the data field is content information. The only time that the control information is used is when it controls an operation in the computer. With reference to Figure 5.1, it is impossible by inspecting the data bus alone to determine that two of the wires convey control information while eight wires convey content information. In fact, the storage system sees no difference. The difference is clear, however, when one inspects the wiring within the arithmetic circuitry of the computer.

Within the brain, different operations are performed, depending on the type of data being processed. How does the brain know what type of data is being processed? One possibility is that some of the information is control information just like the tag bits in the computer just described, and this control information indicates the origin or modality of the content information being processed. As an example, our memories of visual experience contain information which specifies where the particular event occurred. The information that specifies location may be thought of as a tag. Location tags enable access to experiences based on where they occurred.

INFORMATION MODALITY

By **modality** we generally think of one of the major avenues of sensation, such as vision and audition. However, these major distinctions are generally inadequate to characterize the source of information when studying the brain at the neural level. In the visual system, for example, we may analyze various attributes, such as shape, color, and texture. In each case, a different network is used for the analysis, yet the sensory signals for these attributes all originate at the eye. As a result, it is often necessary to qualify the modality: visual pictorial (shape), color, visual texture.

The brain processes numerous different modalities of information as the partial list on the following page suggests. In addition to these modalities, there are numerous internal sensations, such as familiarity and recency. Each one represents a different modality to the brain.

In general, the input patterns to a storage or processing network and the output patterns from the same network have different submodalities. Patterns which are processed during an experience originate externally; patterns which are processed while remembering an experience originate internally. This distinction will play a prominent role later.

SPATIAL ORGANIZATION OF NEURAL PATTERNS

Sensory information is encoded by the sensory organs as two-dimensional patterns. Perhaps this is most obvious in the visual system, where the retina encodes a two-dimensional representation of the ocular image, but in fact two-dimensional patterns occur in all sensory modalities. Two aspects of sensory patterns are of focal importance: their spatial (topographical or pictorial) organization and their temporal organization. I will first discuss spatial organization.

MAJOR MODALITY	QUALIFICATION	EXAMPLES
VISUAL	shape	tree, shoe
	color	red, green
	texture	smooth, fuzzy
	intensity	bright, dim
	change in intensity	getting bright or dim
	distance	near, far away
	size	large, small
	position	2 feet away
	relative position	to the left, above
	motion	5 miles per hour
	relative motion	faster, slower
AUDITORY	sound	speech recognition
	harmony	chords, the key of C
	timbre	harsh, twangy
	relative pitch	higher or lower pitch
	intensity	loud, soft
	distance	near, far away
	location	in front of, behind
TACTILE	shape	round, cubical
	texture	smooth, prickly
	relative position	nearby, touching
	size	large, small
VESTIBULAR	orientation	upright, horizontal
	direction	to the east
	acceleration	speeding up, slowing down
	rotation	spinning
KINESTHETIC, PHYSICAL	muscle sense	
	temperature	hot, cold
	pain	itch, ache
	pressure	
	vibration	
	position	stomach, head
AFFECT	joy	
	fear	
	anger	
	hunger	
	sexual arousal	
	love	
MOTOR	communication	writing, speech
	locomotion	walking, running

It is becoming more and more evident that the receptor topology is preserved throughout all systems that process sensory patterns, and this *preservation of receptor topology* appears to be a fundamental law of brain anatomy. For example, retinal patterns from each eye arrive at the lateral geniculate nuclei relatively undistorted and in perfect registration with one another. (See Figure 7.11.)

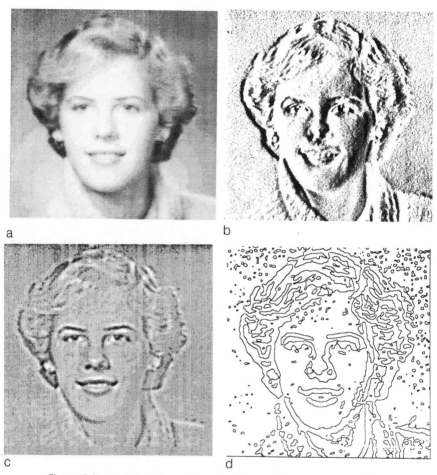

Figure 5.2. a. A sensory pattern. b. The positive component of the x-gradient of the sensory pattern. c. A representation produced by convolving the sensory pattern with the difference of two Gaussian distributions as suggested by Marr (1982, Chapter 2). d. The zero-crossings of the representation shown in d. See Marr for details.

Although it is evident that sensory patterns are two-dimensional, what is not evident is that they are often composed of several independent subpatterns which are all in registration with one another. Although I will illustrate this concept within the visual system, you will see that it pertains to other modalities as well.

Figure 5.2a shows a picture of a face while Figures 5.2b through 5.2d show several different two-dimensional patterns which represent specific attributes of the original figure. To understand the significance of these illustrations, imagine that each figure is printed on graph paper having 10 lines per inch horizontally and vertically. Within each square is a single neuron whose firing rate is proportional to the average brightness of the figure within that grid square. The figure, then, represents the corresponding firing pattern in the two-dimensional collection of neurons. Figure 5.2a represents a sensory pattern while Figures 5.2b through 5.2d represent patterns that can be derived from it. Using a two-cell encoding, Figure 5.2b shows the positive component of the change in brightness while moving from left to right in the original pattern. Figure 5.2c shows the result of convolving the input pattern shown in Figure 5.2a with the difference of two different Gaussian distributions. See Marr (1982) Chapter 2 for details. Figure 5.2d shows the zero crossings of Figure 5.2a as described Marr. Each representation makes explicit a different attribute of the original pattern, and each representation is two-dimensional. In a system which computes these representations, all of them can be computed and transmitted in parallel in different collections of cells, and all of the cells can be in registration with one another.

In each of the above examples, local (neighborhood) operations (transformations) were used to derive the secondary representations from the original pattern. Recent research in computer vision has shown that local transformations are often sufficient to derive complex attributes of the visual field, such as the orientation of surfaces within it. Thus the various computed attributes need not be simple features as illustrated here.

Several questions naturally arise: How can alternative representations of a given sensory pattern be formed? Are the mechanisms for forming alternate representations prewired (genetically specified) or can the system that forms them "learn" to form new representations with experience? Are the pathways that convey the different representations distinct, or are different representations conveyed by the same pathway?

I have already given an answer to the first question. Any network that transforms information changes the nature of the represented information. The transformation performed by a passive or an uncontrolled adaptive network is prewired. The transformation performed by a controlled network depends on the control pattern to that network. If the control patterns are stored in a storage system, then the transformation depends on the control pattern that is being recalled from the storage system. This is illustrated in Figure 5.3. This system can store a new control pattern and later recall it from memory and execute it. The system can therefore "learn" to transform the input pattern in new ways. Learning in this context consists of initially generating the new control patterns (by some unspecified process), storing them in the control store, and later recalling them during sensory processing. (The mechanism for gaining access to the new control patterns is also left unspecified for the present.) The illustrated system is clearly a highly flexible pattern-processing system which can adapt to new sensory environments.

For this system organization, the various encodings of the sensory stimuli are transmitted along the same neural pathways for further processing. This leads to

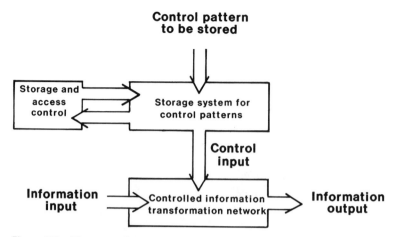

**Control pattern
to be stored**

| Storage and access control | Storage system for control patterns |

Control input

Information input — Controlled information transformation network → **Information output**

Figure 5.3. The essential components of a sensory processing system capable of learning.

one final question: How does the receiving network know what encoding is used to generate the current representation? One possibility is that the control pattern is sent to the receiving network along with the transformed sensory pattern. The control pattern is a "tag" that specifies the representation of the content pattern. I will discuss particular encoding processes in the following chapters, but for now the important issue is that the transformed pattern can encode complex properties of the sensory environment while the tag indicates exactly what it represents. In this system, all of the encodings preserve the topology of the sensory pattern.

One final note: The pathway over which the control pattern is sent may be indistinguishable from the pathway over which the information pattern is sent. This is particularly true if the pathways are in registration with one another.

DIMENSIONALITY OF ENCODED PATTERNS

The dimensionality of a transformed pattern is not necessarily the same as the dimensionality of the original pattern. In the periphery of the eye, for example, there are 100 receptor cells for every cell in the optic nerve. In this case the pattern transmitted by the retina is substantially smaller than the original sensory pattern. When the transformed pattern is smaller, information is lost. As an example, Figure 5.4 shows a transformation of the face of Figure 5.2a in which the dimensionality of the transformed pattern is reduced by a factor of 256. The transformed pattern was formed by averaging the values in each 16-by-16 region of the original figure; hence information was lost. However, the geometrical properties of the original figure are preserved.

When we name things that we see, we are transforming a visual representation into a symbolic representation. The symbolic representation is the internal representation of the name of the object. However, the transformation does not preserve the geometry of the sensory pattern and hence requires a very different type of analysis. Naming is a transformation performed by a mixed modality memory store when it accepts information of one modality and recalls information of a different modality. This type of transformation will be discussed next.

STORAGE NETWORKS FOR ENCODING AND TRANSFORMING INFORMATION

Similarity Encodings

The primary roles of a storage system are storing, searching for, and recalling information. I will show here that these processes are only one aspect of storage processing. Encoding of information is another equally important aspect.

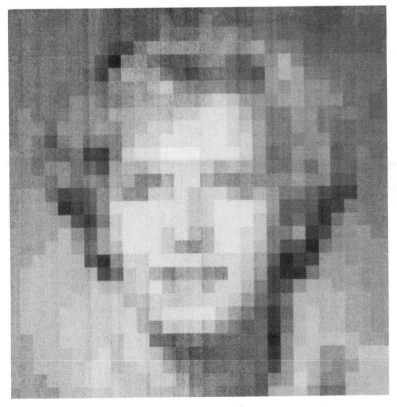

Figure 5.4.   A representation derived from the pattern shown in Figure 5.2a in which information is lost.

Whenever an input pattern is delivered to an associative storage network, each memory location compares that input pattern with its stored pattern. For each storage location, the result of the comparison is a signal that indicates the degree of similarity between input and stored patterns. In Chapter 4, I showed how the similarity signals could be used to activate memory locations and I also showed how memory locations could be organized into a hierarchy for access control. Consider now the pattern conveyed by the cells that compute the similarity values—the similarity pattern. Since there is one similarity cell for each memory location in the memory store, the dimensionality of the similarity pattern is generally greater than the dimensionality of the input pattern. Evidently, the storage system generates information.

What is the spatial nature of the similarity pattern? Clearly there is no relationship between the topology of the input pattern and the topology of its similarity pattern. In the similarity pattern, position corresponds to the place in the memory store where similar information is available. If the storage network is a temporal analyzer (see Chapter 4), then the similarity pattern indicates when the organism experienced similar information. If the storage network is a conceptual analyzer (see Chapter 4) then the similarity pattern indicates regions in the memory store where similar inputs are stored. In either case, the similarity pattern is an encoding of relationships between input pattern and all stored patterns. Similarity patterns can be stored, analyzed, and processed just like any other sensory or secondary patterns, and they are central to many high-level processes, as you will see later.

Associated Encodings

The similarity representation is not the only way that a storage system can encode information. When a mixed modality associative store receives inputs of one modality, one or more memory locations may be activated. When recall is subsequently initiated from an active memory location, recalled patterns of the other modalities are made available. The recalled patterns are therefore encodings of the input pattern. Although there are intervening control functions in an associative store, there are none for an association store (see Chapter 3). Hence an association store converts one representation into another and hence transforms representations. The transformation is an **associative encoding**.

NAMING AND IMAGING

Two types of associative encodings are central to all of brain function: **naming** and **imaging**. Naming is the conversion from sensory to symbolic representations; imaging is the conversion from symbolic to sensory representations. I will not at this time specify the particular sensory or symbolic representations involved; that will come later. The important point here is that the conversion from sensory to symbolic representations or vice versa is effected either by an associative store with appropriate control functions or by an association store, so that the associated output immediately follows or coincides with the corresponding input.

TEMPORAL ORGANIZATION OF NEURAL PATTERNS

The spatial organization of neural patterns derives either externally from the spatial organization of the environment (which is then preserved by the neural circuitry), by the spatial organization of information within the storage systems (which gives rise to specific similarity encodings of the input patterns), or by the spatial organization of the sensory neurons within the body (touch, pain, temperature, muscle tension, etc.). The temporal organization of information likewise derives either from the external environment or from within the neural substrate. I have already discussed several ways that time can be encoded into position within storage systems. This *preservation of temporal information*, like the preservation of spatial information, appears to be a fundamental law of brain function.

Within the time domain, the speed at which sensory signals are transformed from one representation to another varies greatly, and this suggests that perhaps several different storage systems are involved. Speech sounds, for example, must be processed at the phoneme level (milliseconds), at the syllable and word levels (tenths of seconds), at the sentence level (seconds), at the conceptual level (minutes to days), and at the thematic level (years). It is therefore most likely that physically different storage networks, which have different physical characteristics, participate in the analysis and encoding of information at each level of processing.

As a final comment, it might be noted that both temporal and spatial characteristics must be analyzed both for auditory and visual information. Speech sounds are converted by the cochlear networks into patterns of nerve impulses. The cochlear networks consist of two-dimensional arrays of hair receptors which, because of their geometrical structure, are sensitive to different sound frequencies. This will be discussed in greater detail in Chapter 10. The result is a two dimensional pattern where sound frequency is encoded into spatial position.

When reading, the visual patterns vary as rapidly as the auditory encodings do during speech analysis. These observations suggest that several specialized storage systems encode these sensory representations into an appropriate internal format for processing and analysis. Furthermore, this internal representation, upon output, must be transformed into the appropriate motor patterns either for speech or for writing. Hence for output processing we also expect associative encoding networks.

SUMMARY

I have discussed three principal mechanisms for changing patterns from one representation to another: (1) Transforming them with an information transforming network, in which case the spatial organizations of the secondary patterns resemble the spatial organizations of the primary patterns; (2) creating a similarity encoding using an associative memory store, in which case the spatial organization indicates the relationship between the input pattern and the location of associated stored information; and (3) by associative encoding, in which case there is no relationship between the spatial characteristics of the input pattern and the spatial characteristics of its encoding. All three mechanisms of information encoding are fundamental to brain function, as will be seen.

REFERENCE

Marr, D. (1982). *Vision*. San Francisco: W. H. Freeman.

6

INFORMATION
STORAGE AND
HUMAN MEMORY

INTRODUCTION

There is perhaps no aspect of brain function more elusive than memory. There are at least four reasons for this elusiveness. First, there are many different storage systems and hence the single concept of "human memory" is inadequate. Second, although the storage systems are functionally tied together, they are to a great extent independent, and since there is some duplication of function among them, it is extremely difficult to ascribe a particular function to a particular storage system. Third, within a single modality are different types of storage networks (for example, temporary and permanent). These networks are independent to some degree so it is particularly difficult to select one and exclude another for study and analysis. Finally, the memory stores appear to be duplicated from one hemisphere to the other even though the use to which they are put may differ. This adds to the difficulty of studying any one storage system in isolation.

The goal of this chapter is to give insights into the relationship between information storage and human memory. In particular, I will focus on experiential stores, naming stores, and motor control stores and, citing clinical literature as evidence, I will describe the nature of the memory traces and control functions of the memory stores. One must understand the nature of storage before one can hope to understand the computations that underlie language, mental imagery, movement control, and decision making, all of which rely on the storage systems to support their function.

I will not discuss the numerous psychological theories and data that memory researchers have amassed, though I have included a list of suggested readings at the end of the chapter. To explain those data (including item data: thresholds, strengths, attributes; association data: forgetting functions, confidence judgments, repetition effects, symmetry; serial order: retroactive and proactive inhibition, distinctiveness, item order, capacity limitations, chunking; recall:

forgetting, cuing effects, part-to-whole transfer; the affect on recognition and recall of meaningful-versus-nonsense data, serial position, etc.) would require a detailed model not only for the various storage systems, their control systems, and the relationships between them, but also for the affect system and the purposive systems (which I will introduce later). Since, at the present time, we are not even close to such an understanding, I have restricted my coverage in this chapter to those aspects of brain function which I feel give the greatest insight into the functioning of the memory stores and their control systems at the neural level.

Roughly speaking, the human memory stores can be divided into several different classes, depending on the permanence of the memory trace. Sensory buffers hold sensory inputs for a short period of time (up to a few seconds) and are necessary for the initial encoding of sensory data. Temporary memory stores hold information for much longer periods of time—perhaps an hour—but then lose their information suddenly, and permanent memory stores hold information indefinitely. Memory stores can be divided into classes based on the mechanism of trace consolidation. Some memory stores require a single presentation of information to form a trace while other stores require repeated presentations. Memory stores can be grouped according to information modality. Some stores hold sensory patterns or transformed sensory patterns, some stores hold similarity patterns or processed similarity patterns, some hold control patterns which are used to control mental activities, and some hold internally generated motor patterns which control the muscles. Finally, for each memory store, the activation of memory locations is a form of temporary storage which must be considered apart from the stored information itself. The access mechanisms for a memory store determine what can be recalled and when. They must therefore be carefully considered in any discussion of human memory.

THE STORES OF EXPERIENCE

Permanent Storage

This section describes the memory stores which hold the records of conscious experience and presents evidence that they have the following properties: (1) The records of experience are stored continuously in time. Hence trace consolidation occurs during or after a single presentation of the information to be stored. (2) The mechanism for converting between time of input and position in a storage location is an intrinsic property of the storage system. (3) Several seconds of experience are stored in each memory location. This organizes stored information into accessible "packets," a fundamental principle governing the organization of information in experiential memory. (4) Experiential memory stores are associative. This enables immediate access to prior similar stored information. (5) The memory stores are controlled by two functional subsystems: a storage control subsystem which initiates the consolidation process and an access control system which regulates access to stored information and initiates recall of selected information. (6) In part, the records of experience are those auditory and visual patterns which occupy the focus of attention, but additional sensory, affect, and control patterns are also stored as part of each record of experience.

Perhaps the best known evidence for the existence of permanent records of experience comes from the pioneering clinical work of Wilder Penfield and his colleagues ranging over the three decades between 1938 and 1968. This evidence has appeared in the literature in numerous places with one of the most comprehensive being that of Penfield and Perot (1963). I will briefly review the salient points.

Occasionally, for patients with severe epileptic seizures which cannot be effectively controlled by drugs, surgical removal of the focus of epilepsy is the only viable treatment. During surgery, but prior to removal of the pathology, the surgeon probes the brain by stimulating the exposed cortex with a small electrical probe using a mild current that does not harm the neural tissue.[1] The probe is about one millimeter in diameter and does not make direct contact with the neurons; hence a large number of neurons are stimulated.

Two things may happen: (a) Stimulation may interfere with the cortical activity in the region immediately surrounding the surgeon's probe, and (b) One or more cells in the region which are particularly sensitive may be excited and cause activation of cells or groups of cells either nearby or at a distance. When stimulation causes activation, the cells activated by the surgeon's probe appear to be selected at random, probably because they are sensitive at that time due to a pathology, prior activation, or other local conditions.

During this process, the patient is under a local anesthetic and feels no physical pain or discomfort from the process. The patient is fully conscious and responsive to the surgeon. When the surgeon touches the exposed cortex with the probe but the current is off, the patient experiences nothing. However, when the current is turned on, occasionally, and depending on the location of the probe, but independent of its voltage or frequency, the patient may experience a sensation which has been called **second consciousness**. This sensation, as described by the patient, consists of "hearing" or "seeing" some event of his or her past experience. There are also numerous occurrences of spontaneous (nonassociative) recollections of experiences, which are not in the form of second consciousness, occasional feelings of familiarity or *déjà vu*, and occasional dream-like states. The following protocol, taken directly from a

---

[1]By carefully stimulating the exposed cortex, the surgeon is able to localize accurately and outline the speech areas and hence protect them from unnecessary damage during surgery.

surgeon's report, illustrates second consciousness. (The numbers refer to positions of the probe on the exposed brain during the process.)

15.   "I hear singing."
15.   Repeated. "Yes. it is White Christmas." When asked if anyone was singing she said, "Yes, a choir." When asked if she remembered it being sung with a choir, she said she thought so.
16.   "That is different, a voice—talking—a man."
17.   "Yes, I have heard it before. A man's voice—talking."
17.   Repeated without warning. "Yes, about the same."
18.   "There is the sound again—like a radio program—a man talking." She said it was like a play, the same voice as before.
19.   "The play again!" Then she began to hum. When asked what she was humming, she said she did not know, it was what she heard.
19.   Repeated. Patient began to hum. She continued at the ordinary pace of a song. "I know it but I don't know the name—I have heard it before. I hear it, it is an instrument—just one." She thought it was a violin.
15.   Repeated (26 minutes after last stimulation at 15). "White Christmas," she said it was the orchestra playing.
17.   Repeated (24 minutes after last stimulation at 17). "Yes, the play again."
18.   Repeated (21 minutes after last stimulation at 18). "White Christmas."
23.   "The play—they are talking." When asked who, she said, "The men are talking." When asked who they were, she said, "I don't know."
26.   Patient said, "It hurts." Stimulation was stopped. She said, "I see a picture." She added, "It was a face which comes from a picture." (Penfield & Perot, pp. 618-619.)

It is important to understand that second consciousness is only observed under pathological conditions, when the surgeon stimulates the exposed cortex with his electrode. Nonetheless, the vividness and clarity of the experience for the patient cannot be ignored.

Second consciousness is not the only experience patients report. It is also noteworthy that some patients who experience second consciousness also experience stimulation-induced recollections which are not described as second consciousness. This is illustrated below for two different patients:

"Some crazy things ran through my mind; I was younger, at school. I was playing with a polo bat." When asked, he said he remembers doing this when going to school at about the age of 10. (Penfield & Perot, p. 627)

"The world seems awful strange. . . . " When asked why, she said, "You sound distant and I feel strange. A lot of things came back to my memory....There was a boy named Peter Bush. . . . I wonder why these things are being brought to my attention." She added spontaneously, "I know where he lives and can tell you his address. (Ramey & O'Doherty, pp. 171-172.)

Some statements made by Penfield and Perot summarize the content of these experiences:

The times that are summoned most frequently are briefly these: The times of watching or hearing the action and speech of others, and times of hearing music. Certain sorts of experiences seem to be absent. For example, the times of making up one's mind to do this or that do not appear in the record. Times of carrying out skilled acts, times of speaking or saying this and that, or of writing messages and adding figures—these things are not recorded. Times of eating and tasting food, times of sexual excitement or experience—these things have been absent as well as periods of painful suffering or weeping. Modesty does not explain these silences. (Penfield & Perot, p. 687)

The following statements were made by Penfield on another occasion and summarize these findings most eloquently:

When by chance, the neurosurgeon's electrode activates past experience, that experience unfolds progressively, moment by moment. This is a little like the performance of a wire recorder or a strip of cinematographic film on which are registered all those things of which the individual was once aware—the things he selected for his attention in that interval of time. Absent are the sensations he ignored, the talk he did not heed.

Time's strip of film runs forward, never backward, even when resurrected from the past. It seems to proceed again at time's own unchanged pace. . . . (Penfield & Roberts, p. 53)

The experience goes forward. There are no still pictures. The flash-back has strong visual and auditory components, but always it is an unfolding of sight and sound and also, though rarely, of sense of position. . . . (Penfield & Roberts, p. 52)

Every individual forms a neuronal record of his own stream of consciousness. Since artificial re-activation of the record, later in life, seems to re-create all those things formerly included within the focus of his attention, one must assume that the re-activated recording and the original neuronal activity are identical. . . . (Penfield & Roberts, p. 54)

The cortical stimulation data have a natural explanation if we assume there are one or more permanent memory stores which record each person's stream of visual and auditory experience. Our own ability to recognize events, movies, television shows, songs, and so forth, is strong personal support for the assertion that the brain maintains permanent records of the focus of attention throughout our lives.

Temporary Storage

The previous evidence suggests that the brain maintains a continuous permanent record of all conscious experience. The following evidence distinguishes between temporary records of experience and permanent records of experience. The evidence does not, however, distinguish between (a) physically different memory stores, (b) a single memory store having both temporary and permanent memory traces, (c) a single memory store where temporary traces become permanent, or (d) temporary traces in any of the previous cases or permanent traces with temporary access. Nonetheless, the evidence clearly distinguishes between permanent records (once consolidated) and temporary records or temporary access to them, and it motivates several avenues of consideration.

On record are several cases where, because of damage to certain brain structures, the patients appear unable to make (or access) new permanent records of experience even though prior records remain functionally intact. These studies, which will be reviewed briefly, describe a memory disturbance resulting from bilateral damage to the hippocampus and hippocampal gyrus (Milner, 1965, 1970; Milner, Corkin, & Teuber, 1968; Penfield, 1968, 1972; Penfield & Mathieson, 1974). For one patient, known throughout the literature as H. M., the brain damage was the result of surgery performed to relieve severe recurring epileptic seizures. The resulting memory disturbance is similar in many respects to Korsakoff's syndrome (see, e.g., Talland & Waugh, 1969; or Kolb & Whishaw, 1985) and is characterized in part by the patient's inability to remember experiences that occurred after the brain damage. This inability to remember new experiences is called **anterograde amnesia**. Milner described H. M. this way:

> As far as we can tell, this man has retained little if anything of events subsequent to the operation, although his I.Q. rating is actually slightly higher than before. . . . On formal testing, it was clear that forgetting occurred the instant the patient's focus of attention shifted, although in the absence of distraction his capacity for sustained attention was remarkable. . . . Last autumn, more than seven years after the operation, I found him essentially unchanged since 1955, and with the same apparent inability to recall anything once he had been distracted. (Milner, 1965, pp. 104-105)

Analysis of the Evidence

This case suggests the existence of at least two independent storage systems: a system for the temporary storage of experience and a system for its permanent storage. (Later I will show that the same case suggests, in addition, the existence of independent storage systems for controlling visually coordinated movements and for controlling simple movement procedures.) The temporary store holds the records of current experience until the focus of attention shifts at which time the temporary records are lost. I will proceed under the assumption that these systems are independent even though, as I indicated earlier, there are several alternate explanations for the same data.

When the cortical stimulation data and hippocampal damage data are analyzed in terms of an associative storage system of the type described in

Chapter 3, these data have a very simple and natural explanation. Under normal circumstances, the neural patterns which occupy the focus of auditory and visual attention are delivered to the permanent stores of experience. The storage control system determines where to store these current records of experience and generates and delivers the appropriate signals to the selected storage locations to effect storage. Now suppose that the cerebral cortex in the regions surrounding the temporal lobes are the permanent storage systems and the hippocampus and related structures are either the storage control system, a functional subsystem that regulates the storage control system, or a pathway along the avenues of regulation. When the hippocampus and surrounding tissues are removed or damaged, the signals that initiate permanent storage do not reach the intended memory locations. Either they are not generated at all (if the hippocampus contains or is part of the storage control system), or the pathway of regulation is severed. In either case, the effectual signals which initiate storage do not arrive at the intended memory locations. As a result, new permanent traces of experience are never made. As long as the memory stores are undamaged and all information pathways from the sensory organs to the permanent stores of experience are undamaged, prior memories can be accessed and recalled. Hence only anterograde amnesia results.

Returning to the earlier cortical stimulation data, the explanation is equally simple and natural. There are two types of control inputs for every associative memory store: those that initiate storage and those that initiate recall. In addition, there are similarity outputs from the memory locations. When the surgeon's electrode happens to stimulate (either directly or indirectly) a recall command input to an activated memory location, recall is initiated. Since this is not the result of a voluntary command, the patient experiences a spontaneous **recollection** of some prior event. The patient is surprised and wonders why this or that came to mind. When stimulation activates an effectual input that initiates storage, the result is the pathological restorage of a past event which gives rise to the sensation of second consciousness. Finally, when the surgeon's probe happens to activate a similarity output, the result is the unexpected feeling of familiarity or *déjà vu*.

To support these assertions further, note that in each case where stimulation causes second consciousness, the surgeon's probe was located on the patient's temporal lobe. The temporal lobe is just above the hippocampus, where stimulation may activate a cell and send an initiate storage command to a memory location in the permanent experiential memory store. This is consistent with the hypothesis that the hippocampus is part of the storage control system (or contains a pathway along the avenue of control).

It is important to note that I have not suggested that the content patterns of experience pass through the hippocampus or that damage to the hippocampus interferes with the information pathways. If the information pathways to the experiential memory stores are damaged, in addition to anterograde amnesia one would expect amnesia, since the patient would not be able to access prior stored information by association. That simply has not been the case after hippocampal damage.

Organization of Memories into "Packets" of Experience

Let me now return briefly to the assumption that experiential information is organized by the permanent storage system into accessible packets by the memory locations. There is direct evidence that activation of the records of experience progresses at time's normal pace, moving only forward. However, during stimulation, when second consciousness is experienced, the experience always begins at a fixed point in time and then moves forward. If stimulation is stopped and then restarted, the activated event always begins at its beginning, never in the middle. Although stimulation is generally stopped before the experience is completely played out, there are many cases on record where stimulation was not discontinued but the experience ceased on its own. Here are three examples from different patient's reports:

> After a pause the patient said, "I see a machine, one that I have seen before." The machine seemed to disappear before the end of the stimulation. (Penfield & Perot, p. 644)

> When the electrode was applied he said, "I imagine I hear a lot of people shouting at me." This was repeated, the stimulus being applied for two seconds, and she heard the voices for seven seconds. It was repeated a third time and she said, "I hear them again." The duration of the voices with the third stimulation was 14 seconds. (Penfield & Perot, p. 630)

> During stimulation without warning he said, "Yes, there was something." He said he saw it. It was an object. The operator noted that each of these visual experiences seemed to disappear before the end of stimulation. (Penfield & Perot, p. 641)

As indicated, a single activated event may last a few seconds or it may last for as many as 15 or 20 seconds. This suggests that each storage location is capable of storing experiences for as many as 20 seconds, if not longer.

It is noteworthy that damage to the hippocampus and neighboring structures does not appear to interfere with the temporary stores of experience. Earlier I suggested that the temporary and permanent stores might be functionally and physically independent. There are several additional reasons why this might be so. First, one would expect temporary storage systems to hold considerably more detail—have larger patterns—than permanent storage systems. This is so because the neural tissue in a temporary store can be reused. For a permanent store, in contrast, the neural tissue becomes dedicated to the memory traces that it consolidates. Each memory location becomes part of the recognition system for related information and cannot be used for other purposes. Second, the biochemical mechanisms of temporary and permanent storage most likely differ. It would be easier to incorporate different biochemical mechanisms in functionally distinct networks. Third, the control functions differ. In a permanent store, once a memory location is used, it is not reused. This is not so for a temporary store. Also, independent memory stores can store redundant information. This would be advantageous if the system is to be tolerant of traumatic damage. The fact that the patient H. M. reported by Milner was able to live an almost normal life after his surgery is a case in point.

Consolidation of Permanent Traces

Regardless of the underlying biochemical process or transformations that take place during permanent storage, consolidation of permanent memory traces takes time. Current estimates range from a few minutes to as many as 15. According to the neural hypothesis I have been developing here, two distinctly different underlying mechanisms are necessary. First, the neural networks must create the representation to be stored. This is a time-varying spatial pattern that arrives along an input pathway to the store. The input neurons then release their neurotransmitters and the resulting concentrations specify locally the required strengths of the memory traces. Second, an effectual signal must arrive which initiates the consolidation process and "freezes" the parameters into the neural tissue. These two processes together take time. Since consolidation takes time, it follows that signals must not arrive during consolidation at those synapses whose final transmitter chemicals specify the trace parameters. Otherwise the traces would represent more than the intended event. It follows, therefore, that some neural activity in the memory locations undergoing consolidation must be blocked. Now, access to recent events is crucial to normal daily activity. This leads to the possibility that a separate, independent storage system is used to hold temporary representations of the most recent events, at least long enough to allow consolidation of permanent memory traces to conclude. This, I propose, is done in an independent temporary memory store.

The fact that consolidation takes several minutes is supported by a variety of data. After a traumatic event, such as an automobile accident, where the victim is rendered unconscious, he or she often cannot remember the events immediately preceding the accident. This is called **retrograde amnesia**. Retrograde amnesia often covers a period of several seconds and sometimes several minutes or longer prior to the accident. When patients recover, they remember all but the last few minutes, but they rarely remember the accident itself. As a second example, after electroconvulsive shock treatments, patients generally do not remember the few minutes preceding the shock treatment.

There is also evidence that permanent memory traces are blocked from use during consolidation. When dealing cards at a bridge game, for example, the dealer is almost always the person who asks whose turn it is to bid. He or she simply does not remember dealing. Dealing requires little conscious intervention, and when the dealer's focus of attention shifts, temporary memories of dealing are lost. Since his or her permanent traces are undergoing consolidation and are temporarily unavailable for use, the dealer forgets dealing. After consolidation is complete, the memory traces become available and he or she again remembers dealing. As a second example, people who take medicine regularly often forget whether or not they took it, but only when trying to remember shortly after taking it, during those few critical minutes when the permanent memory traces are unavailable for use. If he or she tries to remember later on in the day, the person will do so without difficulty.

What Is in a Memory?

Although visual and auditory components dominate our records of experience, additional types of information are present. First, control information is stored that indicates how the visual patterns were encoded and where they came from in the visual field. Control information is also stored that indicates where sounds originated and how they were encoded. More important, experiences have emotional and motivational (affect) content. I will briefly explore these notions in the next few paragraphs and return to them in subsequent chapters when describing the visual, auditory, and affect systems.

It has been well known for a long time that certain centers in the brain, particularly the hypothalamus, are associated with emotional and mental states. Centers for hunger, thirst, satiation, fear, rage, and so forth, are examples. Other affective states include interest, anger, shame, joy, and sexual arousal. When these brain centers are experimentally stimulated in laboratory animals, the animals behave in interesting and instructive ways. An animal whose hunger center is continually stimulated will eat, regardless of how full it is, and an animal whose satiation center is stimulated will starve to death. When a mouse is placed in a cage with a cat and the cat's fear center is stimulated, the cat becomes frightened and attempts frantically to escape the presence of its now deadly enemy, the mouse!

Now consider a collection of cells that monitor the activity in each of the affect centers and suppose the axons of these cells form an input pathway to a storage system. The pattern of activity in this pathway conveys the affect state of the animal, and the pattern itself is an **affect pattern**. Stored affect patterns record a history of the animal's emotional state and form part of its records of experience.

Affect patterns are part of the encodings of experience, and this is borne out by the cortical stimulation data of Penfield and his colleagues:

She began to sob, "That man's voice again! The only thing I know is that my father frightens me a lot." (Penfield & Perot, p. 626)

"Yes, I felt just terrified for an instant." Stimulation was continued. She was asked if she still felt terrified and she said, "No." She explained that it was the kind of terror she had with her attacks. (Penfield & Perot, p. 642)

The affect pattern is a tag attached to the sensory encoding.

In addition to the affect state, the records of experience are tagged with their time of occurrence and the coordinates of where they took place. If the experiential store is a temporal analyzer (see Chapter 4), then the time of occurrence is encoded in the position of the memory trace within the memory store. Otherwise a time indicator must be stored as part of the experiential record. Second, experiences contain an indication of where the event took place. If the store is a conceptual analyzer and the position of storage corresponds to location of event, then no additional information is required to encode position. Otherwise location indicators must be stored as part of the experiential record. In either case, the time and location indicators are tags attached to the stored record, just as the affect pattern is. There may be other tags attached to the encodings of experience as well, but these examples suggest that the records of experience contain subpatterns of several different modalities and are not simply visual and auditory encodings as one might naïvely assume.

The existence of different tags enables the memories of experience to be accessed by several different associated patterns. For example, it is possible to locate events which took place at a specified location and it is possible to locate them based on the mental state of the individual at the time. These aspects of the experiential memory stores play an essential role in several high-level processes which will be studied in more detail later.

At an organizational level, the picture that begins to emerge is illustrated in Figure 6.1. Visual and auditory patterns are transformed into representations which are suitable for permanent storage. The networks labeled "visual encoding and selection" and "auditory encoding and selection" are responsible for these transformations, which will be described in later chapters. The final visual and auditory subpatterns that become the records of experience are called **permanent visual** and **permanent auditory encodings**. The memory stores which temporarily hold memories of experience are not shown. The pathways which convey the affect and location tags are shown as are the corresponding output pathways. Finally, the two control subsystems that initiate storage and control access are illustrated. Not shown are any of the external pathways that regulate the visual and auditory encoding and selection networks or the storage and recall control subsystems. I will leave until later the task of filling in the details of this system.

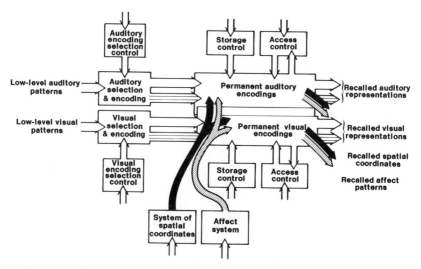

Figure 6.1. The architecture of the low-level visual and auditory systems showing the visual and auditory encoding and selection networks, the visual and auditory stores of experience, and their control networks. Inputs from the affect system and system of spatial coordinates are also shown. The spatial memory system is not shown.

Consciousness and Attention

As a final note, two concepts play an important part in descriptions of our thought processes: consciousness and attention. Although there are currently no universally accepted functional definitions of either concept, the following working definitions agree with intuition and are consistent with generally accepted usage. **Consciousness** is the sensation associated with the storage of information in a memory store, and **attention** is the process of selecting one or another stimulus event or modality (sight, sound, taste, pain, thought, motor function) for storage (and hence consciousness). The **focus of attention** is that part of our sensory encoding that is selected for permanent storage—the part that becomes a permanent record of our experience. Only those events which are selected for storage in one memory system or another enter our consciousness; we remain unaware of those events which are not selected. (Chapter 16 elaborates on these issues.)

NAMING STORES

The stores of experience are the repository for the encodings of our experience. However useful and necessary experiential information is for life's normal processes, it is not the only form of permanently stored information. This

120

section will describe memory stores that transform information from sensory to symbolic representations, and vice versa. These are **naming stores**. They play a fundamental role in all language processing and thought, as you will see later.

In Chapter 5, I defined naming and imaging. I will now elaborate on these notions. **Symbols** are the internal representations for words and are used extensively in most high-level thought processes. The symbol for "ball" is the dynamic pattern that results when we silently read the word "ball", when we see a ball and identify it as "ball", or when we identify a ball from a description such as "the object that gets batted when the Yankees play the Dodgers." It is also the pattern that results when we perceive the spoken word "ball". Likewise the symbol for "red" is the dynamic pattern that is generated when describing the color of something red, and the symbol for "headache" is the dynamic pattern that is generated when naming the corresponding painful sensation. Symbols are the patterns we manipulate when we think symbolically and they are in the modality of our verbal thoughts.[2]

When we describe sensory events we convert from sensory representation to verbal representation and when we speak we convert from verbal representation to vocalization representation. Conversion between modalities is a rapid and automatic process which will be the topic of the next few pages.

In general, **naming** is the process of associating and recalling the symbol for a concept or token when given its nonsymbolic or sensory encoding, and **imaging** is the process of associating and recalling the nonsymbolic encoding of a token or concept when given its symbolic encoding. There are several intermediate control processes involved in imaging and naming. For naming, after the sensory encoding is delivered to the naming store, a decision must be made to recall a piece of stored information.[3] Assuming a control structure similar to the one described in Chapter 4, recall must be initiated from an activated memory location. If more than one memory location is activated, one of them must be selected. If the recalled information has an appropriate symbol for the given sensory encoding, the process can terminate. Otherwise, recall must be initiated from another memory location. Even after a symbol is found, it must be accepted as a correct symbol for the given sensory encoding. This determination is made by the belief system, a system which will be introduced later. In summary, there are several decision and control functions that can potentially mediate between the initial input of an image and the final output of its name. A similar situation holds for imaging.

---

[2]The modality probably differs for different people. For some people the underlying modality may be auditory; for other people it may be visual; for still other people it may be within the motor system. For purposes of this discussion the particular modality is not important.

[3]While reading, the written words are converted into their symbolic form without intervening control. The intermediate processes are automatic. This suggests that an association store is used rather than an associative store.

The importance of these intermediate control processes cannot be overemphasized. If one simply ignores them and attempts to replace the naming store by an association store, then only one response will be given for any sensory encoding. In addition, the recalled symbol would be generated immediately, as soon as the image is presented. This is often not the case. We often do not use the associated name or image; often it is not even recalled. Similarly, we often cannot get at the name of something even though we are sure we know what it is (e.g., the "tip-of-the-tongue" phenomenon). This further supports the hypothesis that intermediate control networks regulate access to the associated information.

Naming takes place continually when we describe a scene, for example, and imaging takes place continually when we imagine a scene which is being described verbally. In each case, naming stores are crucial to the ongoing processes. So are the networks which control the naming stores, which select among activated storage locations, which deactivate them when necessary, and which formulate the descriptions or control the imagery apparatus to name a few. Later I will discuss some of the control networks, but for now, understand that the processes of describing and imaging are subserved by naming stores which are themselves regulated by other high-level networks.

Even keeping in mind the fact that naming stores are controlled by other networks, we are still a long way from understanding them in isolation. We do not know yet the sensory and verbal codes that are used. Hence we do not know how similarity is measured. We do not know how the access parameters are modified. We do not even know how a simple pattern can be recognized when part of it is not given. (This corresponds to finding words like *rea*, where the asterisks can be replaced by arbitrary letters, or recognizing partly occluded objects. Thus although naming and imaging are fundamental parts of human information processing, we are still a long way from understanding them completely.

Examples of Naming

The mechanisms that underlie naming are varied and depend to a great extent on modality. The common thread that binds together the many aspects of naming is the utilization of a naming store to associate a verbal symbol with its nonsymbolic or sensory representation.

Within the visual system we most often regard naming as the assignment of a class token to the image of an object or shape: a square, a circle, a shoe, a tree, a radio. The visual system first encodes the retinal image of the object to be named into an internal representation called a **pictorial pattern**. The resulting pattern is delivered to the naming store for the final assignment of its symbolic name. (Note that there may be several different intermediate stages of encoding in this process.) The naming store finally associates the symbolic encoding with the pictorial encoding and hence can be used both for naming and imaging as defined earlier.

Pictorial naming, however, is only one aspect of visual naming. Our ability to name color is distinctly different from our ability to name shapes, and the underlying encoding mechanisms differ. Color information, as will be seen, is encoded as a set of ratios of firing rates within sensory neurons in such a way that each color has its own unique set of ratios regardless of brightness. Our ability to name colors, then, is a consequence of the sensory encoding and the way the ratios are recognized by a memory store.

Texture is yet another example of a visual attribute that can be named, and our ability to name texture is independent of our ability to name shape or color. In fact, there are several different attributes of a visual object that can easily be named, and each one has a different underlying mechanism of encoding and analysis. Among the nameable attributes are surface shading, relative brightness, surface reflectance, and surface orientation. In each case, naming consists of encoding the stimulus pattern in such a way that the desired attribute is made explicit in the encoding, and then delivering the encoded pattern to a naming store for association. If one or more memory locations in the naming store are activated, then recall of the associated symbolic token completes the process of naming. The sensory encoding process that is necessary for naming is a complex process as you will see. The control processes which (1) regulate the encoding process, (2) control the transmission of encoded patterns to the naming store, and (3) control the naming store itself are likewise complex and involved. The major point here is that for naming to take place at all it is necessary to assign a symbolic token in the verbal modality to an encoded sensory pattern, and the associative storage system that performs the final assignment is not an experiential memory store.

Certain attributes derived primarily through the visual system can also be named, including the distance of an object from the viewer, the relative locations of different objects, movement of objects, rate of change of movement of objects, and so forth. We can name these attributes because we can associate symbolic names to control patterns that regulate computations of the visual system: convergence and focus of eyes, movement of eyes, head, and body, rate of change of eye movement, to name a few. Once again, naming is the result of transmitting the appropriate sensory information to a naming store for analysis and then recalling from an activated memory location the symbolic name of the analyzed pattern: "to the left," "above," "near," "moving to the left," "coming closer," and so forth.

Using the auditory system, we can name items from their sound (bell, whistle, rustling of leaves), we can understand spoken words, we can determine and name the location of a source of sound in the external world, we can identify sound texture (harshness, brilliance, clarity, tone), we can identify specific sound frequencies (the key of C# minor), and we can identify tonal qualities. In each case, naming is the assignment of a symbolic token to a pattern generated by the auditory encoding networks. In each case, naming is accomplished by an associative memory which recognizes an input pattern of one modality and generates its name in the modality of symbolic thought.

Naming also occurs for internally generated signals: pain, hunger, temperature, fear, and so forth. This suggests that the current affect pattern not only forms a part of a person's experiential records, but also makes an input to a naming store.

Artificially Induced Aphasia in the Naming Stores

Although there is little direct clinical evidence for the existence of naming stores, and the evidence is also less convincing than for experiential memory stores, there is, nonetheless, some evidence which deserves review. Penfield and Roberts (1959) have described a technique for mapping the cortical speech areas. This technique, which is similar to the stimulation technique described earlier, also consists of stimulating the exposed cortex during brain surgery. In this case, however, stimulation appears to interfere with the cortical activity in the region surrounding the surgeon's probe. During stimulation, the patient is shown a sequence of pictures of simple objects which are to be named. On occasion, the patient is unable to name an object presented during stimulation, but he or she is able to do so as soon as the stimulation is halted. In some cases, the stimulation appears to arrest the speech process. However, in other cases the stimulation appears simply to block the association between image and symbol. The following statements, taken from the surgeon's report, illustrate this:

23　Stimulation carried out while the patient was talking. He stopped but vocalized a little. After cessation of stimulation, he said he had been unable to speak.

23　Repeated when patient was not trying to talk. There was no vocalization and he observed nothing.

24　Patient tried to talk and mouth moved to the right, but he made no sound.

25　The patient hesitated and then named "butterfly" correctly. Stimulation was carried out then below this point and at a number of points on the two narrow gyri that separate 25 from 24, but the result was negative—no interference with the naming process. The points of negative stimulation are shown by the small circles in Figure VII-5 [not reproduced here].

26　The patient said, "Oh, I know what it is. That is what you put in your shoes." After withdrawal of the electrode he said, "foot."

27　Unable to name tree which was being shown to him. Instead he said, "I know what it is." Electrode was withdrawn then he said, "tree."

28　The patient became unable to name as soon as the electrode was placed here. When asked why he did not name the picture shown, he said, "no." He continued to be silent after withdrawal of the stimulating electrode.

Dr. Jasper reported that the electrograph showed after-discharge which began in a nearby recording electrode and spread to involve the whole temporal region. During this, the patient continued to be unable to name and no longer would answer anything.

The electrographic seizure stopped suddenly and the patient spoke at once. "Now I can talk," he said. "Butterfly." Dr. Pasquet who was acting as observer, had concluded from the patient's expression and movements that he had been trying to answer all through the stimulation and during the after-discharge.

When he bagan to talk he was asked why he had not been able to name the picture, and he replied, "I couldn't get at the word 'butterfly' and then I tried to get the word 'moth.'" (Penfield & Roberts, pp. 116-117)

In more recent studies, care was taken to show that the inability to name a pictorial image was not due to a disruption in the vocalization process or in various thought processes. (See for example, Ojemann, 1978; and Ojemann & Whitaker, 1978.) For example, the patient may be asked to read words printed on one of the cards as well as to name the item shown graphically, or he may be asked to perform mental arithmetic or to recall an item shown or named on a previous card.

Unfortunately, none of the experiments done to date indicate the organization of information within the naming store. The fact that the symbolic encodings for the words "moth" and "butterfly" could not be obtained at the same time suggests a possible organization based on visual category, but no attempt was made to have the patient identify birds, airplanes, and other winged objects. Similarly, when "tree" could not be named, no attempt was made to have the patient identify shrubs, bushes, or specific types of trees (oak trees, maple trees, etc.). Thus, although there is a hint that the naming store for pictorial patterns is a conceptual analyzer, there is not enough evidence at the current time to draw any firm conclusion.

It is also unfortunate that studies have not yet been done in an attempt to discover the existence of naming stores for other than the visual pictorial modality. As I indicated earlier, there are numerous types of patterns involved in naming, including the naming of sensory patterns, control patterns, and affect patterns, and the patterns that can be named are in virtually all modalities. There is clearly a need for additional study here.

I might add that studies have been done to determine the relationships between cortical focus and naming in bilingual patients (Ojemann & Whitaker, 1978). These studies show that sites in the center of the language area of each patient were involved in both languages, but peripheral sites were involved in one language or the other, but not both.

The previous discussion showed that there are several different storage systems having different mechanisms of trace consolidation and different storage and recall policies. In this section I will describe additional storage systems used during skilled behavior. These stores differ both in how they are regulated and in the origin of the memory traces. They also differ in functional architecture, a fact that will be explored in detail in Chapters 12 through 15.

There are clearly many aspects to skilled behavior. We speak, write, walk, drive automobiles, engage in sports, and so forth. One of the fundamental differences between skilled behavior and other activities is that skilled behavior is the result of practice. When we experience an event, our ability to recall that event and describe it does not come from practice; we only experience the event once. We learn skills, however, by repeated execution of efferent motor patterns that are generated internally. Initially the motor patterns are only approximately correct, but with practice, we can improve the skills until the motor patterns can be generated unconsciously—while we are thinking about entirely different things. During the learning process, however, our attention must be directed at learning the skill. Our minds cannot think about anything else.

It is clear that skills improve with practice. This means that changes of some sort occur within the brain during practice. These changes include the formation of memory traces of at least two types: **kinesthetic patterns** and **premotor patterns**. Kinesthetic patterns are sensory patterns that describe the muscles—their lengths, changes in their lengths, and their tensions. Premotor patterns are representations that enable access to motor patterns. Motor patterns are the efferent patterns that activate the muscles. Under some circumstances, kinesthetic patterns may be premotor patterns, but they need not be so. Kinesthetic patterns are used to regulate access to motor patterns during skilled movements. When regulated by suitable control networks, the stores that hold kinesthetic and premotor patterns associate them with motor patterns that control the skilled act.

Execution of a skill consists of several processes. First, the movement must be planned. For example, the words of a sentence to be written or spoken must be formulated by the symbolic processing system, or the desire to walk from here to there must be formulated as a general plan of bodily motion. Plan formation will not be considered here.

After a plan is formulated, it must be converted into a sequence of successive motor acts. The plan may be in terms of symbols if the final act is speaking, it may be in terms of images if the final act is drawing a picture, or it may be in terms of "body images" if the final act is locomotion. In any case, these images or symbols must be translated into premotor patterns, which are further translated into motor patterns—efferent impulses that control the muscles. The

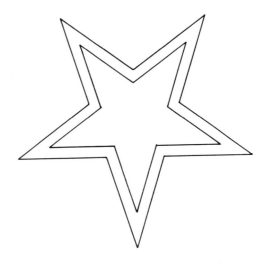

Figure 6.2. An example figure of the type used for studying the learning of hand-eye co-ordination in brain-damaged patients.

memory stores needed for the translation will be described in detail later. A note on the translation process, however, might be insightful. As stated by Luria:

> Before a voluntary movement can be carried out, the visual, vestibular, or acoustic impulses must first be recoded into a definite system of kinesthetic signals. This system forms a three-dimensional grid, enabling efferent signals to be correctly directed to the appropriate muscle groups and at the same time dynamically altering the direction of these signals in accordance with the positions of the muscles and joints in space." (Luria, 1966, p. 174)

When controlling movements, control networks regulate access to the memory stores that translate intentions into premotor and motor patterns. Control networks also join motor patterns together prior to their orchestration so that the movement is a single smooth integrated activation of the original plan. (The cerebellum plays an essential part in this final transformation and integration of constituent motor patterns.)

Execution of hand-eye coordination tasks utilizes associative memory stores to translate visual information into motor information. As an illustrative example, consider the task of following the outline of the five-pointed star shown in Figure 6.2. While following the outline, the pencil point must be kept within the double lines. This is a relatively easy task for most of us to do. We select an arbitrary starting point and place the pencil point there. As we scan the figure, our visual systems determine the spatial direction of each intended movement. Each spatial direction, a premotor pattern, is sent to our motor system where it is translated into the appropriate motor pattern to activate the desired muscles. The translation is done by an associative memory store, and the

127

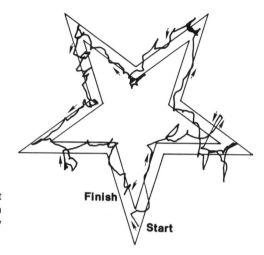

Finish

Start

Figure 6.3. My first attempt at
following the curve shown in
Figure 6.2 while viewing my
own hand through a mirror.

selected motor pattern depends on the current position and orientation of the
hand (among other parameters).

Now consider the same task, only instead of looking at the original figure,
you may only view your hand through a mirror; your hand and the original figure
are blocked from view. Each spatial direction of the intended movement is
reversed by the mirror. When a movement strays outside the lines and you try
to correct it, your correction will be in the wrong direction. Figure 6.3 shows the
result of my first attempt at this task. You might enjoy trying the same
experiment yourself. With practice, you will learn to perform the mirror-
drawing task with little error. What is particularly interesting is that Milner's
patient, H. M., learned to perform this mirror-writing coordination task with a
perfectly normal learning curve (Milner, 1965)! The patient did not, however,
remember performing the task even as his skill improved. For this patient, the
storage system which associates spatial directions with motor patterns remained
intact even though the storage system for the permanent records of experience
did not function correctly. This clearly shows the independence of the motor
stores from the stores of experience.

Interpreting the clinical evidence is not always easy. The patient H. M.,
whom I have mentioned several times already, was studied over a period of many
years and was trained on a variety of tasks. Two, in particular, are much more
difficult to interpret than the other tasks I mentioned. One is finding a path
through a stylus maze. The other is solving the Tower of Hanoi puzzle.

A stylus maze consists of a two-dimensional 10-by-10 square array comprised
of 100 metal bolt heads. One of them is a starting position and a second a
finishing position. Refer to Figure 6.4. There is one path from start to finish,
and the object for H. M. was to discover the path. He used an electrified stylus
which, if he touched it to a bolt head not on the correct path, would ring a

buzzer. To find the path, then, would mean touching the stylus to adjoining bolt heads, in sequence, from start to finish, without ringing the buzzer. H. M. was never able to find the correct path; nor did he show improvement (partial learning) over 215 trials in three days. This is an easy task for normal subjects. What is interesting is that H. M. was able to master a similar though smaller maze, one comprised of a four-by-five array of bolt heads. For the smaller maze, H. M. required 155 trials and made 256 errors. Moreover, two years later he reached the same level of performance in 39 trials, making only 69 errors. One explanation, suggested by Milner, is that the larger maze has 28 choice points, which is a sequence of choices well beyond the span encompassed by temporary memory; the shorter maze, in contrast, has only 8 choice points. Hence a person can hold the decision sequence (left, down, down, etc.) in temporary memory at one time. What is not clear is how H. M. represented the solution in memory once he learned to perform the task. Keep in mind the fact that he never remembered learning the maze on previous trials even after he mastered the maze.

The Tower of Hanoi puzzle consists of a set of three vertical pegs and a set of round disks of different sizes. See Figure 6.5. The disks have holes in their centers and can be placed on top of one another with a peg extending up through them. Initially, all disks are on one peg in pyramid fashion: The largest disk is at the bottom and the smallest disk is on top. The object is to move all

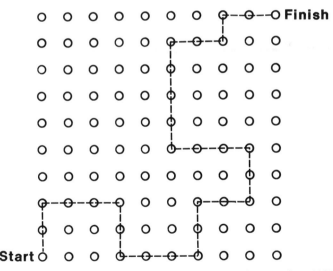

Figure 6.4. The stylus maze problem presented to patient H.M. (Adapted from B. Milner (1965) Memory disturbance after bilateral hippocampal lesions. In P. M. Milner & S. E. Glickman, *Cognitive Processes and the Brain*. New York: D. Van Nostrand Company, Inc.)

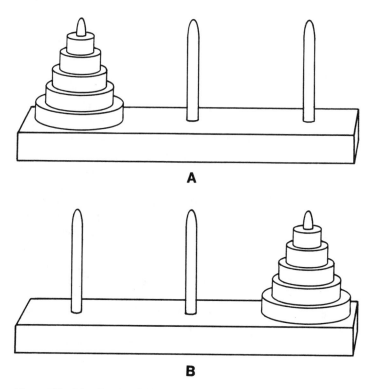

Figure 6.5. The Tower of Hanoi puzzle. a. The starting configuration.
b. The final configuration.

disks from the original peg to the final peg, one at a time, never placing a larger disk on a smaller one. The third peg is used as an intermediate position while solving the puzzle. For this puzzle, the moves comprise a binary sequence; once a solution is found, it is quite mechanical. The patient H. M. was able to solve this puzzle although he did not remember performing the task before. Apparently the storage system, which holds the procedural knowledge for performing this task, remained intact.

At the present time we do not know the relationships between the storage systems used when learning to solve the Tower of Hanoi puzzle, for solving the stylus maze, and for holding the temporary and permanent records of experience as I described earlier in this chapter. Nor do we know if the same storage system is used for both the stylus maze and for the Tower of Hanoi puzzle. Several authors have suggested a procedural memory may be involved (Cohen & Corkin, 1981; Cohen & Squire, 1980), but for the present the evidence must remain a mystery.

SUMMARY

There are numerous storage systems in the brain. They differ in modality, permanence of trace, mechanism of trace formation, temporal characteristics of pattern, and control discipline. This chapter presented evidence for the existence of at least two distinct stores of experience (temporary and permanent), the existence of naming stores, and the existence of stores used for hand-eye coordination.

For the permanent stores of experiences, the traces are consolidated immediately after the experience, and during consolidation, the corresponding memory locations are unavailable for use. The temporary stores of experience are used while the permanent traces undergo consolidation. If a shift in the attention of an individual causes one's temporary memory store to dump its traces before the permanent traces of the same experience are available, a person will experience retrograde amnesia of those events.

Evidence was also presented for the permanent naming stores which associate visual with symbolic data. Stimulation of the exposed cortex caused patients to experience temporary aphasia, an inability to name an object that appears in view. After stimulation ceased, the patient immediately named the visible item. Stimulation of the exposed cortex interfered with the proper operation of the stimulated system; termination of the stimulation enabled the system to resume its normal operation. The one patient's inability to name both "moth" and "butterfly" is slight evidence that the naming stores are conceptual analyzers.

Stores that associate motor patterns with spatial information were shown to be independent of the stores of experience. Patients whose permanent memory stores for experience were damaged retained the ability to learn new hand-eye coordination tasks even though they did not remember learning the skills, and they learned the skills as quickly as normal subjects do.

The relationships between memory and storage are complex. Memory is subserved by a variety of storage systems of different types and a variety of storage control and access control networks with vastly different behavioral characteristics. This chapter barely scratched the surface of those relationships.

REFERENCES

Cohen, N. J., & Corkin, S. (1981). The amnesic patient H. M.: Learning and retention of a cognitive skill. *Neuroscience Abstracts, 7,* 235.

Cohen, N. J., & Squire, L. R. (1980). Preserved learning and retention of pattern analyzing skill in amnesia: Dissociation of knowing how and knowing that. *Science, 210,* 207-209.

_____ (1981). Retrograde amnesia and remote memory impairment. *Neuropsychologia, 19,* 337-356.

Corkin, S. (1968). Acquisition of motor skills after bilateral medial temporal-lobe excision. *Neuropsychologia, 6,* 255-265.

Kolb, B. & Whishaw, I. Q. (1985). *Fundamentals of human neuropsychology* (2d ed.). New York: W. H. Freeman.

Luria, A. R. (1966). *Higher cortical functions in man.* New York: Basic Books.

Milner, B. (1965). Memory disturbance after bilateral hippocampal lesions. In P. M. Milner & S. E. Glickman (Eds.), *Cognitive processes and the brain.* New York: D. Van Nostrand, An Insight Book.

⸺ (1970). Memory and the medial temporal regions of the brain. In Karl H. Pribram & Donald E. Broadbent (Eds.), *Biology of memory.* New York: Academic Press.

Milner, B., Corkin, S., & Teuber, H.-L. (1968). Further analysis of the hippocampal amnesic syndrome: 14-year follow-up study of H. M. *Neuropsychologia,* 6, 215-234.

Ojemann, G. A. (1978). Organization of short-term verbal memory in language areas of human cortex: Evidence from electrical stimulation. *Brain and Language,* 5, 331-340.

Ojemann, G. A. & Whitaker, H. A. (1978). Language localization and variability. *Brain and Language,* 6, 239-260.

⸺ (1978). The bilingual brain. *Archives of Neurology,* 35, 409-412.

Penfield, W. (1968). Engrams in the human brain. Mechanisms of memory. *Proceedings of the Royal Society of Medicine,* London, 61, 831-840.

⸺ (1972). The electrode, the brain and the mind. *Zetschrift Fur Neurologie,* 201, 297-309.

Penfield, W., & Mathieson, G. (1974). Memory. Autopsy findings and comments on the role of the hippocampus in experiential recall. *Archives of Neurology,* 31, 145-154.

Penfield, W., & Perot, P. (1963). The brain's record of auditory and visual experience. A final summary and discussion. *Brain,* 86, 595-696.

Penfield, W., & Roberts, L. (1959). *Speech and brain-mechanisms.* Princeton, NJ: Princeton University Press.

Ramey, E. R., & O'Doherty, D. S. (Eds.). (1960). *Electrical studies on the unanesthetized brain.* New York: Paul B. Hoeber.

Squire, L. R. (1982). The neuropsychology of human memory. *Annual Review of Neuroscience,* 5, 241-273.

Talland, G. A., & Waugh, N. O. (1969). *The pathology of memory.* New York: Academic Press.

SUGGESTED READINGS

In addition to the excellent references listed above, the following references on human memory are a small sampling of the many excellent sources describing human memory.

Adams, J. A. (1967). *Human memory.* New York: McGraw-Hill.

Anderson, J. R., & Bower, G. H. (1973). *Human associative memory.* Washington DC: V.H. Winston & Sons.

Cermak, L. S. (1982). *Human memory and amnesia.* Hillsdale, NJ: Lawrence Erlbaum Associates.

Cofer, C. N. (1975). *The structure of human memory.* San Francisco: W. H. Freeman.

Crowder, R. G. (1976). *Principles of learning and memory.* Hillsdale, NJ: Lawrence Erlbaum Associates.

John, E. R. (1967). *Mechanisms of memory.* New York: Academic Press.

Gurowitz, E. M. (1969). *The molecular basis of memory.* Englewood Cliffs, NJ: Prentice-Hall.

Horel, J. A. (1978). The neuroanatomy of amnesia. A critique of the hippocampal memory hypothesis. *Brain,* 101, 403-445.

Kimble, D. P. (Ed.). (1965). *The anatomy of memory.* Palo Alto, CA: Science and Behavior Books.

⸺ (Ed.). (1967). *The organization of recall.* New York: The New York Academy of Sciences.

Kihlstrom, J. F., & Evans, F. J. (1979). *Functional disorders of memory.* Hillsdale, NJ: Lawrence Erlbaum Associates.

Kintsch, W. (1970, 1977). *Memory and cognition.* New York: John Wiley & Sons.

Klatzky, R. L. (1975, 1980). *Human memory. Structures and processes.* San Francisco: W. H. Freeman.

Melton, A. W., & Martin, E. (Eds.). (1972). *Coding processes in human memory.* New York: John Wiley & Sons.

Murdock, B. B., Jr. (1974). *Human memory: Theory and data.* Potomac, MD: Lawrence Erlbaum Associates.

Norman, D. A. (1982). *Learning and memory.* San Francisco, CA: W. H. Freeman.

Olton, D. S., Becker, J. T., & Hendelmann, G. E. (1979). Hippocampus, space, and memory. *The Behavioral and Brain Sciences, 2,* 313-365.

Pribram, K. H. (Ed.). (1969). *Brain and behavior 3. Memory mechanisms.* Harmondsworth, Middlesex, England: Penguin Books.

Spear, N. E. (1978). *The processing of memories: Forgetting and retention.* Hillsdale, NJ: Lawrence Erlbaum Associates.

Swanson, L. W., Teyler, T. J., & Thompson, R. F. (1982). Hippocampal long-term potentiation: Mechanisms and implications for memory. *Neurosciences Research Program Bulletin, 20,* No. 5. Cambridge, MA: MIT Press.

Talland, G. A. (1968). *Disorders of memory and learning.* Harmondsworth, Middlesex, England: Penguin Books.

Tulving, E., & Donaldson, W. (Eds.). (1972). *Organization of memory.* New York: Academic Press.

Ungar, G. (Ed.). (1970). *Molecular mechanisms in memory and learning.* New York: Plenum Press.

7
THE
VISUAL
SYSTEM

INTRODUCTION

Low-level visual representations are those derived from retinal patterns not using prior knowledge of the visual world. Examples are brightness, color, texture, location, movement, and surface orientation. This chapter will describe some of the low-level representations and encoding networks of the human visual system. Understanding these representations is a first step toward understanding the representations used and stored by the high-level visual networks. I will not describe the visual reflex system in this presentation.

THE ANATOMY OF THE HUMAN VISUAL SYSTEM

The principal networks of the human visual system for fine-grained pattern recognition are illustrated in Figure 7.1. The lenses of the eyes focus images of the world, **ocular images**, on the retinas. The retinas convert and encode these images into low-level visual representations called **primary visual patterns**. The primary visual patterns comprise several different registered subpatterns which describe various temporal and spatial characteristics of the ocular images. The primary visual patterns are transmitted by the optic nerve to the lateral geniculate nuclei, where they are further processed and analyzed. The result of the analysis is transmitted over the optic radiations to the primary visual cortex[1] for additional processing and encoding. The retinas, lateral geniculate nuclei, and primary visual cortex together transform the primary visual patterns into internal representations suitable for storage and analysis. Each of these low-level visual networks will be described shortly.

---

[1]The terms striate cortex and area 17 are synonymous with primary visual cortex.

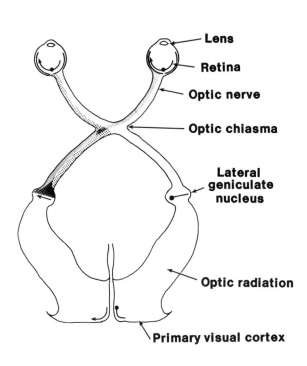

Figure 7.1. The anatomy of that part of the human visual system responsible for fine-grained pattern recognition.

Laboratory Techniques in Low-level Vision Research

Sophisticated experimental techniques and elaborate experiments performed over the last 20 years have given us a great deal of insight into the computational nature of the visual system. At the present time the most common technique for studying the brain's computational activity is to probe it with a microelectrode and record the electrical, hence computational, activity of the contacted cell. When researchers study the visual systems of animals in this manner, they direct the animal's eyes toward a visual display which may contain a stationary or moving visual pattern. The display may also be generated by a computer. During these experiments, the head of the animal is held fixed and the eyes are paralyzed and do not move. A microelectrode is inserted through a surgical opening in the skull and held in a prescribed position by a stereotaxic device which accurately positions the probe in the brain. See Figure 7.2. The probe may be moved by microscopic amounts during experimentation so as to contact

135

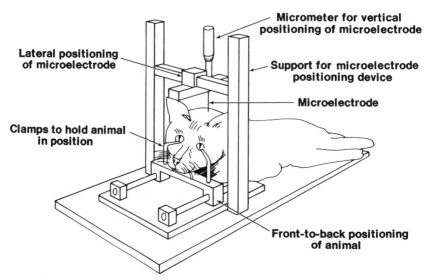

Micrometer for vertical positioning of microelectrode

Lateral positioning of microelectrode

Support for microelectrode positioning device

Microelectrode

Clamps to hold animal in position

Front-to-back positioning of animal

Figure 7.2. A stereotaxic device holds an animal and positions a microelectrode during acute neurophysiological studies of single cell responses to visual stimuli.

in turn several different cells that lie along its linear path of penetration. After all experiments with an animal are completed, the animal is sacrificed and the exact locations of the probe determined at autopsy. Thus the researcher can accurately determine which cells were responsible for the recorded activity. By correlating the cellular response with the visual display, the researcher can accurately determine how the contacted cells reacted to the visually presented stimuli.

These same experimental techniques have been used to determine the functional architecture of the retinal ganglion cells, cells of the lateral geniculate nuclei, and cells of the primary visual cortex. Most experiments have been performed on cats, though some have been performed on monkeys. Most researchers believe that similar cell responses would be found if the experiments could be performed on man.

As a general rule, the visual patterns that are used consist of simple geometrical shapes such as light spots with a dark surrounding region, dark spots with a light surrounding region, edges formed by a dark rectangle adjacent to a light rectangle, or rectangular bars having a specified width and length. Sinusoidal gratings (alternating light and dark stripes) have also been used as well as various forms of time-varying patterns such as flickering spots of light. See Figure 7.3.

The Topography and Connectivity of Visual Projections

As with all sensory modalities, the topographic (somatotopic) arrangement of neurons and nerve fibers in these networks preserves the local geometry of the receptor surface, but in the visual system this is done in an interesting and unexpected way. Information that arrives at the right eye from the right half of the visual field is encoded by the retina and is transmitted along the optic nerve across the optic chiasma (see Figure 7.1) to the left lateral geniculate nucleus; none of the visual information from the right half of the visual field is sent to the right lateral geniculate nucleus. Information that arrives at the left eye from the right half of the visual field is encoded by that retina and is also transmitted along the optic nerve to the left lateral geniculate nucleus. The information from opposite eyes arrives in registration at different layers of the lateral geniculate nucleus. The specific layer of arrival depends, as I will indicate shortly, on the type of information. The situation is similar for the left half of the visual field, which is encoded by the retinas and processed only in the right lateral geniculate nucleus. Thus the visual arrangement of the nerve fibers splits the visual field in half vertically; each half is processed independently, but in parallel, by the opposite side of the brain.

Neurons in the lateral geniculate nuclei process the retinal information and transmit their results to the primary visual cortex for further processing and

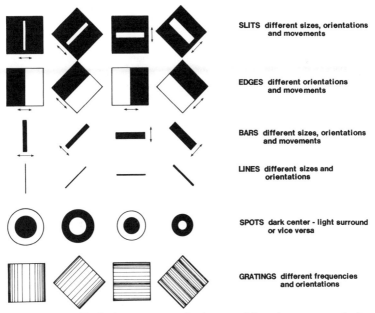

SLITS different sizes, orientations and movements

EDGES different orientations and movements

BARS different sizes, orientations and movements

LINES different sizes and orientations

SPOTS dark center - light surround or vice versa

GRATINGS different frequencies and orientations

Figure 7.3. Typical patterns used when studying the responses of single cells to visual stimuli.

137

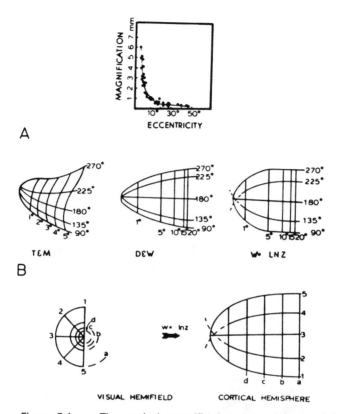

Figure 7.4. a. The cortical magnification data of Daniel & Whitteridge (1961). b. The measured and predicted mappings of visual landmarks in the striate cortex. The left figure shows the data of Talbot & Marshall (1941), the central figure shows the data of Daniel & Whitteridge (1961), and the right figure shows the theoretical predictions. c. The global retinotopic mapping under the logarithmic function. (Reproduced, with permission, from E. L. Schwartz, Spatial mapping in the primate sensory projection: analytic structure and relevance to perception. *Biological Cybernetics*, 25, 1977, 181-194.)

analysis. Finally, the two cortical hemispheres are tied together by an extensive collection of nerve fibers called the corpus callosum. The corpus callosum connects symmetrically opposite points of the two hemispheres together. The role of the corpus callosum in elementary visual processing is not yet known although some suggestions will be forwarded in Chapter 17.

In addition to the major visual projections from retina to lateral geniculate nucleus and primary visual cortex, there is a much smaller system of projections from the retinas to various subcortical structures: the superior colliculus, pretectum, hypothalamus, and accessory optic nuclei. These projections play

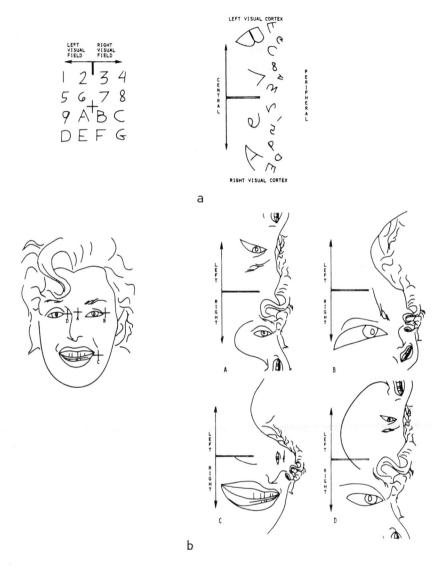

Figure 7.5. Distortions produced by the complex logarithmic mapping. a. An array of numbers as it would appear at the retina and primary visual cortex. b. A face as it would appear at the retina and primary visual cortex for four different fixation points. (Reproduced, with permission, from R. J. Baron, Mechanisms of human facial recognition. *International Journal of Man-Machine Studies*, 15, 1981, 137-178.)

important roles in a diversity of activities such as eating, locomotion, stability of gaze, saccadic eye movements, and various visual reflexes. I will not discuss these functions in this book. (See Fuchs, 1985.)

The connections from retina to lateral geniculate nuclei and then cortex do not form a single visual-processing system as the gross anatomy suggests, but rather, they form a complex of parallel systems which work together to perform distinctly different analyses of the ocular images. These systems become evident when the detailed morphology and physiology of the networks are studied.

Although local regions of the retina innervate local regions of the lateral geniculate nuclei and then local regions of the primary visual cortex, thereby preserving the local geometry of the visual field pattern, the global geometry is modified in such a way that the projections from the center of the visual field (the foveal projections) occupy substantially more area in the primary visual cortex than do the peripheral projections. Figure 7.4 shows how the projections have been mapped and Figure 7.5 shows approximately how retinal patterns appear at the primary visual cortex and how they depend on the fixation point. I will discuss the significance of these projections for pattern processing in the following chapter.

Processing Two-Dimensional Patterns

The depolarization patterns that are generated by the eyes and used by the other visual processing networks are two-dimensional: Position in the neural pattern preserves the spatial relationships of objects in the visual field. The firing rate of a single cell in one of the registered subpatterns represents a particular visual attribute in the encoded subpattern. For purposes of illustration in this book I will use digitized images to represent neural depolarization patterns; black in the digitized image represents the minimum firing rate and white represents the maximum firing rate. As an example, Figure 5.2a showed a digital image consisting of 480-by-512, or 245,760 picture elements (pixels). This represents a neural pattern comprising the same number of neurons. As you will soon see, this corresponds approximately to one of the subpatterns produced by the retina.

LOW-LEVEL VISUAL PROCESSING

This section will discuss the lowest-level visual processing networks to give some insight into the detailed nature of the visual encoding mechanisms.

The function of the low-level visual machinery, including the eyes, lateral geniculate nuclei, and primary visual cortex, is to encode the changing visual patterns into a form and dimensionality suitable for the high-level visual processes. (See Marr, 1976 and 1982, e. g.) Low-level control processes include directing the gaze and selecting meaningful objects or patterns to occupy its center and ultimately the focus of visual attention. The requirements on the low-level control processes are varied, and depending on the particular task, they are subserved by several reflex subsystems which operate in parallel. These subsystems will not be described here.

Low-level networks encode and make explicit specific attributes of the visual world, including but not exclusively, light intensity, color, texture, movement (visual flow), surface orientation, surface discontinuities, and distance of object from viewer. These visual qualities are determined to a great extent without using knowledge about the particular object, but it is well known that low-level processes can be influenced by such knowledge.

Receptive Fields and Cell Types

Assuming that the eyes are looking straight ahead, the **receptive field** of a cell is that portion of the visual field where a visual stimulus may cause it to fire. The **receptive field size** of a cell is the size of its receptive field usually measured in degrees of solid angle. (A 17-millimeter spot at a distance of 1 meter fills approximately 1° of solid angle in the visual field.)

Cells in the visual system have been categorized according to the type of stimuli to which they best respond. **Circularly symmetrical** cells show no preference to the orientation of edges or lines in the visual field. **Simple cells** respond best to edges or lines oriented in a specific direction and at a specific location. Such cells fail to respond when the edge or line is moved to a new position unless its orientation is also changed. **Complex cells** are sensitive to edge or line orientation but less sensitive to position within the receptive field. Their response changes when the length or orientation of the stimulus pattern changes, and they tend to be insensitive to diffuse light. Finally, **hypercomplex cells** are in general similar to complex cells but respond minimally or fail to respond at all if the stimulus extends beyond the region within which the responses are produced.

Retinal Processing

Figures 7.6 and 7.7 show schematic diagrams of the retina in which several different types of cells are identified. (Also see Figure 2.4.) The rods and cones are the receptor cells that convert the light signals into graded neural depolarization potentials, which are ultimately converted by the remaining cell types into a firing pattern in the retinal ganglion cells. The myelinated axons of the retinal ganglion cells form the afferent portion of the optic nerve.

The approximately 125 million rod cells are sensitive to a broad band of light which peaks at about 500 nanometers (green). The rod cells are not direction-ally sensitive and hence respond to scattered light. They can detect light which

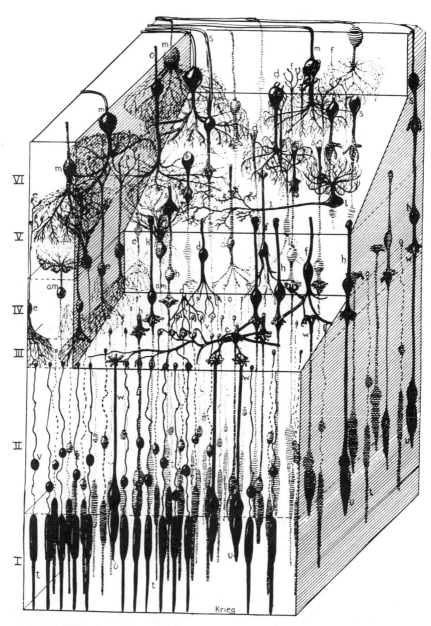

Figure 7.6. The retina of the eye. Layers: I, rods and cones; II, rod and cone cells; III, outer fiber layer; IV, bipolar cells; V, inner fiber layer; VI, ganglion cells. Cells: (am) amacrine; (c) external horizontal cell; (d) bipolar cell of d-type; (e) bipolar cell of e-type; (f) bipolar cell of f-type; (h) bipolar cell of h-type; (l) internal horizontal cell; (m) large ganglion cell; (s) small ganglion cell; (t) receptive part of rod cell; (u) receptive part of cone cell; (v) central process of rod cell; (w) central part of cone cell. (Reproduced, with permission, from W. J. S. Krieg, *Functional Neuroanatomy*. Third Edition. Evanston, IL: Brain Books. Copyright (c) 1966 by the author.)

142

is about 1000 times dimmer than can be detected by the cone cells, but because all rods respond to light colors in exactly the same way, they are not directly responsible for color encoding.

The rod cells are the sensory cells of a system of diffuse connections to horizontal and bipolar cells. The bipolar cells contact the amacrine and ganglion cells, making the final connections that encode the ocular information in this system. There is a convergence from rod cells to ganglion cells of about 100 to 1 at the periphery of the retina. Some cone cells may also make inputs into this diffuse system, which is called the **rod system**. The rod system integrates the light intensity across small neighborhoods of the visual field and because of its greater light sensitivity is responsible for night vision. As you will see later, the rod system appears to play an important support role in color vision and brightness normalization. Finally, because of their greater sensitivity to light, the rod cells recover much more slowly from bleaching light than do cone cells.

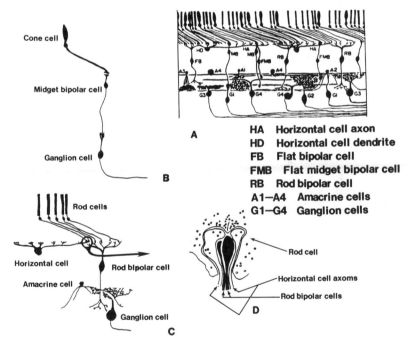

HA	**Horizontal cell axon**
HD	**Horizontal cell dendrite**
FB	**Flat bipolar cell**
FMB	**Flat midget bipolar cell**
RB	**Rod bipolar cell**
A1—A4	**Amacrine cells**
G1—G4	**Ganglion cells**

Figure 7.7. The structure of the primate retina. a. The cells of the retina. (Slightly modified from B. B. Boycott & J. E. Dowling, Organization of the primate retina: Light microscopy. *Philosophical Transactions of the Royal Society of London*, B, 255, 1969, 109-184.) b. The cone system. (Horizontal and amacrine cell contacts are not shown.) c. The rod system. d. Detail of the rod-horizontal-bipolar cell connections (from Boycott & Dowling, 1969). (Compare this figure with Figure 7.6.)

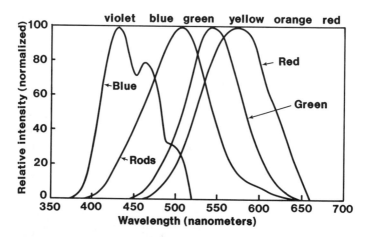

Figure 7.8. Normalized spectral sensitivities of four visual pigments. (Based on Edwin H. Land, The retinex theory of color vision. *Scientific American*, 237, 1977, 108-128. Copyright © 1977 by Scientific American, Inc. All rights reserved.)

The approximately 6 million cone cells are divided into three different color-sensitive groups, depending on the color pigments they contain. These groups of cells appear to form three independent color subsystems. Figure 7.8 shows how the three groups of cone cells respond to light of different wavelengths. The three different color subsystems, which show peak spectral sensitivities at 440 nanometers (blue light), 535 nanometers (green light), and 565 nanometers (red light), encode color information in three different registered subpatterns. Cone cells occupy the vast majority of the the macula, the center of the retina, and are primarily responsible for high-resolution vision, but cone cells appear throughout the retina as well. Unlike the rod cells, the cone cells are sensitive to the direction of the incoming light and hence do not respond well to scattered light. In addition, cone cells are superior to rod cells in their response to small changes in light intensity. The systems of connections from cones to horizontal and bipolar cells and then to amacrine and ganglion cells are called the **cone systems**.

Retinal ganglion cells are circularly symmetrical and respond optimally to approximately circular spots of light whose size depends on the particular cell. If a stimulus spot is larger than the optimal size for a particular ganglion cell, that cell's response decreases. Thus the receptive field organization appears to consist of a central excitatory region surrounded by an inhibitory region. This has been called an **on-center/off-surround** organization when a bright center causes excitation, or **off-center/on-surround** when a dark center causes excitation. For most types of cells with on-center/off-surround organization there also appears to be corresponding cell types with off-center/on-surround organization. These cells appear to be part of a two-cell encoding for the particular attribute of the visual field they represent.

Among the categories of retinal cells having on-center/off-surround or off-center/on-surround organization are x-cells (brisk sustained response), y-cells (brisk transient response[2]), tonic cells (sluggish sustained response), and phasic cells (sluggish transient response). See Rodieck (1979) for an excellent review. Other classes of circularly symmetrical cells have also been observed, but they are a very small percentage of the population of retinal cells. Virtually all ganglion cells appear to be either x-type or y-type cells.

The retinal mechanisms which account for the x- and y-ganglion cells have been the subject of detailed modeling by Fernandez-Escartin and Moreno-Diaz (1978) as well as Richter and Ullman (1980), who have modeled their response as a difference of two gaussian distributions. Richter and Ullman assert that the x-cell response is due to a small excitatory central contribution generated by a single retinal cone cell combined with an inhibitory surrounding gaussian distribution generated most likely by the midget bipolar cells which either contact the bipolar cells or the cone cells. These two contributions have different time constants, which accounts quite nicely for the transient nature of x-cell responses. Figure 7.9 illustrates the wiring model proposed by Richter and Ullman (1980) for the y-ganglion cells and shows some of the responses of several types of retinal cells. The receptive field size of the x-cells varies from .1° to 1.3°, and the x-cells are often color-specific. It therefore appears that x-cells convey the output of the cone systems.

The y-cells respond differently to visual stimuli. When the incident light changes, y-cells give an initial transient response. However, in the absence of any change in stimulus, y-cell activity dissappears completely. Richter and Ullman assert that the y-cell response is due to a derivative-like operation on an x-type signal, taking place in the connections between bipolar and ganglion cells, followed by a rectification in the convergence of these signals. The receptive field size of the y-cells is larger than for the x-cells and varies between .6° and 2.5°. The y-cells tend to respond to a broad band of colors and appear to convey the retinal output of the rod system.

It might be added that the three populations of cone cells are distributed uniformly on an approximately hexagonal grid, with the cells of the different pigment groups arranged like the phosphor spots on a color television picture tube (de Monasterio, Schein, and McCrane, 1981). This highly specific arrangement was suggested by Richter & Ullman when modeling the x- and y-cell responses, and is consistent with their predictions of receptive field sizes.

---

[2]Response dies off when the stimulus does not change.

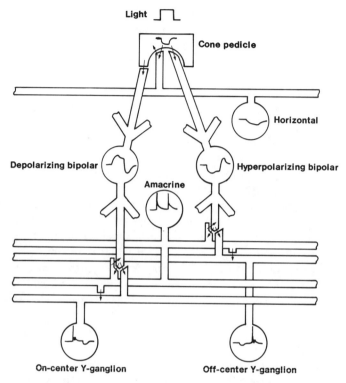

Light ⊓

Cone pedicle

Horizontal

Depolarizing bipolar

Hyperpolarizing bipolar

Amacrine

On-center Y-ganglion

Off-center Y-ganglion

Figure 7.9. Functional and wiring model for a Y-ganglion cell in the retina. (Redrawn, by permission, from J. Richter and S. Ullman, A model for the spatio-temporal organization of the x-type and y-type ganglion cells in the primate retina. Massachusetts Institute of technology A.I. Memo 573, April 1980.)

Unlike an encoding of intensity, which varies from absent (value 0) to some maximum value, gradients have both a positive and negative component. For the x-component of the spatial gradient, an increase in light intensity while moving to the right constitutes a positive gradient value while a decrease constitutes a negative gradient value. For spatial gradients, a cell with on-center/off-surround organization can encode one component of the gradient (say positive) while a cell with off-center/on-surround can encode the other component. Because cells having these organizations appear to be paired, a two-cell encoding for the gradient seems natural and likely.

The transient nature of the visual encodings should by now be obvious. Transients are formed whenever the intensity of light on the retina changes, either due to a change in level of illumination, to an intensity change resulting from the movement of something in the visual field, or to movement of the eyes. Saccadic eye movements (between points of fixation), movement of the body, and ocular tremor are three causes of visual transients. Ocular tremor is a very small but continual movement of the eyes, which displaces the ocular image by a distance of several receptor cell diameters. Evidently, the only place on the retina where a true steady-state pattern is formed corresponds to the interior of a region of the visual field having a constant color and uniform illumination, and then only between saccades.

Both x-cells and y-cells give transient responses due to changing visual patterns. After the transients decay, the y-cells fail to respond at all while the x-cells maintain an approximately uniform value indicative of the light level in the visual field. It is interesting that not only are the conduction velocities of the x-cell and y-cell axons different, with y-cells having a much faster conduction rate, but that the axons terminate in slightly different regions of the lateral geniculate nuclei as described previously. Thus both anatomical and physiological evidence suggests that the differences in x-cell and y-cell encodings are put to different uses in higher stages of visual analysis.

Color Coding.   Color information originates predominantly in the cone receptors of the retina. The three populations of cone cells respond differently, depending on the type of photopigments they contain. However, cells of each pigment type respond to a broad range of wavelengths, with frequency of cell response varying according to the integrated intensity of light. For example, a cell that responds at one frequency when illuminated with red light will respond at the same rate when illuminated with blue light at a different intensity. The firing rate of a single cell clearly does not convey adequate information to describe color in the visual field.

In attempting to discover exactly what external stimulus corresponds to the sensation of color, Land (1977) and his colleagues performed a series of elaborate experiments. Two identical displays consisting of matte-finish colored patches were assembled and each illuminated independently by three narrow-band light sources: 450 nanometers (short-wave light), 530 nanometers (middle-wave light), and 630 nanometers (long-wave light). The color patches resembled those used for selecting paints in a hardware store, only their sizes varied. Figure 7.10 illustrates this. Each of the six light sources could be independently adjusted for brightness, and the intensity of light reflected by a single colored patch from each light source could be determined accurately using a telescopic photometer. When measuring the reflected light from one source, the other light sources were turned off.

Using one of the two displays, the three light sources were adjusted so that the white patch appeared to be a good white while the remaining patches were deeply colored. Focusing on the white patch, the intensity of reflected light for each source of illumination was measured, giving an **intensity triple**. The intensity triples from other colors were also measured in the same way. Using the second display and a patch of unknown color, the light sources for that display

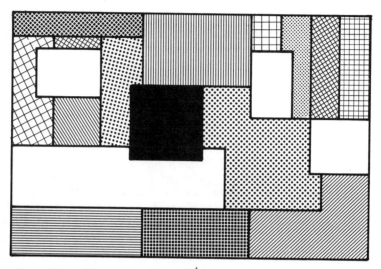

Figure 7.10. The type of pattern used by Land for determining how the eye encodes color information. The various textures in this illustration were different colors in his test patterns.

were independently adjusted so that the intensity triple from the unknown patch exactly matched the intensity triple from the white patch of the first display. When all three light sources for the second display were turned on, however, the color of the unknown patch was easily recognized. This same result was obtained when the lights were adjusted so the intensity triple matched that of any of the other colors of the first display. Clearly the triple of reflected intensity values is not the physical correlate of color. Land and his colleagues tried to find out what it is.

One quantity which enters into the answer is the integrated flux of radiant energy over a broad band of wavelengths. Two measurements can be made: (1) the value of the integrated flux if a patch of white is used, and (2) the value if a patch of color is used. The ratio of these two values is the integrated reflectance, which can be expressed as a ratio of the two quantities. The process of dividing by the integrated flux reflected from the white patch is called brightness normalization. By using color filters that correspond closely with the spectral sensitivities of the color pigments of the eye, Land was able to determine quite accurately the total energy absorbed by each receptor type. This value is the integrated energy density for each color pigment. By scaling these values according to lightness sensation, a final measurable physical quantity called the **scaled integrated reflectance** can be obtained for each color pigment. Because a unique triple is formed for each colored patch regardless of the intensity or color makeup of the light source, these triples of scaled integrated reflectance values appear to be the physical quantity that corresponds to the sensation of color.

Now suppose that the eye forms three independent representations of the visual world, one for each type of photopigment in the cone cells, and further suppose that these three subpatterns are delivered in registration to the brain for analysis. If these subpatterns encode the scaled integrated reflectances, then clearly sufficient information is present to distinguish among different colors. The problem is that although each cone cell can measure the value of the integrated flux for its own photopigment, there is no standard of reflectance available in the visual field (such as the patch of white used for brightness normalization) to measure the brightness of the light source—hence the value of integrated flux if a white patch could be used. How, then, can the integrated reflectance values measured by the cone cells be normalized?

A possible answer to this question was supplied by Richards (1979) and is based on significant physiological differences between rod and cone cells. Richards argued that the level of scattered light in an optical system, in this case the eye, does provide an independent measure of the brightness of the light source. The eye can determine the brightness of the light source provided that two independent measurements can be made, each of which responds differently to the internal optical scatter. Since the rod and cone systems have properties which are ideally suited for these measurements, Richards concludes that the retinas can indeed deliver the required triples of scaled integrated reflectance values.

Lightness Normalization.   Apparently, the retinas are able to normalize surface reflectance measurements. This is important even in the absence of color coding. Our perception of surface brightness remains nearly constant even though the level of illumination often changes by a factor as large as 1000 across a surface. Change in surface illumination occurs, for example, when shadows are present. In fact, a surface for which there is a gradual change in illumination level appears to have a constant brightness unless a sharp discontinuity in brightness is present.

The process of brightness normalization described in the previous section is one possible explanation for how the brain performs that function. Another explanation, suggested by Horn (1975) and others, uses gradient information in areas having no sharp discontinuities of illumination. Regardless of how the computation is performed, brightness normalization is an important low-level process without which visual recognition would be much more difficult.

The Lateral Geniculate Nuclei

Each lateral geniculate nucleus has a layered structure as illustrated in Figure 7.11, which shows a cross section of the lateral geniculate nucleus of a macaque monkey. The layers receive different types of information and from the opposite eye as follows. The ipsilateral (same side) projections from the rod system

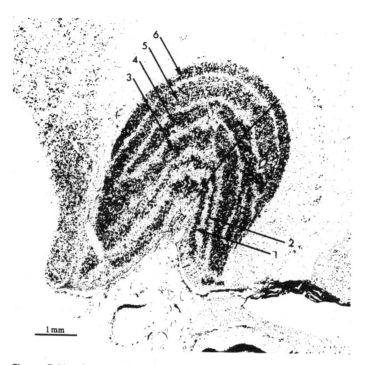

Figure 7.11. A coronal section through the right lateral geniculate body of a normal adult macaque monkey. Cells are divided into six layers as shown. Layers 1, 4 and 6 receive inputs from the left (contralateral) eye. Layers 2, 3 and 5 receive inputs from the right (ipsilateral) eye. The unlabeled arrow indicates a radial axis along which the various retinal representations are in perfect registration. (Reproduced, by permission, from Ferrier Lecture by D. H. Hubel & T. N. Wiesel, Functional architecture of macaque monkey visual cortex. *Proceedings of the Royal Society of London*, B, 198, 1977, 1-59.)

terminate predominantly in layer A1 whereas the projections from the contralateral (opposite side) eye terminate predominantly in layers M and A1. Cells which originate in layers M, A, and A1 of the lateral geniculate nuclei terminate in several inner layers of the primary visual cortex. For the cone system, the ipsilateral projections from the retina terminate predominantly in layer B1 of the lateral geniculate while the contralateral projections terminate in layers B0 and B2. Cells originating in layers B0, B1, and B2 terminate in the outer layer (layer I) of the cerebral cortex. The relationship between the cells having different color sensitivities and layers in the lateral geniculate nuclei, if any, is not known. Figure 7.12 summarizes the pattern of connections.

Throughout the lateral geniculate nuclei, only circularly symmetrical cells are found.

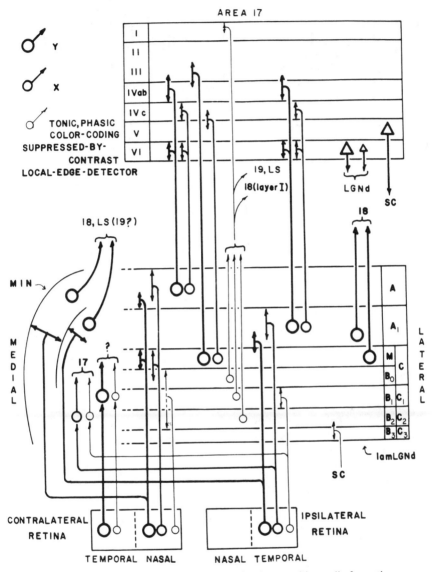

Figure 7.12. Projections of the x, y, and color sensitive cells from the retinas to the striate cortex of the cat. Layers C3, C2, C1, C, A1 and A correspond approximately to layers 1 to 6 in the previous figure. (Reproduced with permission, from R. W. Rodieck, Visual pathways, *Annual Review of Neuroscience*, 2, 193-225. Copyright © 1979 by Annual Reviews Inc.)

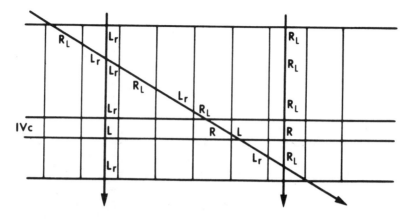

Figure 7.13. Illustration of ocular dominance columns in macaque monkey. (Reproduced, by permission, from Ferrier Lecture by D. H. Hubel & T. N. Wiesel, Functional architecture of macaque monkey visual cortex. *Proceedings of the Royal Society of London*, B, 198, 1977, 1-59.)

The Functional Architecture of the Primary Visual Cortex

Low-level features are combined by the primary visual cortex to make intermediate-level features explicit. This section describes the underlying structure and computations. See Hubel and Wiesel (1977) for additional details.

Cells are said to be **monocular** if they respond to visual patterns projected in one eye only and **binocular** if they respond to patterns projected in both eyes. Binocular cells first appear in the cerebral cortex. Cells in layer IVc, where the inputs from the lateral geniculate nuclei terminate, are almost exclusively monocular, as are the cells in layer IVb, whereas the majority of cells in layers II, III, V, and VI are binocular.

Cells are **right dominant** if they respond preferentially to stimulus in the right eye and **left dominant** if they respond preferentially to stimulus in the left eye. The distribution of right and left dominant cells throughout the primary visual cortex is not at all random but organized in an interesting and methodical way (Gilbert, 1983; Hubel & Wiesel, 1977; Van Essen, 1979). Cells which are right dominant tend to be segregated from those which are left dominant is such a way that vertical penetrations tend to find one or the other type of cell. See Figure 7.13. If one were to paint the surface of the cortex either black or white, depending on the presence of left or right dominant cells underneath, the cortex would appear like a zebra, with black and white stripes. This is shown in Figure 7.14. Each cortical volume of size larger than about 1 millimeter on an edge contains approximately the same number of cells of each dominance.

Now consider the distribution of cells which respond to short oriented lines. As one traverses the cortex in a direction parallel to its surface, the orientation-sensitivity of the cells changes systematically so that within a 2-millimeter traversal there are representatives of cells from each different orientation. If the penetration is taken across the eye dominance columns, the same result is obtained, only the favored eye changes as the penetration leaves the dominance column for one eye and enters the dominance column of the other. This is illustrated in Figure 7.15. If one penetrates the cortex perpendicular to its surface, one detects cells whose orientation-sensitivity is in a fixed direction, but the cells may be circular, simple, complex, or hypercomplex, depending on the layer. This is also illustrated in Figure 7.15. In layer IVc, which is the principal input layer to the cortex, the cells are circularly symmetrical and monocular. This is the primary input layer as described earlier. In other layers the cells are sensitive to stimulation from both eyes but are more sensitive to stimulation from the dominant eye. The cells may be simple, complex, or hypercomplex, as described earlier, but they are most sensitive to lines (edges) having the same orientation.

Within the primary visual cortex, the longest local connections between cells are a few millimeters, with most connections under 2 millimeters. Within each

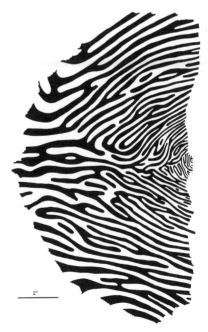

Figure 7.14. A reconstruction of the ocular dominance columns of layer IVc, area 17, of the macaque monkey, translated into the visual field. (Reproduced, by permission, from Ferrier Lecture by D. H. Hubel & T. N. Wiesel, Functional architecture of macaque monkey visual cortex. *Proceedings of the Royal Society of London*, B, 198, 1977, 1-59.)

2°

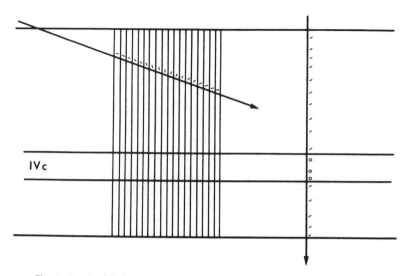

Figure 7.15. Diagram to illustrate orientation columns in monkey striate cortex. (Reproduced, by permission, from Ferrier Lecture by D. H. Hubel & T. N. Wiesel, *Functional architecture of macaque monkey visual cortex. Proceedings of the Royal Society of London*, B, 198, 1977, 1-59.)

vertical column 1 millimeter on an edge are approximately 424,000 cells with roughly the same number of each eye dominance[3]. Furthermore, representatives from all orientations are found. Each small region, therefore, appears to have the same computational power and machinery as every other, and the computational picture that emerges was summarized most clearly by Hubel and Wiesel (1977, p. 17) as follows:

> This [the local connectivity] means that there is little opportunity for signals entering the cortex in one place to make themselves felt at points more than 1-2mm away. As a corollary to this it may be added that the striate cortex must be analysing the visual world in a piecemeal fashion: information about some region in the visual field is brought to the cortex, digested, and the result transmitted on with no regard to what is going on elsewhere. Visual perception, then, can in no sense be said to be enshrined in area 17—the apparatus is simply not made to analyse a percept that occupies more than a small region of the visual field. All of the single cell physiology in fact suggests that area 17 is concerned simply with what may be thought of as building blocks for perception.

Based on the evidence gathered in this and similar studies, the primary visual

---

[3] There are approximately 106 cells per .001 mm³ in area 17 according to Blinkov and Glezer (1968), Table 225 (p. 398). One square millimeter by 4 millimeters thick gives 4000 mm³ or 424,000 cells.

cortex appears to comprise a two-dimensional array of independent computational elements as illustrated in Figure 7.16. Hubel and Wiesel called these computational elements **hypercolumns**, and I will continue to do so here. Within each hypercolumn are a large number of much smaller columns comprising those cells which share the same orientation sensitivity. These smaller columns are called **microcolumns**.

The receptive field sizes of cortical cells vary. Cells at the center of the visual field generally have a small receptive field size (.1°) whereas cells at the periphery generally have a large receptive field size (3°). However, within any one area there are cells having a variety of receptive field sizes. These findings are consistent with anatomical studies showing how the retinal cells are connected together.

INTERMEDIATE-LEVEL VISUAL PROCESSES

The next few sections of this chapter will explore several possible encodings of the visual field suggested by the preceding physiological investigations.

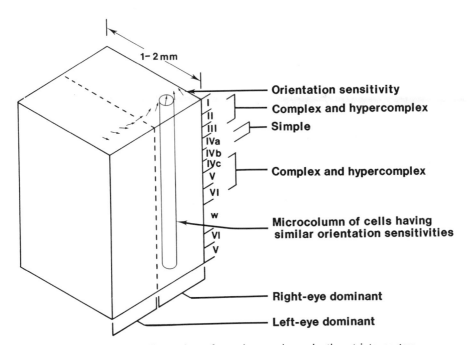

Figure 7.16. An illustration of one hypercolumn in the striate cortex, summarizing the experimental results obtained by Hubel & Weisel.

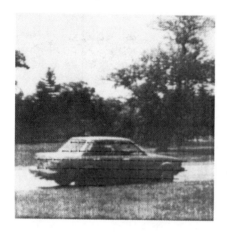
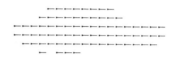

a   b

Figure 7.17.   a. A moving car with its visual flow superimposed. b. The visual flow pattern alone. (Reproduced, with permission, from R. J. Baron, Visual memories and mental images. *International Journal of Man-Machine Studies*, 23, 1985, 275-311.)

Visual Flow

When the visual world is not stationary, either because something moves in the visual field or because the eyes move, that movement is perceived regardless of the nature of the objects involved. Sudden movement of an object in the periphery of the visual field, for example, causes an alerting response to take place which shifts the gaze in the direction of the movement. This reflex is not involved with pattern recognition per se and will not be discussed further. Movement of water in a river or stream is easily perceived as the movement of a fluid, and when walking or driving a car, the world itself appears to flow by: The observer perceives his or her own motion.

Based only on the light intensity images focused on the retina, it is possible to derive a representation of the visual world that encodes movement information, and this representation will be called the **visual flow pattern** (Gafni & Zeevi, 1979; Horn & Schunck, 1981; Lawton, 1982; Ullman, 1979). The visual flow pattern, or visual flow for short, is a two-dimensional pattern of vectors, a vector field, which indicates the direction and magnitude of movement of each point in the visual field. Figures 7.17 through 7.19 give examples. In the figures, the arrows (tails are indicated by dots) point in the directions of movement on the retina of the corresponding points in the visual field, while the lengths of the arrows give the speeds. Figure 7.17 shows the image of a moving car and the resulting visual flow pattern. Figure 7.18 shows the visual flow for a uniform rotation and simple contraction of a visual image. Finally, Figure 7.19 shows the visual flow that results when a person moves toward two planes separated in space as shown above the visual flow pattern (Prazdny, 1980).

There are a few important points to note about visual flow. First, each component of the pattern is a vector and therefore cannot be encoded in the nervous system by the firing rate of a single cell. This is analogous to the inability to encode color by the firing rate of a single cell. For a two-dimensional visual flow pattern, either three or four cells are sufficient to encode the visual flow at each point. Refer to Chapter 5.

Based on the fact that cells in the retina and lateral geniculate nucleus show no directional sensitivity while some cells in the primary visual cortex do, it appears that one role of the primary visual cortex is to compute visual flow patterns. Although at the current time there is no explicit model which shows how the cortex might produce a visual flow pattern, a recent analysis by Horn and Schunck (1981) does show how visual flow patterns can be derived from a sequence of intensity images. Their model is easily implemented in a neural structure and will be briefly described next.

Horn and Schunck first derive the x and y components of the spatial intensity gradient for each point in the visual field. They let Ex and Ey denote the x- and y-components of the spatial intensity gradient at a given point, so that the vector (Ex,Ey) denotes the spatial intensity gradient. Just like visual flow, the spatial intensity gradient is a pattern of vectors. It therefore requires a code using three or four neurons to express visual flow at each point in the visual field. Given a sequence of intensity patterns, it is also possible to determine the temporal gradient of intensity at a given point. The temporal gradient represents

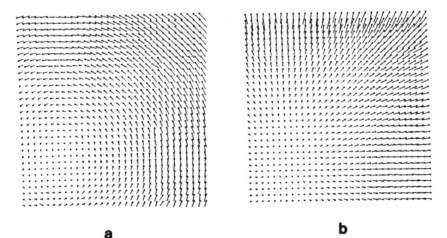

a   **b**

Figure 7.18. Visual flow patterns computed for simple rotation and simple contraction of a brightness pattern. (Reproduced, by permission, from B. K. P. Horn & B. G. Schunk, Determining optical flow. *Artificial Intelligence*, 17, 1981, 185-203.)

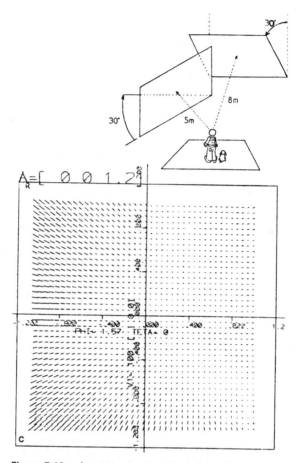

Figure 7.19. An example visual flow field produced on a
planar retina, while moving toward two planes in space.
(Reproduced, with permission, from K. Prazdny, Egomotion and relative depth map from optical flow. *Biological
Cybernetics*, 36, 1980, 87-102.)

the rate of change of light at a given point as a function of time. Temporal
gradient will be denoted Et. If we let P = (Px,Py) denote the local flow vector,
then (Ex,Ey) • (Px,Py) = −Et, where '•' denotes the vector dot product. From
this equation one can compute the component of visual flow in the direction of
the spatial gradient (Ex,Ey). However, without an additional constraint it is not
possible to determine the component in the direction at right angles to the
spatial gradient. Horn and Schunck point out, however, that neighboring points
on objects have similar velocities and therefore the velocity fields of the
brightness patterns vary smoothly except at object boundaries. This constraint
can be expressed as the minimization of the sum of squares of the Laplacians of

the x- and y-components of the flow. Horn and Schunck, in a final step, show how the flow vectors can be computed iteratively, based on the sequence of intensity patterns. Such an iterative computation can be carried out in a layered neural network like the cerebral cortex, using only local information.

One certainly cannot conclude that one of the computations performed by the primary visual cortex is the creation of an explicit representation of the visual flow. In fact, movements in space are three-dimensional quantities, not two-dimensional. Nonetheless, computing visual flow is an important step in determining three-dimensional movement vectors. This argues strongly on behalf of making visual flow explicit. Prazdny (1980) shows that both the relative depth map of the stationary environment and the movement parameters of the observer can be computed directly from the visual flow pattern. Clearly the importance of visual flow for locomotion cannot be overlooked.

Distance Information

Distance (depth) information can either be low-level or high-level, depending on its source. Low-level distance information is derived only from the intensity encodings regardless of the context or situation. High-level distance information, in contrast, depends on the nature of the visual scene. For a situation where neither the viewer nor objects in the visual scene move, low-level information comes primarily from two sources: (1) the disparity between the images received by the two eyes and, less importantly, (2) internally generated signals which control the convergence, divergence, and focus of the eyes. Figure 7.20 illustrates a stereo image pair called a random dot stereogram (Julesz, 1965) in which only low-level information is available. When viewed with a stereoscope, the stereogram in Figure 7.20 appears to have the surface contour shown in the accompanying isometric plot. High-level information comes from a number of sources, including our knowledge of the sizes of objects as a function of their distance, the nature of the texture gradient as a function of distance, and convergence and divergence of parallel lines in the visual world. See Figure 7.21. When we allow for movement of objects or the observer, we get additional distance information from the visual flow pattern.

Numerous workers have studied the process of determining distance from stereo image pairs such as the two retinal images (Barnard & Martin, 1982; Forshaw, 1979; Hannah, 1974; Julesz, 1971; Marr, Palm, & Poggio, 1978; Marr & Poggio, 1979; Mayhew & Frisby, 1981; Trehub, 1978). The computation of distance consists first of determining which points in the two visual patterns correspond to one another, and second, determining the distance of the point based on the convergence angle of the eyes. The majority of the research to date has been directed toward efficient computations for determining corresponding points in stereo image pairs. Once the correspondence is determined, the remainder of the computation is easy.

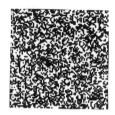

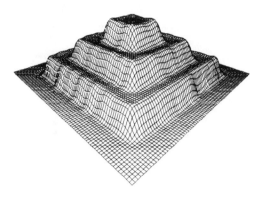

Figure 7.20. A random dot stereogram comprised of low-level depth information only. The lower figure shows the structure of the encoded object. (Reproduced, with permission, from W. E. L. Grimson, *From Images to Surfaces*. Copyright © 1981 by The MIT Press.)

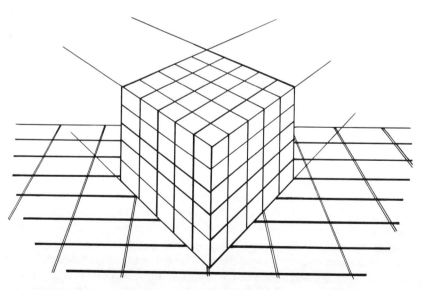

Figure 7.21. Depth information can be derived from texture gradients as well as convergence of parallel lines in the image.

For two stereo images, if one object is closer to the observer than a second object, there will be a set of points on the distant object which will only occur in the left image; they will be occluded from view in the right image by the left edge of the intervening object. Similarly, there will be a set of points that only appear in the right image. Refer to Figure 7.22. For the more distant object, there will be two sets of points near the edge of the occluding (closer) object which appear in both images. The change in focus and convergence of the eyes as they look at distant objects visible to both eyes and then points on close objects can be used to determine the distance of the closer object. We do not yet know how this is done.

Small differences between the visual encodings generated by the two eyes give rise to a **disparity pattern** as illustrated in Figures 7.23 and 7.24. Such disparity

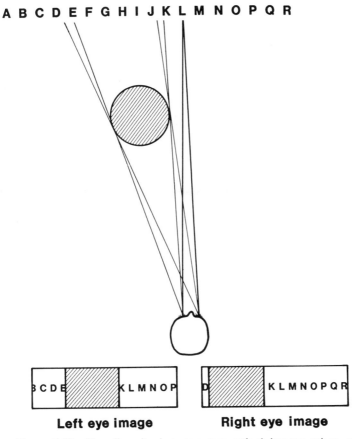

Left eye image   **Right eye image**

Figure 7.22. The disparity between two retinal images when an occluding object is present in the foreground.

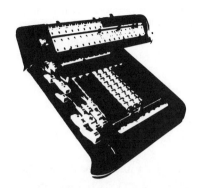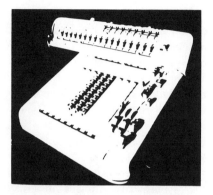

Figure 7.23. A positive and negative stereo pair. (Reproduced, with permission, from R. L. Gregory, *Eye and Brain: The Psychology of Seeing.* Copyright (c) 1966 by McGraw-Hill Book Company.)

patterns can easily be obtained by subtracting intensity values from the patterns produced by each eye. When the eyes are focused on a particular object, the two images of that object will be nearly identical and in registration at the lateral geniculate nucleus and beyond. In contrast, the images of the background will be out of registration. Because the representations generated by the eyes remain in registration at the lateral geniculate nuclei, the computations of disparity between the patterns produced by the two retinas can easily be performed by the lateral geniculate nuclei. For a given object, the width of the disparity pattern at its edge gives a direct indication of its distance from the viewer, a fact which was illustrated. Once again, we do not know the details of these computations.

Using one of the many available techniques for computing the distances of points in the visual field, one can generate a **depth representation**, an encoding of the distance from the viewer of each point in the visual world. Each point in the depth representation is a positive value and hence can be encoded in a neural network using a single set of neurons. For example, lack of firing can represent an infinite distance, while maximum firing can represent close proximity—touching. Figures 7.25a and 7.25b show a visual scene and its corresponding depth representation.

The depth representation makes distance information explicit, just as the visual flow pattern makes movement information explicit. As with the visual flow pattern, information in the depth representation is useful for several functions, including navigation, protection, and hand-eye coordination. Furthermore, the temporal gradient of the depth representation is an explicit representation of movement toward or away from the observer, and this is particularly useful for manipulating and avoiding moving objects. It should be clear that distance information is extremely useful and no doubt computed at an early stage of visual processing. Knowledge of how the brain computes depth information awaits research.

162

Just as there are several ways that distance values can be computed from low-level information, there are several ways that high-level information can be used for computing distance values. Our expectation and knowledge about the absolute and relative sizes of objects plays a direct role in our analysis of distance, and numerous psychological experiments and illusions have shown this directly. However, I will defer until later a discussion of how high-level information can be used to determine distance.

Normal Gradients and Surfaces

The final visual representation to be described here indicates for each point in the visual field the orientation of the surface containing that point and hence is called the **surface orientation pattern**. Like the visual flow pattern, the surface orientation pattern consists of vectors and hence requires a multicell encoding. Since surface orientation vectors are three-dimensional, three signed values must be encoded and hence six cells could be used for each component of such a pattern. A four-cell encoding analogous to the three-cell encoding described for visual flow can also be used. Figure 7.26 gives an example of a scene and its corresponding surface orientation pattern.

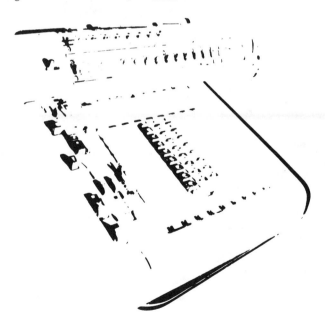

Figure 7.24. The disparity image obtained by placing Figure 7.23a on top of Figure 7.23b. This is equivalent to subtracting intensity values in stereo image pairs. (Reproduced, with permission, from R. L. Gregory, *Eye and Brain: The Psychology of Seeing.* Copyright © 1966 by McGraw-Hill Book Company.)

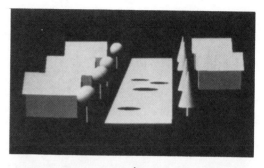

A

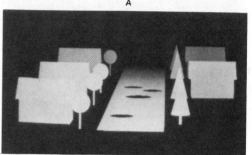

Figure 7.25. Intensity and depth (range) images. (Reproduced, by permission, from D. H. Ballard & C. M. Brown, *Computer Vision*. Copyright © 1982 by Prentice-Hall, Inc.)

B

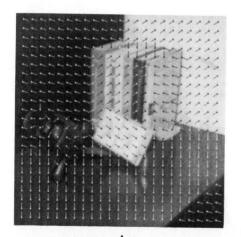

A

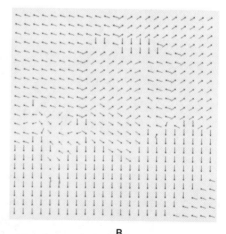

B

Figure 7.26.   A. A visual scene with surface orientation representation superimposed. B. The surface orientation representation alone. (Reproduced, with permission, from R. J. Baron, Visual memories and mental images. *International Journal of Man-Machine Studies*, 23, 1985, 275-311.)

164

As with all visual representations described in this chapter, there are several different computational techniques that can be used to produce surface orientation vectors, and these can be categorized as low-level and high-level techniques, depending on the source of information. Low-level techniques depend only on the general nature of the visual world and rely primarily on the local values in the intensity (color) representations (Grimson, 1981; Stevens, 1981). When shadows are formed in a visual scene, the statistical properties of those shadows are a result of distortions produced by the skewed angles the surfaces make with respect to the source of light and the viewer. Horn (1977) and Witkin (1981) have suggested particular computational techniques for recovering orientation vectors, based on the statistics of the local intensity patterns. In contrast, high-level information comes primarily from regularities in the way specific shapes are transformed when viewed from different points of view (Kanade, 1981; Kanade & Kender, 1980; Mackworth, 1973, 1977; Stevens, 1981). For example, parallel lines appear to converge at the horizon, and the angle of convergence gives a direct indication of the orientation of the surface containing the two lines. As another example, a circle drawn on a flat surface is projected onto the retina as an ellipse whose angle and elongation give a direct measure of the orientation of the surface itself. Information of this type is high-level and requires more global knowledge than contained in a small neighborhood of the orientation pattern. Nonetheless, the brain appears quite able to use this information to determine surface orientation.

At the present time there is no computational model showing how the brain might produce a surface orientation pattern. In an effort to discover how surface orientation might be determined from high-level information, Mackworth (1973, 1977), Kanade (1981), and Kanade and Kender (1980) have begun to study the mathematical properties that describe the relationships between shapes in the visual world and the shapes of their images when projected onto an image. In due time this research should lead to a computational model.

Just as with visual flow and distance measurements, the orientation pattern makes explicit the relationships between surfaces in the visual world and the viewer. This information is useful and necessary for tasks involving the manipulation of objects. Picking up an object involves determining both the direction of approach of the hand and the orientation of the fingers relative to the surfaces of the object. This is precisely the information that is made explicit in the orientation pattern. Although there is no direct evidence that an orientation pattern is generated, the utility of such a representation is clear.

SUMMARY

I have described several low-level representations of the visual world. Each representation makes explicit a particular attribute of the scene which is useful when interacting with the environment. In his pioneering studies on vision,

Marr (1982) has given the name "primal sketch" to the low-level representation of the visual world produced during early stages of visual analysis. I will continue to use his terminology. By primal sketch I mean the set of representations produced by the retinas, lateral geniculate nuclei, and primary visual cortex as a result of low-level visual computations. During formation of the components of the primal sketch, the cortex may either perform all of the computations in parallel in different collections of cells or it may perform some subset of these computations as dictated by other high-level control networks. Furthermore, the computations may take place in registration or in networks that are spatially distinct. Regardless of how the primal sketch is formed, the ability of the high-level networks to extract and use the appropriate representation for the task at hand is an important capability, and it is precisely that capability that I will explain in the following chapter.

REFERENCES

Ballard, D. H., & Brown, C. M. (1982). *Computer vision.* Englewood Cliffs, NJ: Prentice-Hall.

Barnard, S. T., & Martin, A. F. (1982). Computational stereo. *Computing Surveys, 14,* 553-572.

Blinkov, S. M., & Glezer, I. I. (1968). *The human brain in figures and tables.* New York: Basic Books.

Boycott, B. B., & Dowling, J. E. (1969). Organization of the primate retina: Light microscopy. *Philosophical Transactions of the Royal Society of London B, 255,* 109-184.

Daniel, P. M., & Whitteridge, D. (1961). The representation of the visual field on the cerebral cortex in monkeys. *Journal of Physiology, 159,* 203-221.

Churchill, R. V. (1969). *Complex variables and applications.* New York: McGraw-Hill.

Fernandez-Escartin, V., & Moreno-Diaz, R. (1978). A Spatio-temporal model of cat's retinal cells. *Biological Cybernetics, 30,* 15-22.

Forshaw, M. R. B. (1979). The cooperative stereo algorithm: An empirical approach. *Biological Cybernetics, 33,* 143-149.

Frisby, J. P. (1980). *Seeing. Illusion, brain and mind.* New York: Oxford University Press.
This beautifully illustrated book is a particularly good and up-to-date presentation of all aspects of the human visual system. I recommend it highly.

Fuchs, A. F. (1985). Brainstem control of saccadic eye movements. *Annual Review of Neuroscience, 8,* 307-337.

Gafni, H., & Zeevi, Y. Y. (1979). A model for processing of movement in the visual field. *Biological Cybernetics, 32,* 165-173.

Gilbert, C. D. (1983). Microcircuitry of the visual cortex. *Annual Review of Neuroscience, 6,* 217-247.

Gregory, R. L. (1966). *Eye and brain. The psychology of seeing.* New York: World University Library.

Grimson, W. E. L. (1981). *From images to surfaces.* Cambridge, MA: MIT Press.

Hannah, M. J. (1974). Computer matching of stereo images. Stanford Artificial Intelligence Laboratory Memo AIM-239, Computer Science Department, Stanford University, Stanford, CA.

Horn, B. K. P. (1975). Image intensity understanding. MIT A.I. Memo 335, Laboratory for Artificial Intelligence, MIT, Cambridge, MA.

Horn, B. K. P., & Schunck, B. G. (1981). Determining optical flow. *Artificial Intelligence, 17,* 185-203.

Hubel, D. H., & Wiesel, T. N. (1962). Receptive fields, binocular interactions and functional architecture in the cat's visual cortex. *Journal of Physiology, 160,* 106-154.

Hubel, D. H., & Wiesel, T. N. (1977). Ferrier Lecture. Functional architecture of macque monkey visual cortex. *Proceedings of the Royal Society of London B, 198,* 1-59.

Julesz, B. (1965). Texture and visual perception. *Scientific American, 212,* 38-48.

———. (1971). *Foundations of cyclopean perception.* Chicago: University of Chicago Press.

Kanade, T. (1981). Recovery of the three-dimensional shape of an object from a single view. *Artificial Intelligence, 17,* 409-460.

Kanade, T., & Kender, J. R. (1980). Mapping image properties into shape constraints: Skewed symmetry, affine-transformable patterns, and the shape-from-texture paradigm. (Tech. Rep. CMU-CS-80-133), Computer Science Department, Carnegie Mellon University, Pittsburgh.

Kaneko, A. (1979). Physiology of the retina. *Annual Review of Neuroscience, 2,* 169-191.

Krieg, W. J. S. (1966). *Functional Neuroanatomy, (3d ed.).* Evanston, IL: Brain Books.

Land, E. H. (1977). The retinex theory of color vision. *Scientific American, 237,* No. 6, 108-128.

Lawton, D. T. (1982). Motion analysis via local translational processing. (Tech. Rep. 82-23), Computer and Information Sciences, University of Massachusetts, Amherst, MA.

Mackworth, A. K. (1973). Interpreting pictures of polyhedral scenes. *Artificial Intelligence, 4,* 121-137.

——— (1977). How to see a simple world: An exegesis of some computer programs for scene analysis. In E. W. Elcock & D. Michie (Eds.), *Machine Intelligence, 8.* Edinburgh: Edinburgh University Press.

Marr, D. (1976). Early processing of visual information. *Philosophical Transactions of the Royal Society of London B, 275,* 483-519.

——— (1974). An essay on the primate retina. Artificial Intelligence Memo 296, Artificial Intelligence Laboratory, MIT, Cambridge, MA.

——— (1982). *Vision.* San Francisco: W. H. Freeman.

Marr, D., Palm, G., & Poggio, T. (1978). Analysis of a cooperative stereo algorithm. *Biological Cybernetics, 78,* 223-229.

Marr, D., & Poggio, T. (1979). A computational theory of human stereo vision. *Proceedings of the Royal Society of London B, 204,* 301-328.

Mayhew, J. E. W., & Frisby, J. P. (1981). Psychophysical and computational studies toward a theory of human stereopsis. *Artificial Intelligence, 17,* 349-385.

de Monasterio, F. M., Schein, S. J., & McCrane, E. P. (1981). Staining of blue-sensitive cones of the Macaque retina by a fluorescent dye. *Science, 213,* 1278-1281.

Poppel, E., Held, R., & Dowling, J. E. (1977). Neural mechanisms in visual perception. *Neurosciences Research Program Bulletin, 15,* No. 3. Cambridge, MA: MIT Press.

Poggio, G. F., & Poggio, T. (1984). The analysis of stereopsis. *Annual Review of Neuroscience, 7,* 379-412.

Prazdny, K. (1980). Egomotion and relative depth map from visual flow. *Biological Cybernetics, 36* 87-102.

Richards, W. (1979). Why rods and cones? *Biological Cybernetics, 33,* 125-135.

Richter, J., & Ullman, S. (1980). A model for the spatio-temporal organization of X and Y-type ganglion cells in the primate retina. A.I. memo No. 573, Artificial Intelligence Laboratory, MIT, Cambridge, MA.

Rodieck, R. W. (1965). Quantitative analysis of cat retinal ganglion cell response to visual stimuli. *Vision Research, 5,* 583-601.

——— (1979). Visual pathways. *Annual Review of Neuroscience, 2,* 193-225.

Schwartz, E. L. (1977). Spatial mapping in the primate sensory projection: Analytic structures and relevance to perception. *Biological Cybernetics, 25,* 181-194.

Sterling, P. (1983). Microcircuitry of the cat retina. *Annual Review of Neuroscience, 6,* 149-185.

Stevens, K. A. (1981). The visual interpretation of surface contours. *Artificial Intelligence, 17,* 47-73.

Talbot, S. A., & Marshall, W. H. (1941). Physiological studies on neural mechanisms of visual localization and discrimination. *American Journal of Ophthalmology*, *24*, 1255-1263.

Trehub, A. (1978). Neuronal model for stereoscopic vision. *Journal of Theoretical Biology*, *71*, 479-486.

Ullman, S. (1979). *The interpretation of visual motion*. Cambridge, MA: MIT Press.

Van Essen, D. C. (1979). Visual areas of the mammalian cerebral cortex. *Annual Review of Neuroscience*, *2*, 227-261.

Witkin, A. P. (1981). Recovering surface shape and orientation from texture. *Artificial Intelligence*, *17*, 17-45.

8

VISUAL
EXPERIENCES
AND MENTAL IMAGERY

INTRODUCTION

The low-level sensory representations created by the retinas are varied and complex as the previous chapter showed. Once formed, they are processed by the intermediate-level visual networks which form intermediate-level representations of the world and objects in it. The intermediate-level representations make explicit various features such as position, surface orientation, surface quality, and movement of the scene and objects in it. The set of intermediate-level representations comprises the primal sketch. The intermediate-level representations are further analyzed and high-level representations are formed which make explicit salient features of the scene and objects in it. Features of selected objects include their locations, orientations in space, surface orientations, contact and connectivity points, movements, and so forth.

We do not yet know very much about these high-level representations. We do not know what coordinate systems are used, what specific features are represented, how the features are represented, what types of storage systems hold and process the representations, how the various storage systems which process them communicate with one another, or how they communicate with other systems of the brain. Still, one can gain some insights into the representations and networks that process them by analyzing various psychological and clinical aspects of vision.

The goals of this chapter, then, are twofold. First, I will analyze selected clinical and psychological aspects of vision and, based on the evidence, suggest what some of the encoding strategies are. Second, I will present a specific model for how visual information might be represented in temporary and permanent memory. In particular I will suggest how permanent visual memories might be represented in storage and how the static stored representations might be converted back into the dynamic mental images of the scenes and objects they depict.

MODES OF VISUAL RECOGNITION

On the one hand we instantaneously recognize objects by their total appearance—the face of a friend, a book, an automobile. The term **gestalt** refers to form or configuration as a whole, unanalyzable from its parts, and **gestalt recognition** denotes that instantaneous process of visual recognition which occurs when we see something familiar. In contrast, under many circumstances, recognition is not based on a single instantaneous impression. We look at objects in question and explore them with our eyes until we gather enough information to identify them. Figure 8.1 illustrates how a determination is made which requires movements of the eyes. **Sequential recognition** denotes any recognition process which is based on the sequential analysis of selected features and their relationship to one another.

Regardless of the recognition process, visual images must be encoded for storage in such a way that the resulting **storage representations** can be recognized by the storage systems. It should by now be apparent that the low- and intermediate-level visual machinery make explicit certain attributes of the visual field. The intermediate-level networks, in particular, create storage representations by explicitly encoding attributes such as size, shape, surface orientations, component connectivity and so forth to depict accurately the objects they represent. A storage representation that depicts a single object is an **object representation**. At the present time, we do not know very much about object representations or the systems that create, process, or store them.

The permanent visual memory stores perform three functions: (1) They convert dynamic storage representations into static memory engrams. (2) They compare all incoming storage representations with all existing engrams and locate similar stored information. And (3), if commanded to do so, they generate dynamic output patterns. Output patterns are synthesized copies of earlier storage representations.

Just as the low-level and intermediate-level visual networks transform sensory representations into storage representations, the visual imagery system transforms storage representations back into iconic representations in a temporary storage system called **spatial memory**. The reconstructed representations, **mental images**, can be combined, transformed, and inspected by the mind's eye. Moreover, they can be used during a variety of thought processes, including mental rotation, predicting the outcomes of physical events, and sequential recognition. The appendix to this chapter presents a neural network model for spatial memory and introduces the mathematics suitable for analyzing its computational properties.

As I stated earlier, object representations are one type of storage representation. When an object representation is recalled and the resulting synthesized image placed in spatial memory, the recalled object is seen in the mind's eye. There is some evidence, now under current intensive investigation, which

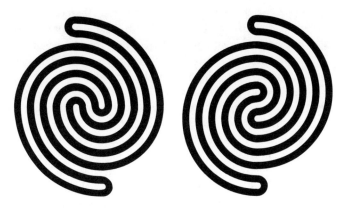

Figure 8.1. Connectivity cannot be determined by gestalt (instanta-neous) recognition. (Suggested by the cover of Minsky & Papert, *Perceptrons. An Introduction to Computational Geometry*. The MIT Press, 1969.)

suggests that object representations can also be recalled and placed in temporary storage and processing networks called **object buffers**. Object buffers can transform the representations in a variety of ways and make available to spatial memory mental images of the transformed representations. The transformations correspond to the operations we mentally perform on objects such as rotating them in space, squeezing them (if soft), stretching them, or breaking them. Thus object buffers are the networks which enable us to simulate mentally the physical properties of objects and the physical interactions between objects. The structure and functioning of object buffers is currently unknown.

The following section presents a brief discussion of selected syndromes resulting from damage to different parts of the human visual system. Visual syndromes give a great deal of insight into the computations which underlie the intermediate-level and high-level processes. The remainder of the chapter focuses first on the networks which convert low-level visual representations into storage representations and second on the networks which convert storage representations into visual images. The nature of the storage representations and the nature of visual images will be explored in detail.

SYNDROMES OF THE VISUAL SYSTEM

One paradox of a complex computational system whether computer or brain, is that observing it when damaged often gives more insight into its logical nature than does observing it when working properly. Errors in a computer program

171

often tell us more about the nature of the computation than do the results when the program works properly, and studying brain-damaged people often tells us more about the logic and organization of the brain than does studying normal people. The syndromes summarized below give a great deal of insight into the computational organization of the human visual system.

Damage to the visual system causes syndromes of two types: those that impair the use of language (e.g., inability to name, inability to read) and those which do not (e.g., inability to recognize objects, colors, faces). Loosely speaking, the left hemisphere appears to be involved most directly with language function: Damage to the visual areas of the left hemisphere tends to impair the use of language. The right hemisphere, on the other hand, seems to be involved with gestalt recognition: Damage to the visual areas of the right hemisphere tends to impair recognition but not (directly) language function. I will start with a brief discussion of the syndromes which do not impair the use of language and conclude with a brief discussion of those which do.

Agnosia is the inability to recognize objects as a result of brain damage, even though the sensory impressions are intact. Thus **visual object agnosia** is the inability to recognize objects by sight, **acoustic** or **auditory agnosia** is the inability to recognize sounds (e.g., a bell, a whistle, the rustling of leaves), and **tactile agnosia** or **astereognosia** is the inability to recognize objects by touch. These forms of agnosia are functionally independent: A patient with visual object agnosia cannot recognize objects by their gestalt appearance even though he or she can recognize them by touch if allowed to handle them. In fact, patients with visual object agnosia can sometimes learn to recognize objects by tracing their outline with their eyes, thus "feeling them" as if by touch. This shows a definite shift from the gestalt to the sequential mode of visual recognition and suggests that different underlying mechanisms are responsible for each process.

Prosopagnosia or **agnosia for faces** is the inability to discriminate between different faces by sight, even those of close friends or relatives (or oneself in a mirror). In prosopagnosia, the sensation of familiarity for the gestalt image is lost. However, patients with prosopagnosia can easily recognize friends and relatives by voice if they are allowed to speak. This illustrates the independence of the visual and auditory modes of recognition. In addition to faces, patients with prosopagnosia appear unable to distinguish between similar objects of other types from their gestalt appearance, although some objects can be distinguished by certain features. One farmer who was diagnosed as having prosopagnosia was unable to distinguish his cows from one another, an easy task for a normal farmer. Another patient, unable to recognize her own car in the parking lot, simply looked for a car with the correct license plate number (Damasio, Damasio, & Van Hoesen, 1982).

Color agnosia is the inability to recognize colors although similar colors differing only slightly in hue can easily be distinguished. A patient with color agnosia might know that red is the correct color of a fire engine but be unable to select a card "the same color as a fire engine" from among a set of different colored cards. To a patient with color agnosia, a picture of a friend with hair painted blue might look strange—something wrong with the color of the hair, but be unable to identify the problem. It is interesting to note that patients with prosopagnosia often suffer from color agnosia as well.

As mentioned earlier, visual perception and recognition consist not of a single process which can be isolated from other brain functions but of a system of highly interdependent tasks which together perform a complex analysis of the visual world. Among the fundamental processes are: (1) directing the gaze toward the object of interest, (2) generating the neural encoding of the selected object, (3) isolating and extracting the representation of the selected object from its background, and (4) transmitting the final visual encoding to the appropriate storage networks for analysis and recognition. During sequential recognition, the basic process is repeated many times with the final result determined by the combined analyses of the pictorial encodings and the control encodings that direct the gaze and focus the attention. Several syndromes which relate to the control and extraction processes will now be discussed.

One syndrome that illustrates the complexity of object selection is **simultaneous agnosia** or **simultagnosia**, which is the inability to perceive more than one object at a time. Luria (1966) described a patient with simultaneous agnosia this way:

> When the field of vision contained two objects (for example, a needle and the flame of a candle) the patient could see only one of them; if he looked at the needle, the flame of the candle in the background disappeared, and vice versa. The narrowing of the field of vision in this case was thus expressed not in units of space but with the number of simultaneously perceived objects. (p. 141).

Perhaps the most revealing feature of this narrowing of vision is that it is independent of the size of the object.

It is not clear whether the syndrome of simultaneous agnosia is the brain's way of compensating for the patient's inability to control his or her gaze consciously[1], or whether the patient is unable to control his or her gaze because of his perceptual disability, which may have several origins. For example, the patient may be able to extract an object representation from its background and therefore perceive it, but he or she may be unable to store background information in spatial memory and therefore not perceive other objects in the visual field. This may be due to a defect in the spatial memory system or it may be due to a defect in the storage control system. Or the patient may suffer an attention disorder, where he or she is unable to focus on more than one

---

[1]The inability to control the gaze intentionally is called **optokinetic alexia**.

object at a time. In either case, the patient's inability to look intentionally from one object to another graphically illustrates the close relationship between the mechanisms which direct the gaze and those which select one part of the visual field for analysis. More important, this syndrome indicates that objects (rather than areas) are extracted for analysis.

Object extraction is a fundamental property of the visual system. Object extraction means first of all, that the background is eliminated or **masked** from the visual pattern by the selection networks, and second, some form of size standardization takes place. **Size standardization** is the process of modifying the representation of the selected object to a dimensionality suitable for transmission to the storage networks for analysis and recognition.

A person with simultaneous agnosia is severely impaired. Although he or she can recognize individual objects by sight, the inability to direct the gaze intentionally from place to place in the visual field means that he or she cannot create an integrated model of the world from sight alone. He or she also cannot determine spatial relationships between objects. As a corollary we find that an essential aspect of visual perception is the ability to extract and use knowledge about the location and size of the selected objects. This ability is severely impaired for patients with simultaneous agnosia.

To understand the syndrome of simultaneous agnosia better, imagine that your only form of visual input is from a television screen. The images that appear on the screen come from around the room, but the camera is only turned on when it is not moving or zooming closer to or farther away from the selected objects. Finally, only objects can be sensed by the camera; not their background. What you see on the TV screen, then, is a sequence of randomly selected images; however, you have no idea how big they are or where they come from. Of what use is the knowledge? Although you can state that certain objects are present, you cannot locate them or determine their relationship to one another. Quite simply, you cannot create an integrated model of the room. In contrast, imagine exactly the same situation with one difference: You control the movement and focus of the camera.[2] Now you can scan the room in an intentional way, select exactly what you wish to focus your attention on, know how large it is, and know exactly where it is in the room. When you control the camera, you gain enough information, in addition to the images, to construct an internal model of the room.

Two related syndromes which further illustrate selection and masking are

---

[2]In recent research with blind patients, a similar phenomenon was observed. A two-dimensional array of tactile stimulators was strapped to a patient's back. The elements in the array were driven by a computer to vibrate in accordance with the light intensity that arrived at a corresponding position in the visual field. With practice, the patient could learn to recognize very simple objects such as a coffee cup and a telephone. However, it was essential that the patient controlled the movement and focus of the camera; only then could the patient learn to recognize the selected objects.

visual extinction and **visual completion**. A patient with visual extinction is unable to detect the presence of a visual stimulus when a second, competing stimulus is present in the same position of the opposite visual field. This occurs whether or not the patient concentrates on the object which subsequently becomes invisible. Just as in the case of simultaneous agnosia, the size of the competing object is unimportant. Completion is a seemingly opposite syndrome. For some patients who have a blindness in one half of the visual field (**hemianopia**), that part of an object which cannot be sensed because of the blindness is mentally filled in. As described by Heaton (p. 122), "If the patient is asked to fix on the examiner's entire face, and a black card is then slowly moved across the patient's hemianopic side; in many cases the patient is unaware of any change." The relationship between extinction and completion is summarized by Heaton this way (p. 122):

> There is a dynamic relation between extinction and completion. Extinction is most pronounced on prolonged exposure of a figure. But if the same areas of the field are stimulated by rapid tachistoscopic exposure of the figure (maximum effect 1/100 to 1/150 second), extinction is prevented and completion of the figure occurs. Some field defects are a result of processes of extinction rather than permanent loss of function; for with rapid tachistoscopic exposures the defects in these fields can be reduced.

Objects, once selected for analysis, appear to be close to the viewer or far away, large or small, depending on where they are located in the environment. Several syndromes alter the sensations of size or proximity while leaving intact the ability to recognize the selected objects. **Macropsia** is the condition in which objects appear larger than they really are while **micropsia** is the condition where they appear smaller. **Teleopsia** is a related disorder where nearby objects appear to be far away, as if viewed through the wrong end of a telescope. Each of these syndromes illustrates that the perceptual processes not only operate on pictorial representations of the selected objects, but also on control information which indicates how the pictorial representations are formed. The perception of size and distance are distinctly different processes from the recognition of the objects themselves.[3]

The records of visual experience contain not only pictorial components but also control components that specify how the pictorial components were formed and from where in the visual field they arose. The syndromes described herein amply show the existence of the control components. The syndromes also show that damage to the subsystems that control the gaze or to the subsystems that

---

[3]Similar modifications to the interpretation of the sensory data are reported under various drug-induced states. A person might report that a particular object initially seemed far away, but when noticed, it suddenly seemed to move closer and assume its usual appearance. Similar sensations have also been reported in states of near sleep.

select objects for further analysis can selectively interfere with later analyses and sensations that depend on their normal operation.

I will now describe several syndromes of the visual system that are related to language function (and hence are generally the result of damage to the left hemisphere). **Alexia** or **word blindness** is the total inability to read handwritten text and an almost total inability to read printed text. Patients with alexia may retain the ability to read individual letters, although sometimes by tracing their outlines with their eyes. Patients with alexia also generally retain the ability to read numbers, and in pure alexia, patients retain the ability to write. The inability to write is called **agraphia**, and patients with alexia without agraphia cannot read what they have just written. Many patients have both alexia and agraphia and therefore can neither read nor write. Some patients retain the ability to read words although they cannot recognize the individual letters, and some patients retain the ability to read words although they cannot understand complex text (**semantic alexia**). The inability to recognize letters suggests a malfunction with the gestalt machinery, whereas the inability to read words or understand sentences suggests a malfunction in sequential recognition or in a subsequent language processing network.

The apparent independence of the various mechanisms underlying reading as distinct from the other visual recognition processes suggests that different neural circuitry is used. The existence of different circuitry is supported by the fact that linguistic functions tend to be localized in the left hemisphere. Also, some nonlinguistic functions such as emotions and gestalt recognition, tend to be localized in the right hemisphere. Another clear example of the separation between linguistic and nonlinguistic function is the inability of some patients to name visually recognized objects, a syndrome called **object anomia**. (A patient with object anomia can pick up and use a fork and spoon, for example, but be unable to name them.) This disability points out that recognition of objects for manipulation and recognition of them for use require different underlying neural circuitry. The distinction between visual recognition and naming was most graphically illustrated in the previous chapter by the naming disability induced by electrical stimulation to the exposed cortex during surgery—"I couldn't get at the word 'butterfly' and then I tried to get at the word 'moth.'" Clearly the butterfly was recognized.

MENTAL IMAGERY

Mental images are those mental representations which we create and manipulate in our "mind's eye." They are not only the representations retrieved or formed from memory but also the stable representations actively formed during our daily activities. Mental images are dynamic temporary representations which we use to simulate mentally all those activities which we cannot or need not perform in reality: movements of furniture when planning to rearrange a room, movements of objects in the refrigerator when making space for a sack of groceries, holding figures temporarily when performing mental arithmetic.

Mental images are held and processed by spatial memory. Spatial memory performs a variety of computations on them, and since it is implemented in neural circuitry, it has properties and limitations which can be determined experimentally. The following few paragraphs describe some properties of the imagery system—spatial memory—and give insights into the relationships between mental images and the memories of visual experience.

Spatial memory has a fixed spatial extent; Images which are shifted beyond its borders are lost. Mental images which occupy the center of spatial memory have higher resolution than those which occupy its periphery. Mental images fade and must be refreshed or re-created to remain visible in the mind's eye. The time it takes to create a mental image increases with the complexity of the image and with the number of components in the image. Complex images are often coded in terms of the names of subsidiary parts; locating objects explicitly named in the images is faster than locating objects which are not explicitly named (refer to Kosslyn, 1980; and Reed, 1974).

The time it takes to create an image is proportional to the complexity of the image, and locating an object that has already been named in the image is easier than locating an object not explicitly named. Kosslyn (1980) had subjects create mental images of geometric shapes which were described to some subjects as two overlapping rectangles and to other subjects as five squares. Subjects whose instructions involved two rectangles required less time to construct the images than the other subjects; the time was, in fact, proportional to the number of subsidiary parts. Moreover, subjects found it easier to locate the parts they had been asked to imagine: rectangles for that group of subjects, squares for the other. Reed (1974) also found subjects had an easier time locating objects which were part of the description from which the image was built.

The time it takes to scan between different objects in an image is proportional to their distance apart. Kosslyn (1973) had subjects memorize line drawings containing several different objects. Subjects were then asked to focus on a particular place in the image and were then asked if a particular object was present. The time subjects took to determine if a named object was present or absent was proportional to the distance of the object from the current focus of attention in the mental image. This effect was absent when the subjects were instructed to view the entire mental image. Kosslyn, Ball and Reiser (1978) found similar results in an experiment in which subjects memorized a row of upper- and lower-case letters. In this experiment, subjects were asked to scan along the row to determine the case of a named letter. The determination time was proportional to the number of intervening letters (and hence distance). In another experiment, subjects memorized a stylized map which they were to then

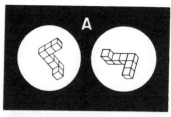

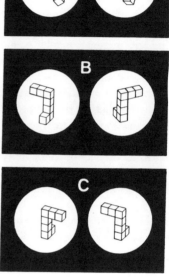

Figure 8.2. The types of figures studied by Shepard & Metzler (1971) and Cooper & Shepard (1973) in their pioneering studies on mental rotations. (Reproduced, with permission, from J. Metzler & R. N. Shepard, Transformational studies of the internal representation of three-dimensional objects. In R. L. Solso (Editor), *Theories of Cognitive Psychology:* The Loyola Symposium 1974. Copyright © 1974 by Lawrence Erlbaum Associates.)

imagine moving a black speck from one object to another in the image. Once again, the scan time increased linearly with the distance between objects.

Images held in spatial memory can be transformed so the imagined objects appear from different points of view. Once transformed, the images can be compared with current visual stimuli to determine sameness. Thus, a ". . . subject makes the determination of sameness of shape by carrying out some internal analog of an external rotation . . ." (Shepard & Cooper, 1982).

Shepard and Metzler (1971), Metzler and Shepard (1974), and Cooper and Shepard (1973) presented subjects with pairs of images and asked the subjects if the two images represented the same object. See Figure 8.2. In some presentations the objects were the same only seen from a different point of view. In other cases the objects differed: They were mirror images of one another. When the objects were the same, the time it took subjects to make the determination was linearly proportional to the magnitude of the underlying spatial rotation. This linear relationship held true regardless of whether the rotation was in the picture plane, in depth, or a mixed rotation. Two experiments by Cooper (1975) came to similar conclusions. Subjects memorized a set of random shapes (having no linguistic meaning) which were presented in an upright position. Subjects were then given a test shape to identify, which was either a rotated instance of one of the memorized set or its mirror image. When it was a rotated instance, the time required to determine that the figure belonged to the memorized set was linearly proportional to its angular displacement from upright.

In the second experiment, Cooper presented subjects with a shape followed by an angle representing the upright direction for the test pattern which would follow. The subjects were instructed to press a button when they were ready for the test pattern. The time it took subjects to prepare for the test pattern varied linearly with the angular displacement of the arrow from upright; the time it then took the subjects to determine whether the test pattern was the memorized stimulus or its reflection was constant. (One mechanism for performing the determinations described herein will be presented later in this chapter when discussing hypothesis verification.)

Components of mental images can be spatial or symbolic and they can be individually moved within the image. When used in this way, spatial memory becomes the mind's scratchpad on which notes can be written, moved, modified, and eliminated. In a series of experiments, Hayes (1973) presented subjects with flash-cards on which arithmetical and algebraic expressions were printed. The subjects were then asked to perform certain operations in their heads. For example, subjects were asked to solve for X in the equation $6 + X = 12$ and to subtract 964 from 1315. Subjects reported visualizing the answers (Hayes, p. 183 and p. 185):

> The answer, when it was visualized (and sometimes even when it was not—see below), was placed in a well-defined location with respect to the original problem. The digits of the answer were lined up with the columns of the problem card and placed immediately below them in the addition and subtraction problems and above them in the addition problem.
>
> and
>
> In the addition and subtraction problems (Problems 7 and 8), most subjects worked from right to left, processing each column in turn and storing the result. The results were announced in left to right order. Thirteen of the subjects reported that they stored the results of column processing in images. Subject 3 said that the important thing about generating "imaginary figures is that they stay while you move to the left to do more calculation." . . . Three subjects volunteered that they had to read the answer quickly because the image faded rapidly.

From the previous discussion it should be clear that the sensory encodings that occur at the retina, the internal regulatory functions that control the gaze, and the internal regulatory functions that control the encoding and selection processes are functionally distinct. It should also be clear that the brain maintains temporary representations, mental images, which appear to be analog spatial representations of currently or previously perceived objects. The system that maintains mental images can manipulate them in a variety of ways but has both physical and computational limitations.

The remainder of this chapter, and parts of the following chapter, explore specific encoding mechanisms, storage system organizations, and computational networks for processing the mind's representations of visual memories and mental images. The models proposed suggest in detail the underlying mechanisms of visual storage and mental imagery.

I will now change the focus of this discussion and center on the encoding mechanisms of the visual system. Keep in mind the fact that there are several low-level representations which make specific visual attributes explicit, and those representations may either be in registration or in isolation.

VISUAL STORAGE REPRESENTATIONS

In this section and the following few sections I will present one particular model for a sensory buffer. The sensory buffer not only holds the low-level representations for a short time, but it also converts them into a suitable representation for the permanent storage networks. The primary visual cortex will be implicated in this function.

Studies of the brain's records of visual experience suggest that the brain places in permanent experiential memory a time-varying representation of all those things upon which the focus of attention was directed at the time—a dog, a man, a pencil, and so forth. These experiences always appear to be based on meaningful physical quantities such as objects, features of objects, or groups of objects, and the experiences always contain information that specifies the location of the object in the world. (I will use the generic term "object" to denote any meaningful unit of visual information.) The brain's ability to extract objects rather than arbitrary visual fragments from the low-level representations was further illustrated in this chapter by the syndrome of simultaneous agnosia.

Temporary storage systems and object buffers also record the current visual representations. Spatial memory maintains the mind's active representation of the world—mental images of those objects in the immediate vicinity and their relationship to one another and to the body. Object buffers maintain the mind's representations of objects on which the attention was recently focused. For the present I will focus on those permanent memory stores which store representations that enable gestalt recognition—those associative memory stores which enable access to related experiences based on the visual appearance of objects and scenes.

In order for an associative storage system to recognize visual representations, the visual system must create storage representations which are independent of distance from object, viewpoint, and lighting conditions. This does not mean that the representation of an object when seen from the front must be identical to its representation when seen from behind, but it does mean that a building should appear the same when seen straight on or when seen from an oblique angle, even though the retinal patterns will differ. A **canonical storage representation** is one which has these properties. This section describes neural networks which locate objects and form canonical storage representations of them.

Size And Rotation Invariant Visual Representations

The visual system can compensate for different lighting conditions either by normalizing reflectance values (see Land, 1977), by representing only the outlines of objects, or by representing objects independent of their surface quality. There is considerable evidence for all three types of processing, and a later section describes in particular how objects can be represented independent of their surface quality. The visual system can compensate for differences in size and orientation[4] by transforming the retinal patterns into size and orientation independent representations. I will now show how this can be done.

Figure 8.3 illustrates the topology of the transformation from retina to primary visual cortex. This transformation has several important features. It is nonlinear: Projections from the centers of the retinas to the primary visual cortex occupy a much greater part of the cortex than projections from the surrounding retinal areas. It preserves local topology but not global topology: The representations of lines which are perpendicular at the retina are also perpendicular at the cortex; however, a given shape at the retina has a different shape at the cortex. As Figure 8.3 shows, lines radiating from the center of the retina are projected onto parallel strips of the cortex, while circles centered on the retina are projected onto perpendicular parallel strips. Finally, circles which are exponentially farther apart at the retina project to cortical strips which are a constant distance apart.

I will convey the nature of this transformation by using a fiber optics system as an analogy to the neural system. In the fiber optics system, the individual fibers correspond exactly to axons in a neural system. Hence bundles of fibers correspond to neural pathways.

Imagine that two parallel image planes are connected together by a dense bundle of optical fibers. The lower image plane will be called the **input plane** and the upper one the **output plane**. This is illustrated in Figure 8.4. Assume that corresponding points are connected. Each fiber will be labeled by its coordinates on the input plane. If the input and output planes are labeled with xy coordinates, then point (x,y) in the input plane is connected to point (x,y)

---

[4]The transformation described here can only compensate for rotations about the line of sight; not for differences in the appearance of three-dimensional objects when looked at from different viewpoints. Additional research is necessary to discover networks which can compensate for changes in perspective.

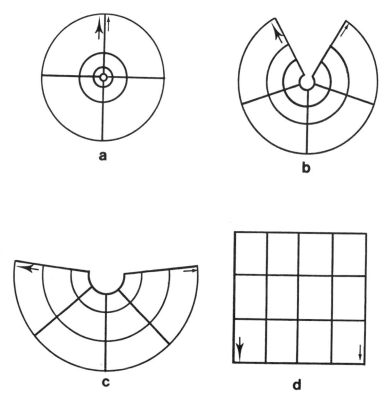

Figure 8.3. The complex logarithmic mapping can be approximated by splitting the upper half of the retinal pattern and unfolding it as shown here. Central points must be expanded during the unfolding process to fill in the available space. (Reproduced, with permission, from R. J. Baron, Visual memories and mental images. *International Journal of Man-Machine Studies*, 23, 1985, 275-311.)

in the output plane. As a result, the pattern in the input fibers formed by placing an image beneath the input plane will be seen undistorted in the output plane.

The fiber-optics system is now modified as follows. First, let the **transform plane** be that plane lying halfway between the input and output planes. Without breaking the connections between the input and output planes, the fibers are rearranged in the transform plane to conform to the topology of the retina-cortex projections. During the rearrangement, the fibers are made thicker or thinner to fill available space in the transform plane. Figure 8.5 shows this rearrangement. If points in the input plane have xy cartesian coordinates and points in the transform plane have uv cartesian coordinates, then a fiber originating at coordinates (x,y) in the input plane passes through coordinates $(u, v) = (\ln (\sqrt{x^2 + y^2}), \tan^{-1} (y/x))$ in the transform plane. Using the terminology of complex variables, if z designates the xy plane and w designates the uv plane, then the transformation between input plane and transform plane is $w = \ln(z)$. This transformation is called the complex logarithm, and the system being constructed will be called the "logmap system." Schwartz (1977) first identified this transformation in the visual systems of vertebrates, while mathematical details can be found in Churchill (1960).

Now suppose that after the fibers are rearranged in the logmap system they are encased in plastic and frozen in position. An image placed below the input plane will still be undistorted in the output plane, since the geometry of the output image is determined only by the actual connections and not by the topology of the pathway. Next, suppose that the system is cut in half through the transform plane. The lower half will be called the **input subsystem** and the upper half the **output subsystem**. Although each subsystem now has its own distinct set of optical fibers, each fiber will retain the label it originally had. Fibers of the input subsystem are **input fibers**, and those of the output system are **output fibers**. These fibers are in one-to-one correspondence, with corresponding fibers having the same labels. Since the optical fibers are frozen in position, the output will still be identical to the input.

An important question may now be asked: How would the output appear if the input and output systems were to be shifted in the transform plane? Note that a shift systematically changes the connections between input and output fibers, but since the fibers in the transform plane have different sizes because of the logmap transformation, the changes in connections are not linear. The answer depends on the direction of the shift. If the shift is parallel to the lines in the transform plane which represent radii in the input plane, the output will

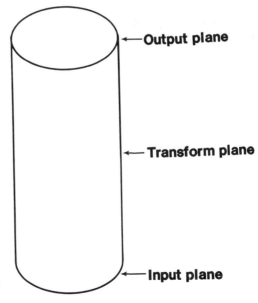

Figure 8.4. A dense bundle of optical fibers connecting an input plane with an output plane. (Reproduced, with permission, from R. J. Baron, Visual memories and mental images. *International Journal of Man-Machine Studies*, 23, 1985, 275-311.)

←—**Output plane**

←—**Transform plane**

←—**Input plane**

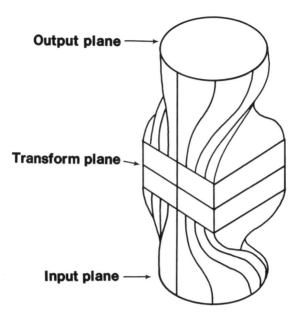

Output plane ⟶

Transform plane ⟶

Input plane ⟶

Figure 8.5. The bundle of optical fibers shown in Figure 8.3 rearranged in the transform plane to produce the complex logarithmic mapping of an input image which is placed in the input plane. (Reproduced, with permission, from R. J. Baron, Visual memories and mental images. *International Journal of Man-Machine Studies*, 23, 1985, 275-311.)

look like the input, only magnified or reduced in size, depending on the direction of the shift. If the shift is in the perpendicular direction, the output image looks like the input image, only rotated clockwise or counterclockwise.[5] An arbitrary shift would result in a combined rotation and scale change, as illustrated in Figure 8.7.

The optical system can standardize the appearance of a rotated or magnified image and produce a canonical representation. Consider the appearance of the output of the optical system if a photographic reduction of a given picture is placed in the input plane. If the input and output subsystems are unshifted, the output will be the same size as the input (and hence smaller than the original

---

[5]Since some of the output fibers have no corresponding input fibers, information is lost. The result is the absence of the output image in a wedge-shaped part of the output plane. This loss can be eliminated by splitting the input fibers and having the input pathway duplicated circularly as shown in Figure 8.6. In the brain, each half of the input pathway is implemented in a different cortical hemisphere. It is not known how the brain combines the two halves of the transformed pattern; hence it is not known whether or not duplication of part of the transformed pattern is even necessary.

image), but if the input and output subsystems are shifted to magnify the image, the output can be made to appear exactly as if a full-sized image were placed in the input plane. By linearly shifting connections between input and output fibers in the transform plane, the system can compensate for a change in size of the input. The same is true for a rotation or a combination of magnification and rotation. Like a zoom lens which can magnify or reduce an optical image, the fiber-optics system can also magnify or reduce an image, but it uses a very different physical process. In addition, it can rotate the image, a transformation not possible with a zoom lens. By analogy, it follows that both scale changes and rotations can be performed in a neural system—the brain.

The fiber-optics system shares several important properties with the human visual system. The connections between points on the input plane (corresponding to the retina) and transform plane (corresponding to the primary visual cortex) are fixed. In both systems, values of individual components of dynamic patterns are transmitted along fixed conductors: axons in the brain and optical fibers in the optical system. Pattern conductors in both systems have "inherent" labels based on their geometrical position on the receptor surface. Finally, with reference to the input and output patterns in the optical system, there is an intuitive notion of when an output pattern equals an input pattern: Under the natural correspondence between input and output fibers having the same labels, the output pattern **equals** the input pattern provided the light value in each output fiber equals the light value in its corresponding input fiber. A similar definition was already made in Chapter 2 for neural patterns.

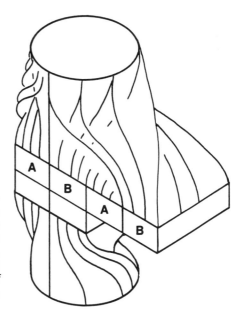

Figure 8.6. Duplicate circuitry must be included if information is not to be lost when an image is rotated. (Reproduced, with permission, from R. J. Baron, Visual memories and mental images. *International Journal of Man-Machine Studies*, 23, 1985, 275-311.)

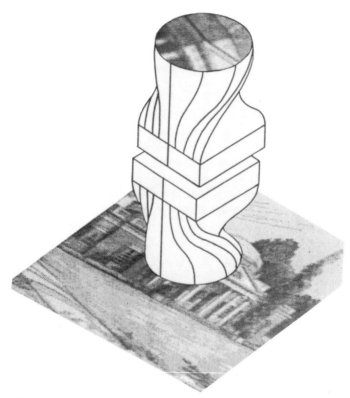

Figure 8.7. The logmap system shown enlarging and rotating part of an image. (Reproduced, with permission, from R. J. Baron, Visual memories and mental images. *International Journal of Man-Machine Studies*, 23, 1985, 275-311.)

A notable property of the logmap system is that the output pattern always "looks like" the input pattern: It an **iconic representation** of the input pattern. In contrast, the pattern in the transform plane of the logmap system is not an iconic representation of the input pattern. The notion of an iconic representation is illustrated in Figure 8.8. The retina, which is an example of an iconic processing network, forms the convolution of its input pattern with a gaussian distribution. This was described in the previous chapter.

We may assume that the eyes and other low-level visual networks encode information from the visual field and create a set of representations in which light intensity, gradient of light intensity, and color information are made explicit. We may also assume that the set of retinal patterns is further processed to create at least four representations: a pictorial pattern (color, brightness), a depth pattern, a visual flow pattern, and a surface orientation pattern. I will now describe how canonical storage representations can be formed from these representations.

Networks which Create Canonical Storage Representations

A **visual buffer,** illustrated in Figure 8.9, is a storage system that produces a representation which is independent of the surface quality of an object. The visual buffer consists of a two-dimensional array of storage locations called **buffer locations** and it receives information from two places. First, it receives the low-level visual representations, which are locally distributed to the buffer locations: Each buffer location receives a small part of them. Global distribution obeys a complex logarithmic map. Information centered at position (x,y) on the retina is centered at position $(\ln(\sqrt{x^2 + y^2}), \tan^{-1}(y/x))$ in the visual buffer. The visual buffer also receives a single **test pattern,** which is sent to all buffer locations. The test pattern describes a particular texture and color and is the neural encoding of a small patch of surface. The test pattern therefore encodes surface quality. All buffer locations are similar and hold patterns which are the same size as the test pattern. The buffer locations have adaptive memory traces, and shortly after the sensory patterns arrive, the traces adapt to store them. Each buffer location compares its part of the sensory pattern with the test pattern, and the single resulting correlation value from each buffer location indicates how similar the sensory pattern is to the test pattern. Hence each correlation value

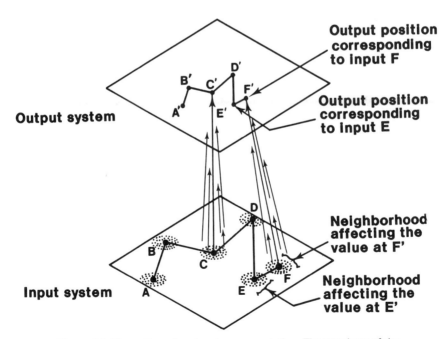

Figure 8.8. The notion of an iconic representation. The topology of the transformed pattern must not be changed even though its local characteristics may be modified.

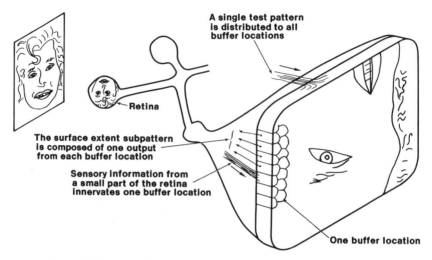

Figure 8.9. The visual buffer receives low-level visual information from the retinas by way of the lateral geniculate bodies and produces multiple representations which are independent of lighting conditions and surface quality of the represented object. Compare with Figure 7.5.

indicates the presence or absence of a surface having the same quality as the test pattern. The set of similarity values from all buffer locations is the **surface extent subpattern,** a spatial representation which is much smaller than the sensory pattern from which it is derived. If, for example, each buffer location holds a pattern comprised of 500 values, then the reduction ratio is 500 to 1.

Intuitively, one role of the sensory buffer is to form a representation of an object which is independent of lighting and surface appearance (such as color and texture). Although not always the case, objects can be characterized by their bounding surfaces: They have a single color or distribution of colors, a single texture, a limited spatial extent, and often are bounded by uniform surfaces. If the eyes are directed toward a particular surface of an object, the visual machinery must be able to extract quickly a canonical description of the object comprised by that surface. Said another way, the visual system must be able to **segment** the sensory representation into regions representing objects. One way to segment the representation is to select a surface patch, a test pattern, from the center of the visual focus and then compare it with all other parts of the visual field. The resulting pattern of correlation values, the surface extent subpattern, indicates the extent (hence shape) of the region having the selected surface quality. The surface extent subpattern can then be used to mask out all parts of the visual field which do not comprise the selected surface. The presence of the selected surface is represented by the surface extent subpattern while its quality is represented by the test pattern. The crucial point is that the surface extent subpatterns will be similar for objects which differ only in surface quality: A red cube, a blue cube, and a cube composed of bricks will all have similar surface extent subpatterns. Hence the resulting representation is closer to the desired canonical representation than the original sensory pattern.

The control system does not need to select the test pattern from the center of the visual focus. The test pattern may be a stored test pattern from a prior experience. When looking for a yellow object, for example, the control system may recall a test pattern representing the color yellow. The low-level visual system is then "tuned" to yellow and will immediately respond (generate similarity values) when yellow objects are present.

Creating canonical storage representations of objects requires first that they be found in the visual field, and second that the representations formed by the encoding networks be canonical. Objects can be found by analyzing the correlation patterns produced by the sensory buffer. The surface extent pattern isolates objects and can be used both for extracting representations from the primal sketch and for masking the background. Even after an object is found, however, the form of the resulting representation depends on the position selected for the center of the logmap transformation, and this depends in part on where the eyes are looking. This follows from the previous description of the logmap system. The problem of creating a canonical representation, then, becomes one of directing the eyes toward a particular point on the selected object and selecting the proper subpattern from the surface extent representation.[6] Directing the eyes and selecting a subpattern from the surface extent representation is called **focusing the attention**, and I will hereafter assume that control networks (which will not be described) focus the attention and create a canonical representation whenever the same object is seen. The pathway that conveys the selected part of the surface extent pattern is the **pictorial pathway**, and for simplicity I will assume that the depth, surface orientation, and visual flow patterns are also transmitted along the pictorial pathway. Figure 8.10 illustrates the various computational networks and pathways of the low-level visual system. Compare with Figures 6.1 and 8.18. A **storage representation** consists of six subpatterns: the test pattern, which describes the surface quality of the represented object; four spatial representations: surface extent, depth, visual flow, and surface orientation; and the control pattern. The background is masked in each of the spatial representations. The control pattern indicates exactly how the storage representation was formed by indicating the fixation point of the eyes relative to appropriate internal and external frames of reference, by indicating which subpattern of the surface extent pattern was selected, and by indicating the source of the test pattern. A storage representation always has all six components.

---

[6] There are some storage systems which can recognize a pattern even though it is shifted within the input pathway. If such a storage system is used, this selection operation may not be necessary.

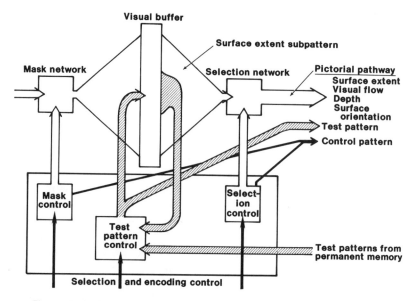

Figure 8.10. The computational architecture of the low-level visual networks, showing both control networks and information pathways. Compare with Figure 6.1.

The storage representations formed by the low-level visual networks are the only visual representations that the high-level networks receive. All visual recognition and all high-level descriptive processes are based on only these representations. A storage representation explicitly encodes the shape of an object (surface extent pattern), its surface characteristics (surface quality and surface orientation subpatterns), its location in space (depth together with control pattern), its size (control pattern), and whether or not it was moving (visual flow subpattern). As a consequence, associative storage systems can base similarity on shape (square, round), surface characteristics (fuzzy objects, red objects, flat objects), movement (objects which rotate, objects which squirm), and even on how the object was processed (scan path). Even though storage systems use template matching, recognition depends on a variety of characteristics, not just the similarity of the retinal projections.

When a person looks about, his eyes are directed from one fixation point to another while his focus of attention shifts from one object to another. The resulting storage representation is stored continuously in time and is the only stored record of that visual experience.[7] Moreover, the storage system compares

---

[7]Verbal thoughts about the event and verbal tokens representing attended objects are also stored, but they are stored in a completely different storage system. This discussion deals only with the representations derived through the visual system.

each component of the storage representation with all previously stored components and immediately locates any similar stored information. This, after all, is the reason for forming a canonical representation of each selected object in the first place. The recall system may then recall the related events.

Intuitively, the global transformations used in forming a storage representation are identical to those in the input subsystem of the logmap system. A storage representation can by formed in the logmap system by placing a bundle of large optical fibers over the transform plane as shown in Figure 8.11. This bundle will also be called the pictorial pathway since it corresponds to the pictorial pathway in the visual system. There is a fundamental difference, however. The logmap system deals only with a single input pattern and only with light intensity values; the visual system merges two different input patterns (the two retinal images) and computes (makes explicit) position, visual flow, and surface orientation. This is all in addition to the formation of the surface extent pattern. Although both systems perform the same topological transformation, the visual system performs an incredible amount of local processing on the visual representations and is therefore vastly more complex.

The process of directing the attention in the visual system corresponds to centering a picture under the input plane of the logmap fiber-optics system (selecting a fixation point). There is, of course, no test pattern in the optical system since it only processes intensity information.

MENTAL IMAGES

Just as the low-level visual system transforms sensory representations of objects into storage representations, the system for visual imagery transforms storage representations back into iconic representations. With reference to the logmap fiber-optics system, I have already pointed out that the low-level visual system corresponds to the input subsystem. The system for visual imagery corresponds approximately to the output subsystem. I also showed that the image of an object in the logmap system can be transformed into a storage representation by placing a bundle of large optical fibers, the pictorial pathway, over the transform plane of the input subsystem. An iconic representation of the object can be reconstructed in the output plane by placing the output subsystem over the pictorial pathway as shown in Figure 8.12. Figure 8.13, a slightly modified optical system, illustrates more closely the architecture of the visual system. Each fiber is divided in half, with one half forming an input pathway to a storage system and the other half forming the pictorial pathway. The output fibers from the storage system merge with the fibers in the pictorial pathway. Connections are specific: Only fibers having the same labels (intrinsic coordinates) are merged. As a result, patterns that arrive at the output subsystem either come

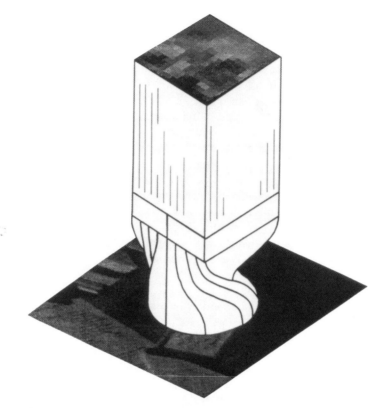

Figure 8.11. The storage representation formed by the input subsystem of the logmap system. Compare with Figures 8.14 and 8.15. (Reproduced, with permission, from R. J. Baron, Visual memories and mental images. *International Journal of Man-Machine Studies*, 23, 1985, 275-311.)

directly from the input subsystem or from the storage system. The output subsystem cannot distinguish between these two sources and will reconstruct an iconic representation from either source.

In the fiber-optics system, information is lost during the formation of a storage representation and therefore the appearance of the reconstructed pattern in the output plane differs from its appearance in the input plane. Information is lost because the pictorial pathway has fewer fibers than the input or output pathways and light values are averaged upon entry to the large optical fibers. Nonetheless, the reconstructed image is an iconic representation of the input pattern. How does a reconstructed image appear? Its center appears identical to the center of the original image, but as one looks farther and farther away from the center, the reconstructed image appears progressively less detailed. The center of the input image occupies a much larger percentage of the transform plane than the perimeter, so that more information is averaged at the perimeter. Specifically, because of the logarithmic transformation, exponentially more information is lost as a linear function of the distance from the center. Figure 8.14a shows an input pattern, Figure 8.14b shows a storage representation resulting from a single fixation point, and Figure 8.14c shows its reconstructed representation for the optical system.

Information is also lost in the visual system. The optic cord has about a million fibers; storage representations, in contrast, have only a few hundred components. (This assumes that storage takes place in associative storage networks of the type described in Chapter 3.) A parallel can therefore be drawn between the fiber-optics system and the visual system when the test pattern represents uniform brightness. In that case, the surface extent pattern represents the average brightness encoded by each buffer location, and to the extent that each fiber in the pictorial pathway of the logmap system also encodes average brightness, the two systems are similar.

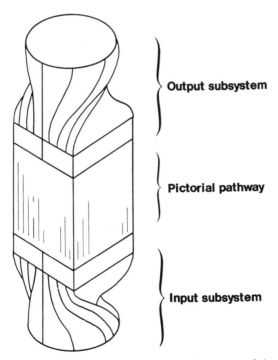

Output subsystem

Pictorial pathway

Input subsystem

Figure 8.12. The input and output subsystems of the logmap system are connected by the pictorial pathway. (Reproduced, with permission, from R. J. Baron, Visual memories and mental images. *International Journal of Man-Machine Studies*, 23, 1985, 275-311.)

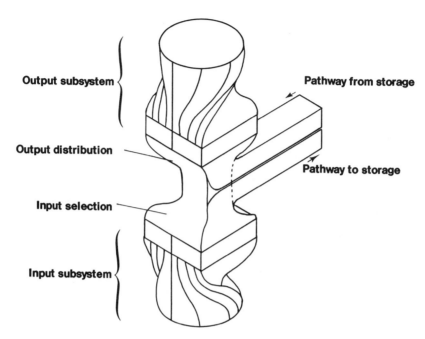

Output subsystem

Pathway from storage

Output distribution

Pathway to storage

Input selection

Input subsystem

Figure 8.13. The major components of the low-level visual system consist of an input subsystem, which computes the complex logarithm of an input pattern; an input selection network, which selects those patterns to be represented; pathways to and from a storage system; an output distribution network, which controls magnifications and rotations of the output pattern; and an output subsystem, which computes the complex exponential of the storage representation. (Reproduced, with permission, from R. J. Baron, Visual memories and mental images. *International Journal of Man-Machine Studies*, 23, 1985, 275-311.)

Within the visual system, the representation of an object is derived from a sequence of fixation points, and hence, during reconstruction it is necessary to reconstruct each pattern in the sequence. Since each pattern may represent a different fixation point and focus, each individually reconstructed pattern must be placed in its correct position relative to other patterns in the reconstruction. Finally, in order to hold the patterns during reconstruction, a temporary storage system is required.

Within a neural system, physical connections are fixed. In particular, the pictorial pathway, which delivers recalled patterns from the permanent storage system to the imagery system, has fixed connections. These connections cannot be changed as a way of placing the reconstructed patterns in their correct relative positions to one another. In order to reconstruct a single composite representation from the sequence of patterns in a storage representation,

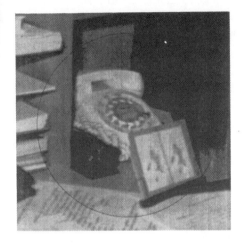
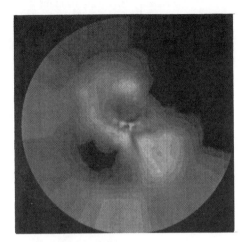

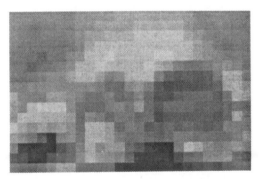

Figure 8.14. a. An input pattern showing the extent of the region selected for the focus of attention while deriving b and also Figure 8.11. b. The storage representation of the pattern shown in c. c. A reconstruction of the storage representation shown in a. (It is best to hold these figures at a distance of six to ten feet for the comparison.) (Reproduced, with permission, from R. J. Baron, Visual memories and mental images. *International Journal of Man-Machine Studies*, 23, 1985, 275-311.)

therefore, a special temporary storage system, **spatial memory**, is required which can internally shift information during the reconstruction.

Spatial Memory

Spatial memory is a temporary storage system and pattern processor which combines, shifts, and transforms patterns of neural activity. The patterns of activity, mental images, are iconic representations of the structures they represent and the control system for spatial memory determines how the mental images will be shifted and transformed. The appendix to this chapter will present a neural network model for spatial memory and indicate its relationship to the cerebral cortex. The appendix will also present the mathematics of mental transformations. The following discussion describes conceptually how spatial memory works.

Spatial memory resembles a large classroom filled with students who are holding flashlights. Each storage location in spatial memory is represented by one of the students, and the flashlight represents the activity in the corresponding storage location. Suppose that most of the flashlights are off and the few that are on appear like the letter A. The pattern of lights is a dynamic iconic representation of the letter A. If the teacher tells the students to turn on their light if the person's light on their left is on, and to turn it off otherwise, then the representation of the letter A will move to the right. The teacher corresponds to the control system and the students correspond to the storage locations in spatial memory. The teacher can clear the system by telling all students to turn off their flashlights, and the teacher can enter a representation into the system by holding up a chart (corresponding to permanent memory) and then telling the students to turn on their flashlights if the chart says to do so.

Each spatial location receives inputs from all neighboring spatial locations within a fixed radius, and each one may select a neighboring location as a **source** of information, a location from which to receive information. In addition, each spatial location receives a control input, a **shift vector**, which specifies the neighboring spatial location to be used as a source. The source location is specified by giving its direction and distance away. If the value of a shift vector is zero, the spatial location retains its previous patterns during a shift operation. If the shift vector specifies a direction and distance for which there is no source location, for example, at the edge of spatial memory, that spatial location enters the null (zero) pattern. The null pattern is also called the **background value**. Shift vectors may all be different, but they may also be the same. If all shift vectors are the same, the entire representation in spatial memory is linearly shifted. The set of all shift vectors to spatial memory is a control pattern called the **shift pattern**, and the operation of shifting information between spatial locations is a **shift operation**.

External input patterns to spatial memory arrive over the pictorial input pathway and are distributed to spatial locations, as shown in Figure 8.15. Just as the input pathway in the logmap system transforms patterns by performing a complex logarithmic mapping on their spatial representation, the pathway to spatial memory performs the inverse mapping: a complex exponentiation. Connections in the center of the transformation are one-to-one but toward the perimeter they are one-to-many. Thus many spatial locations receive exactly the same input value. If (u,v) are the labels of a cell in the input pathway, then $(x,y) = (\exp(u)\cos(v), \exp(u)\sin(v))$ are the labels of the cell in the center of its output field.

Spatial memory holds two distinctly different patterns: the **information**

Input pathway

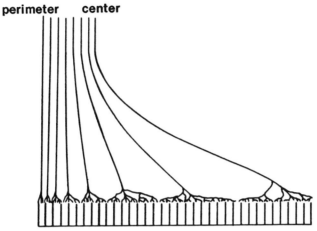

perimeter   center

Spatial locations representing the perimeter of the input pattern

Spatial locations representing the center of the input pattern

Figure 8.15. An illustration showing how the input pathway to spatial memory distributes information to central and peripheral memory locations. (Adapted from R. J. Baron, Visual memories and mental images. *International Journal of Man-Machine Studies*, 23, 1985, 275-311.)

pattern consisting of **mental images,**[8] and a control pattern called the **fidelity pattern**.

The reasons for these names will soon become clear. Mental images are reconstructions of storage representations, either the ones representing the current visual field, or ones recalled from permanent memory. Hence they have four spatial components: surface extent, surface orientation, depth, and visual flow. Each spatial location holds one component of each of these subpatterns.

The fidelity pattern consists of a single value in each spatial location, and each value indicates how much of the information at that location was lost during the formation of the storage representation. Each fidelity value may be used as a control signal to control when a spatial location should accept new

---

[8]Mental images are patterns held in spatial memory. The term "image" indicates a reconstructed visual pattern, which may be an iconic representation but is not required to be. Mental images, regardless of type, can be manipulated by spatial memory in a manner to be described later.

information. The fidelity values are generated by the spatial locations when they accept new external patterns as follows. The unique spatial location in the center of spatial memory always generates the fidelity value zero, representing maximum fidelity. Each other spatial location generates a fidelity value which is proportional to the exponent of its distance away from the center of spatial memory. The distance of a spatial location from the center of spatial memory can be computed since each spatial location has its own unique intrinsic coordinates or **address**, a structural property of each spatial location. The proportionality constant is a control value externally supplied by the spatial memory control system in a manner to be described later.

Three control signals issued by the spatial memory control system synchronize information transfers. The first control signal is the **clear signal**. It simultaneously clears the patterns in all spatial locations: All fidelity values are set to their maximum value (representing minimum fidelity) while all information patterns are set to zero. The clear signal **initializes** spatial memory: All prior information is lost. The second control signal is a **transmit signal**. It causes information to be shifted among the spatial locations. Upon receiving the transmit signal, each spatial location accepts internal information from the source location specified by its shift vector. Both internal patterns and fidelity values are shifted during a transmit operation. The third control signal is a **conditional acceptance signal**. It causes pictorial input patterns to be accepted conditionally by the spatial locations. Input patterns are only accepted in case the proportionality constant, an external parameter, times the distance of the spatial location from the center of spatial memory is smaller than the fidelity value currently being held by that spatial location. It follows that if the proportionality constant is specified as zero, spatial locations unconditionally accept new external input patterns. The fidelity values generated by the spatial locations are inserted when they accept new information. The utility of the fidelity values will become clear shortly.

The Reconstruction of Storage Representations

Here is how spatial memory can be used to reconstruct a storage representation. The clear signal is first issued. It initializes spatial memory: All prior stored patterns are cleared. The first component of a storage representation is then transmitted over the input pathway and the conditional acceptance signal issued by the control system. All spatial locations accept the new information and insert fidelity values which are proportional to their distances from the center of spatial memory. Assume for the present that the proportionality constant is one. A shift pattern is then issued which specifies how the partly reconstructed mental image is to be shifted among the spatial locations. The partly reconstructed image must be linearly shifted (all shift vectors are the same) relative to the next component so that the two patterns remain in registration: The shift must compensate exactly for the shift in the focus of attention during the formation of the storage representation. Using the control pattern of the storage representation, which describes the fixation point of the eyes, the networks that control spatial memory determine the proper shift pattern and send the transmit signal to initiate information transfer. Upon arrival of the shift pattern and transmit signal, all mental images and fidelity values are simultaneously shifted. The shift pattern and transmit signal are then turned off and the next component of the storage representation is transmitted over the input pathway. The conditional acceptance signal is once again given to initiate the information transfer. This time, because there is a fidelity pattern in spatial memory, the only storage locations which accept new information are those whose distances from the center of spatial memory are less than their fidelity values. Reconstruction of a storage representation is accomplished by repeating this sequence of shift and accept operations until the entire storage representation is processed. Figure 8.16a illustrates a reconstructed image whose storage representation consists of a sequence of 41 patterns formed at 41 fixation points, and Figure 8.16b shows the final fidelity pattern for the reconstruction. Figure 8.16c shows the original image and scan path encoded by the storage representation. In this example, the storage representation consists of 41 patterns having 400 components while the original image has 245,760 components. Therefore, the storage representation holds 15% of the amount of information in the original image.

The visual images reconstructed in spatial memory differ from sensory representations because the information contained in the test pattern is not used during the reconstruction. The surface extent subpattern isolated objects in the storage representations, and when reconstructed, the presence of objects is once again indicated. However, the fact that one object may have been yellow while another one red is lost during the reconstruction. (High-level networks can analyze the test patterns during reconstruction to determine the surface characteristics of reconstructed objects, but surface characteristics cannot be determined only from the images in spatial memory.)

The Use of the Fidelity Values During Reconstruction

I will once again rely on the logmap fiber-optics system to explain intuitively both how reconstruction takes place and the role of the fidelity values during reconstruction. In the fiber-optics system, a storage representation can be formed by placing an image under the input plane and moving it to several different positions. Each position corresponds to one fixation point, and the resulting sequence of images in the transform plane corresponds to the pictorial component of the storage representation. During this process, each reconstructed image in the output plane is an output image. As a medium for reconstruction, suppose that a piece of photosensitive glass is placed in contact

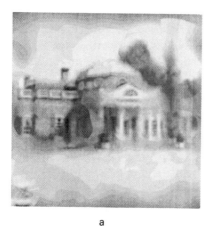
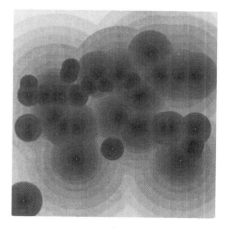

a   b

Figure 8.16 a. A reconstructed representation of the pattern shown in Figure
8.15c. b. The fidelity pattern derived during the reconstruction shown in a. c. An
input image with superimposed scanpath
used in creating the storage representations used for creating b and c. Note that
the fixation points do not tell how large
the focus of attention is at each fixation
point. (Reproduced, with permission,
from R. J. Baron, Visual memories and
mental images, *International Journal of
Man-Machine Studies*, 23, 1985, 275-311.)

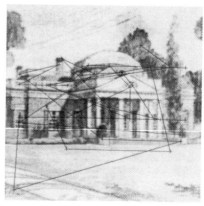

c

with the output plane as shown in Figure 8.17 and allowed to adapt to the first
output image. As Figure 8.14 already showed, the center of a reconstructed
image is very detailed but fidelity decreases as a function of distance from the
center. Now suppose that the input image is shifted to the second fixation point.
In order for the second image to remain in registration with the first image in the
reconstruction, the photosensitive glass must be shifted. Once shifted, it must
be allowed to adapt to the second image. The new center, having more detail
than the surrounding area, will become more faithful to the original image.
However, that part of the reconstructed image that was previously in the center
will lose detail since it is no longer in the center of the second fixation point.
In order to reconstruct a composite image having the highest resolution at every
possible point, the photosensitive glass must selectively adapt to each new
image. Each place where the resolution of the current image is higher than the
resolution of the previous image must adapt while each place where the current

image has less resolution must not adapt. Since the fidelity of each point in the incoming image is inversely proportional to its distance from the center of the system, distance information can be used to determine when new information should replace old information. In particular, new information should replace old information when it comes from a place which is closer to the current center than previous information was to the center when it was reconstructed.

Although there is no simple way to prevent the photosensitive glass in the optical system from adapting, the fidelity values in the visual system serve exactly that purpose: They allow new information having higher fidelity to replace old information having lower fidelity, but not vice versa. This is the reason for conditional acceptance of new information.

Pathways of the Visual Imagery System

Figure 8.18 suggests the organization of the pathways that deliver information to and from spatial memory and to and from the permanent stores of visual experience. The pathway from the visual buffer to spatial memory is a dense bundle of fibers which transmits a detailed representation of the visual field to spatial memory. This is the representation produced by the visual buffer. The pathway performs a complex exponential mapping of the representations produced by the visual buffer, thereby delivering an iconic representation to spatial memory. Spatial memory can therefore maintain a stable iconic representation of the visual world, as I will shortly show. Two pathways deliver information to and from the permanent visual memory stores, and two distribution networks are also required as shown in the figure. A **selection network** extracts information from spatial memory, and a **distribution network** sends information to spatial memory. A neural network model for the selection network was presented in Chapter 2; a distribution network can be built the same way. The selection network extracts information from spatial memory to occupy the focus of attention. The distribution network enters information into spatial memory in a shifted position and therefore controls magnification and rotation during reconstruction. Clearly, the entry of information in the pictorial pathway must be coordinated with the shifting of information in spatial memory during reconstruction.

The pathways between the visual buffer and the permanent visual memory stores correspond exactly to the pathways shown in Figure 8.13. In Figure 8.13, the input selection network is shown as an output network from the visual buffer (the transform plane of the optical system). In Figure 8.18, the input selection network is shown as an output network from spatial memory. However, the connections made at spatial memory are direct: The pattern entering the pathway to the input selection network is exactly the pattern described earlier that is created by the visual buffer. Thus the fact that the connections are made

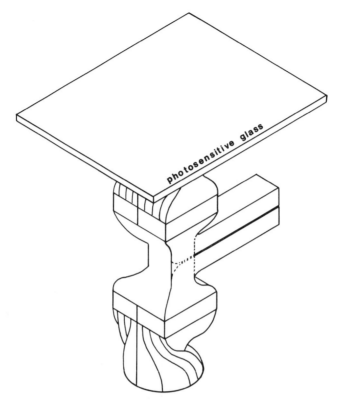

Figure 8.17. A piece of photosensitive glass can be used as an analog model of spatial memory. (Reproduced, with permission, from R. J. Baron, Visual memories and mental images. *International Journal of Man-Machine Studies*, 23, 1985, 275-311.)

at spatial memory rather than at the visual buffer is not relevant to the computational structure of the system.

The Mind's Eye

Patterns sent from spatial memory to the high-level visual networks for storage and analysis are "seen in the mind's eye." Figure 8.18 shows the pathway from spatial memory to the permanent visual storage system. This pathway conveys the only information from spatial memory that can be analyzed by the high-level visual networks, and it performs the logarithmic transformation required for storage. Only the patterns in the center of spatial memory enter this pathway, so the only way a pattern in spatial memory can be analyzed is by being shifted to the center. During a shift operation, the pattern arriving at the center is transmitted to the high-level visual networks for subsequent analysis. That pattern is "seen in the mind's eye," which is why the representations processed by spatial memory are called mental images.

Spatial memory does not distinguish patterns arriving from permanent memory from those that represent the current field of view. The permanent visual memory stores do not distinguish between current sensory representations and representations held and transformed by spatial memory.[9] As a consequence, permanent storage locations which hold memories of an experience may also hold patterns which were formed in spatial memory or transformed by spatial memory. Suppose, for example, that while viewing the picture of Monticello (Figure 8.16), the permanent storage system enabled access to memories containing representations of the Capitol. (The dome of Monticello, when selected for the focus of attention, may cause high correlation signals in storage locations containing representations of domed buildings—the Capitol, the National Gallery of Art, the Jefferson Memorial, and so forth.) If, during the experience, memories of the Capitol were recalled and reconstructed in spatial memory, and hence seen in the mind's eye, then permanent storage

---

[9] The high-level control networks, which regulate transmission over the various pathways, certainly do distinguish between information sources, and the control patterns, which are part of each storage representation, indicate the source of the stored information.

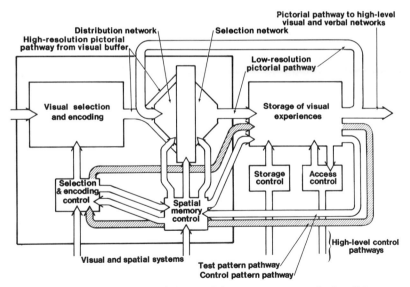

Figure 8.18. a. Pathways of the spatial memory system. b. Possible functional relationships between spatial memory and the low-level visual systems illustrated in Figure 8.10. Also see Figure 6.1. (The affect system and system of spatial coordinates are not shown here.)

locations holding the records of Monticello would also hold representations of the Capitol. Later, while recalling the memories of Monticello, memories of the Capitol may also be recalled and described. The resulting descriptions, then, would include the thoughts of the Capitol which were brought to mind while viewing the picture of Monticello.

Associative Access to Items in Spatial Memory

Images of selected objects can be individually manipulated in spatial memory. If you imagine a boy running after a dog with a house and trees in the background, the house and trees remain fixed in the background. Two questions immediately come to mind: What types of control functions are necessary for restricting operations to individual objects, and how might they be implemented? The first question can easily be answered. During a shift operation, (1) new information should be accepted provided the source location holds the representation of part of the desired object (an object is moving in the foreground), or (2) condition (1) holds and the depth component of the source location is smaller than the depth location of the destination location (the object is becoming partly hidden by moving behind a closer object). Since depth information is already part of the iconic representation, comparing depth values can easily be done. The problem therefore is, how does a spatial location signal the fact that it contains part of the representation of an object?

Locations in spatial memory holding the representation of part of an object can be identified provided (1) spatial locations are associative, (2) they compare their current representations with an externally supplied test pattern, and (3) the resulting similarity values are made available to the spatial memory control system. As noted earlier, objects typically have a limited spatial extent (hence approximately constant depth pattern), they are typically rigid (and hence have a relatively uniform visual flow), they have a small number of surfaces (and hence limited surface orientation values), and they have a constant surface quality (hence the surface extent subpattern has a limited set of values).

Thus an object can be identified associatively in spatial memory by presenting a test pattern representing its salient features. The resulting similarity pattern limits the extent in spatial memory of the object and can therefore be used by the spatial memory control system to identify spatial locations holding parts of the object. Once identified in this way, the control networks can restrict operations to those spatial locations. Referring to the classroom analogy presented earlier, imagine that each student holds a flashlight which can shine red, blue, or green, and the students are told to turn on the color red and turn off any other color provided that their neighbor's light shines red. Otherwise they are instructed to do nothing. The color red corresponds to the test pattern, and a pattern of red lights corresponds to the representation of a specific object. The additional neural circuitry required to make spatial locations associative, for distributing a test pattern to spatial locations, and for comparing depth values is all part of the iconic control system and is not presented here.

Reconstructions at Different Sizes and Orientations

Reconstruction in spatial memory can be performed at any arbitrary magnification and rotation. In the fiber-optics system, the input and output subsystems were not shifted during reconstruction. Suppose, however, that they are shifted so that each reconstructed image is exactly twice the size of its original image. (Refer to Figure 8.7.) The same process of reconstruction can still be used, but now the photosensitive glass must now be shifted twice as far for each fixation point. In this way, each component of the reconstructed image remains in registration with other components, and the only difference during reconstruction is the amount and direction of shift of the photosensitive glass. Notice that the glass never has to be rotated during a reconstruction, even when the reconstructed image is rotated. The capacity of the system to reconstruct a magnified or rotated representation is a function of the topological transformations performed by the system, not by any changes in its connectivity. By analogy, patterns of any size and orientation can be reconstructed in spatial memory. The two requirements are: (1) the reconstructed representation must be shifted in the pictorial pathway to enable the correct magnification or rotation and (2) the appropriate shift patterns must be presented to spatial memory during the reconstruction.

A Stable Representation of the Visual World

Spatial memory can create and maintain a stable representation of the visual world. (See Epstein, 1977.) Whenever the eyes are moved from one fixation point to another and the attention is directed toward a selected object, a storage representation is formed and delivered to spatial memory. If that representation is accepted by spatial memory, and if the representation in spatial memory is shifted to remain in registration with the current visual representations, then a dynamic up-to-date spatial representation of the visual world is maintained. Although the representation shifts whenever the focus of attention shifts, nonetheless it is stable and spatial. This is very unlike the retinal patterns, which change whenever the fixation point of the eyes changes. It is precisely the independence of the spatial representation from the network itself which stabilizes it and distinguishes it from the sensory representations.

The representations in spatial memory can be scanned just as if the scene being represented were in plain view. There is, of course, less information available in spatial memory. Objects in spatial memory are seen in the mind's eye when they are centered during a shift operation, and shifting the iconic representation corresponds exactly to shifting the gaze. Keep in mind the fact that the high-level control networks which regulate the gaze also determine the shift vectors to spatial memory. During ordinary viewing, shifts in the gaze are coordinated with shifts in spatial memory. However, when sensory representations are unavailable (e.g., the eyes are closed), then the high-level networks simply analyze the iconic representations held in spatial memory, and shifts correspond to **scanning the mental images**.

Patterns lost from spatial memory can no longer be seen in the mind's eye. If, for whatever reason, patterns in spatial memory are lost or degraded, the resulting high-level interpretation is one of not remembering what is in the visual field. If an object never entered the focus of attention, the representation of that object will not be a canonical representation; it will therefore not be recognizable by the high-level networks and the interpretation will be one of not having noticed the object. Figure 8.19a shows a chess configuration while Figure 8.19b shows its reconstruction in spatial memory. Notice that the pawns located in rows 3 and 6 of column 1, row 4 of column 4, and row 6 of column 6 do not appear in the reconstruction. They never entered the focus of attention and hence were not noticed. Figure 8.19c shows the fidelity pattern that resulted during the reconstruction, while Figure 8.19d shows the scan path.

The Addition of New Mental Images to Spatial Memory

I have already showed how spatial memory can be used to reconstruct a dynamic up-to-date representation of a single scene. In addition, the representations of objects not currently present can easily be added to the current representation. If the representation of an object is recalled from permanent memory and sent to spatial memory, and if spatial memory is not cleared first, then the result is the addition of the new representation to the current one. Used in this way, spatial memory becomes a tablet onto which iconic representations of arbitrary objects can be placed. Moreover, they can be inserted at any size and orientation and they can be extracted for analysis by the high-level networks: They can be inspected by the mind's eye.

Mental images of objects whose representations are held in object buffers can also be placed in spatial memory. As mentioned earlier, objects appear to be the units represented by the mind. We can hold, rotate, move, squeeze, and break objects in the mind's eye, and these operations suggest that representations of those objects can be manipulated as independent entities. Previously I indicated how the representations of individual objects might be identified and manipulated directly by spatial memory. Those same representations might be manipulated outside of spatial memory and images of them, as seen from the appropriate viewpoint, generated and sent to spatial memory. At the present time we do not know which of these alternatives, or perhaps both, actually occurs, but researchers are currently investigating both possibilities.

Spatial memory can be used during the analysis of spatial relationships as a

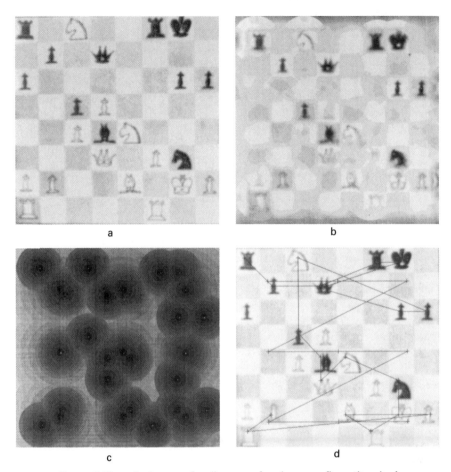

Figure 8.19. a. An image of a diagram of a chess configuration. b. A reconstructed representation of the chess configuration illustrated in a. c. The fidelity pattern generated during the reconstruction shown in b. d. The scan path used in forming the storage representation used for the reconstructed image shown in b. (Reproduced, with permission, from R. J. Baron, Visual memories and mental images. *International Journal of Man-Machine Studies*, 23, 1985, 275-311.)

temporary storage device. Consider how a person might analyze the following situation: A house has two trees in its front yard, an oak tree to the left, and a maple tree to the right. A young boy, chasing his dog, runs from the oak tree toward the maple tree. Which direction did he run? When analyzing the description of the scene, the verbal system enables access to the images of a house, trees, a dog, etc. (Details will be presented in Chapter 11.) The verbal system also analyzes the "to-the-left-of" and "to-the-right-of" relationships and enables access to control patterns that move the eyes, and hence can be used to control shifting in spatial memory. A mental image of the scene can therefore be constructed which is similar to one that would be created if a similar scene were being viewed. When the boy is imagined running from the oak tree to the maple tree, the iconic representation must be shifted to keep the boy in the center of focus. The same shift pattern would be used to maintain a stable image in spatial memory if a running boy were being tracked by the eyes. Consequently, the verbal system can analyze the shift pattern used for controlling spatial memory to answer the question.

The Manipulation of Mental Images Already in Spatial Memory

Not only can arbitrary patterns be placed in spatial memory, but representations currently held there can be modified, distorted, or transformed by various shift operations. The only shift patterns considered so far were uniform: The entire representation in spatial memory was uniformly shifted. If a nonuniform shift pattern is presented, the result may be the rotation, magnification, or distortion either of the entire representation in spatial memory or of a single object in it. Figure 8.20 shows a shift pattern that would cause the entire representation in spatial memory to be rotated, whereas the shift pattern illustrated in Figure 8.21a would cause the face illustrated in Figure 8.21b to smile as shown in Figure 8.21c. [10] The shift pattern superimposed on the cube illustrated in Figure 8.22a would cause the representation of the cube to rotate about a vertical axis through its center. Figure 8.22b shows the resulting rotated representation of the cube while Figure 8.22c shows the original representation superimposed on the rotated representation.

Just as with the smiling face, arbitrary shift patterns cause arbitrary distortions to the representation in spatial memory. If the representation were to be printed on a sheet of rubber, the effect of an arbitrary shift pattern would be the same distortion of the sheet of rubber that would yield the corresponding visual flow pattern, and hence the image on it. A shift pattern can be viewed as a visual flow pattern which specifies the desired movement of each part of the image.

Mental Rotation

Mental rotation is the process of transforming the mental image of a three-dimensional object to represent the same object as if seen from a different point of view, and the question may be asked, how are the individual shift vectors determined for performing the transformation? An equally important question

---

[10] Since visual flow patterns are part of visual storage representations, the storage system can recognize changes in facial expressions. Moreover, such changes are independent of the appearance of the individual. This, then, may in part account for our ability to recognize emotional states.

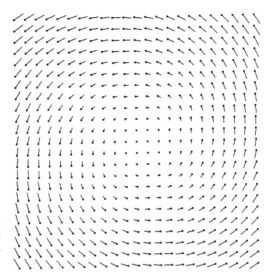

Figure 8.20. A shift pattern which will cause a uniform rotation of the pattern held in spatial memory.

is, how are the surface orientation and depth subpatterns transformed to reflect the changes in the surface orientations of the represented object? This problem is discussed in detail in the appendix to this chapter so I will only present the conceptual issues here. The problem of determining shift vectors can be reformulated as follows. Suppose a real object is placed in the field of view so that its spatial representation is as shown in Figure 8.22, and suppose it is physically rotated about the indicated axis. Each point on the object moves during the rotation and as a result the representation of each point in spatial memory moves. The result of the movement is a visual flow pattern. If, for each spatial location, the visual flow can be computed that would result if the real object were to be rotated in space about the indicated axis, then those visual flow vectors are the required shift vectors to transform the current iconic representation into the rotated representation.

In order to compute the visual flow pattern resulting from the rotation of an object in space, several facts must be known: (1) the coordinates of each point on the object; (2) the axis of rotation; and (3) the rate of rotation. Given a spatial location, the coordinates of each point on the object are implicitly represented in the control pattern and depth subpatterns of the object's representation. The axis and speed of rotation are input parameters to the system. Hence the parameters required for computing the visual flow at each spatial location would be present if the rotation parameters were present. The rotation parameters are the same for all spatial locations and can easily be transmitted to them simultaneously. Each spatial location could, under these circumstances, compute the required visual flow to effect the desired transfor-

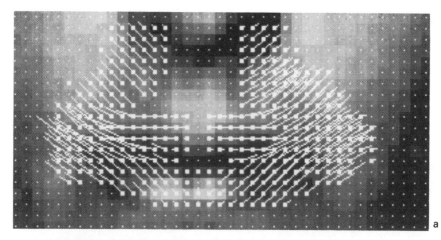
a

Figure 8.21. a. A shift pattern that will cause the unsmiling face shown in b to smile as shown in c. b. A representation of a face which is not smiling. c. The representation generated in spatial memory by applying the shift pattern shown in a to the representation shown in b.

mation. Once the visual flow vectors are determined, each spatial location can inform its destination location of the correct shift vector, and therefore the iconic representation of a three-dimensional object can be transformed just as if the object were actually being rotated in space. (Neural networks for performing these computations are currently under investigation.)

Mental images can also be rotated without using the shifting apparatus of spatial memory. When the rotation is through a sufficiently large angle, mental rotation can be performed by reconstructing a brand new iconic representation with the depicted object in its new orientation. When reconstructing a rotated representation, various features of the current representation are individually transformed, as illustrated in Figure 8.23. Each feature is recognized and then reconstructed in its new orientation, and when placed in spatial memory, the newly reconstructed features are placed in their correct spatial relationships to one another as shown in the figure. This is analogous to the way an artist would sketch the figure on paper.

SUMMARY

This chapter suggested one way that visual information might be represented in permanent storage and how storage representations could then be reconstructed. The reconstructed storage representations, mental images, are held as temporary dynamic patterns in spatial memory. Spatial memory is not only a temporary storage device which holds dynamic patterns, it is also a pattern processor which

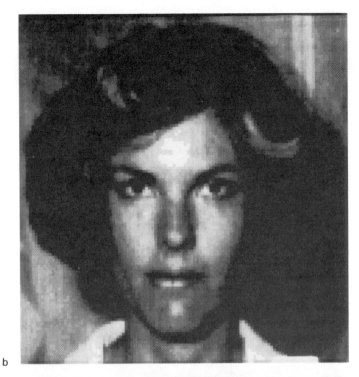

b

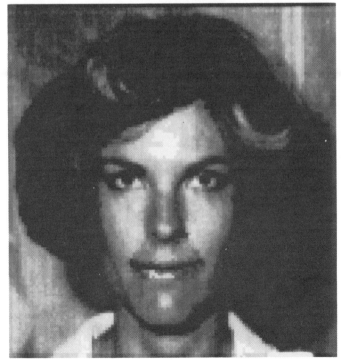

c

211

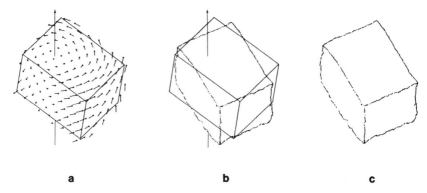

a   b   c

Figure 8.22. a. The spatial memory representation of a cube shown with a superimposed shift pattern and axis of rotation. b. The result of applying the shift pattern in a to the representation of a cube it is superimposed on. c. The original and rotated representations of the cube illustrated in a. (Reproduced, with permission, from R. J. Baron, Visual memories and mental images. *International Journal of Man-Machine Studies*, 23, 1985, 275-311.)

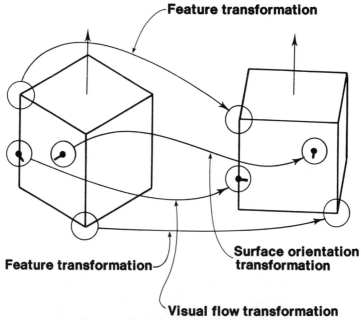

Figure 8.23. During a mental rotation, features must be transformed, surface orientation vectors must be transformed, and visual flow vectors must be transformed. All three types of transformations are illustrated here. (Slightly modified from R. J. Baron, Visual memories and mental images. *International Journal of Man-Machine Studies*, 23, 1985, 275-311.)

can add new images to the existing ones, shift them, rotate them, and distort them in relatively arbitrary ways. Spatial memory can maintain a stable active representation of the current visual world, which can then be scanned in the absence of visible inputs, and it can be used as a temporary storage device during a variety of mental operations.

Spatial memory creates and manipulates mental images. Because spatial memory is a fixed physical network, it has a specific shape and limited spatial extent. Moreover, images which are shifted beyond its edges are lost—they fall off, so to speak. Because there is a fixed pathway from spatial memory to the high-level visual system, and because of the logarithmic transformation on the spatial representations, images have high resolution in the center and decreasing resolution toward the edges. The need in the human imagery system for refreshing the images would be modeled by setting particular trace parameters in spatial memory; parameters whose values were not specified for this presentation. These properties of spatial memory have all been noted in the human imagery system. For further details about mental imagery, the reader is directed to the references of this chapter.

The relationship between spatial memory, the permanent stores of experience, visual naming stores, and other high-level visual processes was suggested in Figure 8.18 and will be explored in greater detail in the next chapter.

REFERENCES

Baron, R. J. (1981). Mechanisms of human facial recognition. *International Journal of Man-Machine Studies, 15,* 137-178.

———— (1985). Visual memories and mental images. *International Journal of Man-Machine Studies, 23,* 275-311.

Block, N. (Ed.). (1981). *Imagery.* Cambridge, MA: MIT Press.

Chase, W. G. (Ed.). (1973). *Visual information processing.* New York: Academic Press.

Churchill, R. V. (1960). *Complex variables and applications.* New York: McGraw-Hill.

Cooper, L. A. (1975). Mental rotation of random two-dimensional shapes. *Cognitive Psychology, 7,* 20-43.

Cooper, L. A. & Shepard, R. N. (1973). Chronometric studies of the rotation of mental images. In W. G. Chase (Ed.). *Visual information processing.* New York: Academic Press.

Damasio, A. R., Damasio, H., & Van Hoesen, G. W. (1982). Prosopagnosia: Anatomic basis and behavioral mechanisms. *Neurology, 32,* 331-341.

Epstein, W. (Ed.). (1977). Stability and constancy in visual perception: Mechanisms and processes. New York: John Wiley & Sons.

Hayes, J. R. (1973). On the functioning of visual imagery in elementary mathematics. In W. G. Chase (Ed.). *Visual information processing.* New York: Academic Press.

Heaton, J. M. (1968). *The eye. Phenomenology and psychology of function and disorder.* London: Tavistock.

Julstrom, B. A., & Baron, R. J. (1985). A model of mental imagery. *International Journal of Man-Machine Studies, 23,* 313-334.

Kosslyn, S. M. (1973). Scanning visual images: Some structural implications. *Perception and Psychophysics, 14,* 90-94.

———— (1980). *Image and mind*. Cambridge, MA: Harvard University Press.

Kosslyn, S. M., Ball, T. M., & Reiser, B. J. (1978). Visual images preserve metric spatial information: Evidence from studies of image scanning. *Journal of Experimental Psychology: Human Perception and Performance, 4*, 47-60.

Kosslyn, S. M., & Pomerantz, J. R. (1977). Imagery, propositions, and the form of internal representations. *Cognitive Psychology, 9*, 52-76.

Kosslyn, S. M., & Schwarz, S. P. (1977). A simulation of visual imagery. *Cognitive Science, 1*, 265-295.

Land, E. H. (1977). The retinex theory of color vision. *Scientific American, 237*, 108-128.

Luria, A. R. (1966). *Higher cortical functions in man*. New York: Basic Books.

Metzler, J. (1977). Mental transformations: A top-down analysis. In J. Metzler, (Ed.), *Systems neuroscience*. New York: Academic Press, 1-24.

Metzler, J., & Shepard, R. N. (1974). Transformational studies of the internal representation of three-dimensional objects. In R. L. Solso, (Ed.), *Theories of cognitive psychology: The Loyola symposium*. Potomac, MD: Lawrence Erlbaum Associates.

Paivio, A. (1979). *Imagery and verbal processes*. Hillsdale, NJ: Lawrence Erlbaum Associates.

Reed, S. K. (1974). Structural descriptions and the limitations of visual images. *Memory and Cognition, 2*, 329-336.

Schwartz, E. L. (1977). Spatial mapping in the primate sensory projection: Analytic structures and relevance to perception. *Biological Cybernetics, 25*, 181-194.

Shepard, R. N., & Cooper, L. A. (1982). *Mental images and their transformations*. Cambridge, MA: MIT Press.

Shepard, R. N., & Metzler, J. (1971). Mental rotation of three-dimensional objects. *Science, 171*, 701-703.

The foregoing references present excellent discussions on visual imagery and visual information processing. The reader might also like to consult literature on eidetic images (Coltheart, 1975; Haber, 1969, 1979, 1980, 1983; and Holding, 1975), which are related in some yet unknown way to the low-level visual networks, and to the literature on eye movements during visual perception (Carpenter & Just, 1972; Corcoran & Jackson, 1977; Gould, 1967, 1969, 1973; Howe, 1969; Jonides, 1981; Just & Carpenter, 1977, Kaufman & Richards, 1969; Prinz, 1977; and Senders, Fisher, & Monty, 1978), which relate to the formation of storage representations. Several additional references on visual imagery may also be of interest (Beck, 1982; Bishop & Henry, 1971, Dick, 1976, Lee, 1978; Kosslyn, et al., 1979; Roitblat, 1982; and Ullman, 1980).

Beck, J. (1982.) *Organization and representation in perception*. Hillsdale, NJ: Lawrence Erlbaum Associates.

Bishop, P. O., & Henry, G. H. (1971). Spatial vision. *Annual Review of Psychology, 22*, 119-159.

Carpenter, P. A., & Just, M. A. (1972). Semantic control of eye movement during sentence-picture verification. *Perception and Psychophysics, 12*, 61-64.

Coltheart, M. (1975). Iconic memory: A reply to Professor Holding. *Memory and Cognition, 3*, 42-48.

Corcoran, D. W., & Jackson, A. (1977). Basic processes and strategies in visual search. In S. Dornic, (Ed.). *Attention and performance, VI*. Hillsdale, NJ: Lawrence Erlbaum Associates, 387-411.

Dick, A. O. (1976). Spatial abilities. In H. Whitaker, & H. A. Whitaker, (Eds.). *Studies in neurolinguistics, Vol. 2*. New York: Academic Press, 225-268.

Gould, J. D. (1967). Pattern recognition and eye movement parameters. *Perception and Psychophysics*, *2*, 399-407.

———— (1969). Eye-movement parameters and pattern discrimination. *Perception and Psychophysics*, *6*, 311-320.

———— (1973). Eye movements during visual search and memory search. *Journal of Experimental Psychology*, *98*, 184-195.

Haber, R. N. (1969). Eidetic images. *Scientific American*, *220*, 37-44.

———— (1980). Eidetic images are not just imaginary. *Psychology Today*, *14*, 72-82.

———— (1979). Twenty years of haunting eidetic imagery: Where's the ghost? *Behavioral and Brain Sciences*, *2*, 583-629.

———— (1983). The impending demise of the icon: A critique on the concept of iconic storage in visual information processing. *The Behavioral and Brain Sciences*, *6*, 1-54.

Holding, D. H. (1975). Sensory storage reconsidered. *Memory and Cognition*, *3*, 31-41.

Howe, J. A. M. (1969). Eye movement and visual search strategy. (Tech. Rep. MIP-R-69), Department of Machine Intelligence, University of Edinburgh, Edinburgh, Scotland.

Jonides, J. (1981). Voluntary verses automatic control over the mind's eye's movement. (Tech. Rep. No. 15), Cognitive Science, University of Michigan, Ann Arbor, MI.

Just, M. A., & Carpenter, P. A. (1977). *Cognitive processes in comprehension*. Hillsdale, NJ: Lawrence Erlbaum Associates.

Kaufman, L., & Richards, W. (1969). Spontaneous fixation tendencies for visual forms. *Perception and Psychophysics*, *5*, 85-88.

Kosslyn, S. M., et al. (1979). On the demystification of mental imagery. *The Behavioral and Brain Sciences*, *2*, 535-581.

Lee, D. N. (1978). The functions of vision. In H. L. Pick, Jr., & E. Saltzman, (Eds.). *Modes of perceiving and processing information*. Hillsdale, NJ: Lawrence Erlbaum Associates, 159-170.

Prinz, W. (1977). Memory control of visual search. In S. Dornic, (Ed.). *Attention and performance, VI*. Hillsdale, NJ: Lawrence Erlbaum Associates, 441-462.

Roitblat, H. L. (1982). The meaning of representation in animal memory. *The Behavioral and Brain Sciences*, *5*, 353-406.

Senders, J. W., Fisher, D. F., & Monty, R. A. (1978). *Eye movements and the higher psychological functions*. Hillsdale, NJ: Lawrence Erlbaum Associates.

Ullman, S. (1980). Against direct perception. *The Behavioral and Brain Sciences*, *3*, 373-415.

APPENDIX 3: A NEURAL REALIZATION OF SPATIAL MEMORY[11]

The body of this chapter described how spatial memory operates. This appendix describes how spatial memory can be constructed out of neurons in a network which resembles the primary visual cortex.

Three categories of neurons are required for constructing spatial memory: information neurons, regulatory neurons, and store-now control neurons. **Information neurons** hold and transfer information between one another. They are self-excitatory and continue to fire at a constant rate until they receive an effectual **store-now control signal** from a store-now control neuron. Upon

---

[11]This appendix is reprinted, in part, from R. J. Baron (1985) Visual memories and mental images. *International Journal of Man-Machine Studies*, 23, 275-311, and from B. A. Julstrom and R. J. Baron (1985) A model of mental imagery. *International Journal of Man-Machine Studies*, 23, 313-334.

receipt of the signal, their firing rates change and become proportional to the current algebraic sum of inputs from all presynaptic information neurons.[12] As a consequence, the set of all information neurons forms a temporary storage system which adapts to an input pattern upon receipt of a store-now control signal. Moreover, both static and dynamic representations of information are present. The static pattern is the pattern of neural self-coupling parameters that enables the information neurons to fire at a particular rate; the dynamic pattern is the firing pattern of the information neurons themselves.

Regulatory neurons control the coupling between all information neurons that make contacts within their regulatory field, but they do not directly modulate the firing rates of information neurons. (Refer to Chapter 2.) In order for information neurons to be functionally connected they must make contacts within the regulatory field of an active regulatory neuron.

Store-now control neurons, like regulatory neurons, do not directly modulate the firing rates of information neurons. Store-now control neurons have effectual coupling which initiates changes in the self-coupling parameters of information neurons. Store-now control neurons therefore determine when information storage occurs—the time of temporary consolidation.

Information neurons are labeled according to which low-level representation they hold, and they only contact other information neurons having the same subpattern label. For example, the neuron in one spatial location holding the vertical component of the visual flow pattern only contacts information neurons in neighboring spatial locations that hold the vertical component of the visual flow pattern. As a result, all subpatterns in spatial memory retain their identity during shift operations, and spatial memory should be thought of as a collection of parallel independent processors, one for each component of the mental image.

Contacts between information neurons are systematically organized. Each spatial location is functionally divided into concentric cylindrical shells as shown in Figure 8.24. Inputs from neighboring spatial locations terminate within the cylindrical shell, which is proportional to its distance away.[13] Moreover, the terminations are restricted to the pie-shaped segment which is in

---

[12]The traces in spatial memory are those biological parameters which determine how fast a neuron will fire. I have assumed that iconic traces do not decay, but studies on visual imagery suggest that indeed they do decay. Since the structure of spatial memory is independent of the trace parameters, I chose nondegrading traces for simplicity.

[13]I have assumed a linear relationship for simplicity. A better, and biologically more plausible assumption, is that inputs from neighboring spatial locations terminate in the cylindrical shell which is proportional to the logarithm of its distance away. This would enable shifting over arbitrary distances. However, if the regulatory neurons are a fixed size, then information would be averaged during a shifting operation, and more information would be lost for large shifts than for short shifts. Since this type of detail is not essential for understanding the general nature of spatial memory, I chose the simpler assumption.

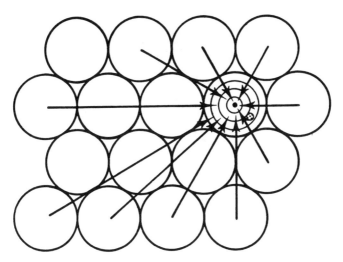

Figure 8.24. Arrival of information from adjacent spatial memory locations is systematic. All information from a single different spatial location arrives within the same microvolume. (Reproduced, with permission, from R. J. Baron, Visual memories and mental images. *International Journal of Man-Machine Studies*, 23, 1985, 275-311.)

line with the source location. Finally, representatives of all subpattern components contact their counterparts within the same microvolume.

The regulatory fields of regulatory neurons are restricted to vertical microcolumns, as shown in Figure 8.25. As a result of this organization, each regulatory neuron determines a source location at a specified distance and direction away. The spatial memory control system analyzes the shift vectors described earlier and activates the correct regulatory neuron to establish the coupling.

The physiology of spatial memory resembles that of the primary visual cortex. Consider the activity that results in the model when the fixation point of the eyes shifts. Because of the shifting sensory pattern on the retinas, a visual flow pattern will be computed by the low-level visual networks. This visual flow is uniform, and hence each component will have a similar value. In order to keep the current iconic representation in registration with the changing sensory pattern, the spatial representation must be uniformly shifted. Moreover, the shift pattern must be identical to the computed visual flow pattern. Hence the visual flow pattern, which is computed by the low-level visual networks, could be used as a shift pattern to control spatial memory.

Now consider the resulting activity in spatial memory when the eyes shift by a fixed amount. For a given shift, a particular regulatory cell in each spatial location must fire, which in turn enables the spatial representation to be shifted

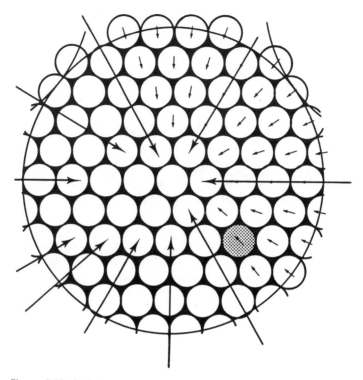

Figure 8.25. A diagram of one spatial memory location showing the microvolumes used for regulating information transfers from nearby spatial locations. Compare this figure with Figure 8.24. (Reproduced, with permission, from R. J. Baron, Visual memories and mental images. *International Journal of Man-Machine Studies*, 23, 1985, 275-311.)

in registration with the sensory pattern. It follows that the microvolume of spatial memory containing the regulatory cell must be sensitive to sensory patterns moving in a specific direction. Moreover, because of the systematic arrangement of regulatory cells required to implement arbitrary shifting of patterns in spatial memory, one would observe a systematic change in the directional sensitivities as one penetrates spatial memory in a direction parallel to its surface. Refer to Figure 8.26, and compare it with Figures 7.15 and 7.16. This is similar to the organization of the orientation-sensitive complex cells in the primary visual cortex (Hubel & Wiesel, 1977), and it is tempting to wonder whether complex cell activity is a consequence of an organization which maintains a stable representation of the visual world. (Complex cell activity by its very nature is already implicated in the computation of visual flow.)

The mechanism of connecting spatial locations together should now be clear. The question remains, how does the spatial memory control system generate the appropriate shift vectors for various operations?

THE CONTROL OF SPATIAL MEMORY

A single **spatial memory control system** controls spatial memory. The control system informs the spatial locations of the transformation they must perform, it initiates the steps of the transformation, and it directs exchanges of data with permanent visual memory. Communications pathways connect the control system directly to each spatial location. The control system always broadcasts control information to all spatial locations simultaneously; it does not select any particular locations to receive control signals or to be excluded from receiving them.

The control system broadcasts to the spatial locations two types of signals: **control signals** and **transformation control patterns**. A control signal directs all

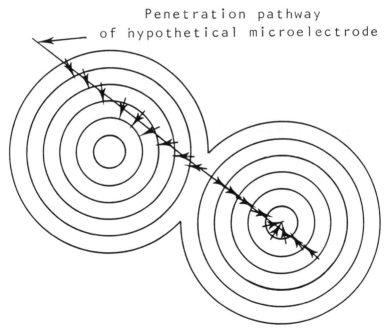

Figure 8.26. Directional sensitivities of microvolumes in spatial memory are a consequence of its microstructure. This figure illustrates how directional sensitivities change along a linear penetration. (Reproduced, with permission, from R. J. Baron, Visual memories and mental images. *International Journal of Man-Machine Studies*, 23, 1985, 275-311.)

spatial locations to perform, in unison, one of six actions. A transformation control pattern specifies the parameters of the transformation each spatial location must perform on its information.

There are six control signals to each spatial location. A **conditional acceptance signal** commands each spatial locations to accept conditionally new information arriving over its input pathway from memory or the low-level visual networks. In response, each spatial location compares the fidelity value of the information it is holding with its own distance from the center of spatial memory. If its distance is smaller, it accepts the incoming information. Otherwise it retains its old information. The remaining five control signals tell the spatial locations how to manipulate the images they are holding. The first of these, **prepare for transformation**, notifies the spatial locations that they will be performing a transformation and to accept the parameters given by the transformation control pattern (to be described next). The **compute destination** control signal tells each spatial location to compute the address of the spatial location it will send information to during the pending transformation. The **broadcast destination** control signal causes each spatial location to broadcast to all neighboring spatial locations an indication of which one will receive its transformed surface patch. It also instructs the spatial locations to analyze the broadcasts of other spatial locations and determine from which one it will receive information. The **transform** control signal tells each location to transform its information according to the pending transformation. The **transmit** control commands each spatial location to do two things: (1) broadcast its transformed information to all neighboring locations and (2) to accept new information from the location it determined in response to the broadcast destination control signal.

The four **transformation control patterns** specify the type of transformation (shifting, scaling, or rotation) and give its parameters. The transformation control pattern that specifies a shift contains two parameters: the horizontal and vertical components of the shift. The transformation control pattern that specifies a scaling transformation contains three parameters: the center of the scale change on spatial memory (two parameters) and the magnitude of the change. The transformation control pattern that specifies a two-dimensional rotation contains three parameters: the center of the rotation (two parameters) and its magnitude. The transformation control pattern that specifies a three-dimensional rotation contains seven parameters. The first three give the axis of rotation in the 2½-D coordinates of the spatial image; the fourth, fifth, and sixth components describe a point through which the axis passes, in those same coordinates; and the last component gives the magnitude of the rotation. Figure 8.27 illustrates the parameters of this transformation.

The six control signals and four transformation control patterns enable spatial memory to translate, scale, rotate in two dimensions, and rotate in three dimensions the spatial image of an object.

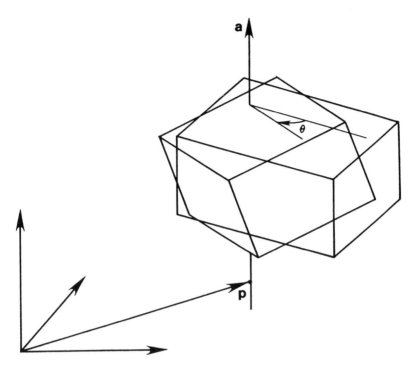

Figure 8.27. Seven parameters specify a rotation in space: three parameters specify a point on the axis of rotation, p; three parameters specify the direction of the axis of rotation, a; and one parameter specifies the angle of rotation, theta. (Reproduced, with permission, from B. A. Julstrom & R. J. Baron, A model of mental imagery. *International Journal of Man-Machine Studies*, 23, 1985, 313-334.)

Transforming the Image Held in Spatial Memory

If spatial memory encodes an up-to-date spatial image of an object and the object is moved in space—shifted relative to the viewer or rotated about an axis—the representations of the visible surfaces of the object must shift among the spatial locations of spatial memory. In addition, the vectors describing each surface must be modified, depending on the transformation. For example, if the image rotates in the image plane, all surface orientation and visual flow vectors must undergo the same rotation, as Figure 8.28 shows.

A **mental transformation** is a transformation performed by spatial memory directly on the representation it holds. During a mental transformation, spatial memory modifies the spatial image of a visible object so that the new representation is the same as if a new image had been created after a physical modification of the visible object. For example, a mental rotation of an object's spatial image is a transformation which directly modifies the mental image as if

221

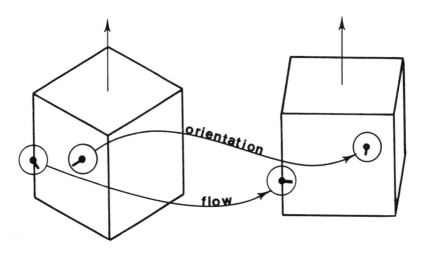

Figure 8.28. Both surface orientation and visual flow are transformed in the same way during a three-dimensional rotation. (Reproduced, with permission, from B. A. Julstrom & R. J. Baron, A model of mental imagery. *International Journal of Man-Machine Studies*, 23, 1985, 313-334.)

the object itself were rotated about some axis in space. Each visible surface element on the object is represented by the surface patch at one spatial location before the transformation and generally at a different spatial location after the transformation. For a particular surface element, the spatial location which holds it before a transformation is its **source location** and the one that holds it after a transformation is its **destination location**.

Mental transformations are governed by a sequence of control signals broadcast by the control system to all spatial locations and proceed in several steps. The control system begins a mental transformation by broadcasting to all locations the prepare for transformation control signal and the transformation control pattern for the transformation. The control signal instructs them to accept the transformation parameters.

Next, the supervisor transmits the compute destination control signal. Upon receiving it, each spatial location computes the address of the destination of its current surface element under the pending transformation. The supervisor next transmits the broadcast destination control signal. In response, each spatial location broadcasts the address of its destination location to all spatial locations within its communications radius.

As Figure 8.24 illustrated, input connections from neighboring locations arrive at specific microvolumes within each spatial location. Among those inputs are ones which carry the address of the destination location. Cells within each microcolumn compare the arriving address with its own address. If the two values match, the control neuron which establishes the communication link is activated. This establishes the communication pathway. See Figure 8.29. Thus in response to the **broadcast displacement** control signal, the spatial locations prepare the communications pattern necessary to carry out the transformation.

Next, the supervisor transmits the **transform** control signal. Upon receiving this control signal, each spatial location transforms its current information according to the specified image transformation. For example, if the image is to be rotated in the image plane, each surface orientation and visual flow vector must be similarly rotated. In general, these transformations are similar to those which compute the address of the destination location, though they are often simpler.

Finally, initiated by the **transmit** control signal from the control system, all spatial locations broadcast their transformed information. All of the transformed information patterns are received simultaneously, and each spatial location now holds part of the transformed image. Because the terminals have established a communications pattern corresponding to the transformation, it follows that each part of the image moves from its current spatial location to its appropriate destination location. Any spatial location which is not the destination for any information replaces its current information with the background value. The entire spatial image is now transformed.

In summary, this sequence of commands from the control system controls every mental transformation in spatial memory:

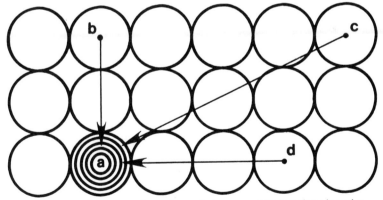

Figure 8.29. The connections shown between spatial locations b and a, c and a, and d and a determine which location sends information to location a. (Similar connections from other spatial locations to location a are not shown.) These connections are regulatory; they determine which information pathways will be active during a transformation but not what information will be transformed. (Reproduced, with permission, from B. A. Julstrom & R. J. Baron, A model of mental imagery. *International Journal of Man-Machine Studies*, 23, 1985, 313-334.)

prepare for transformation
transformation control pattern
compute destination
broadcast destination
transform transmit

Note that using these commands, spatial memory can shift the spatial image of an object within spatial memory without fundamentally altering that image. Thus the representation of an object is independent of its location in spatial memory.

Translation, Scaling, and Rotation in the Image Plane

The simplest transformation performed by spatial memory is **translation**, a rigid shift of the image within spatial memory. The transformation control pattern of a translation consists of its horizontal and vertical displacements in the coordinates of spatial memory, and these values are the displacement values broadcast by the spatial locations. No further computations are necessary, and the components of the surface patches are left unchanged.

In a **scaling** transformation, the image in spatial memory is shrunk or expanded about a given spatial location and the spatial locations must compute the destinations for their surface patches. The transformation control pattern of a scaling transformation describes the center of the transformation (x_c, y_c) and the scaling factor f. The scaling factor determines how much the image shrinks or expands, and the surface patch held in a spatial location (x_o, y_o) has as its destination the location (x, y), where

$$x = f(x_o - x_c) + x_c = x_o f + x_c(1 - f), \text{ and}$$
$$y = f(y_o - y_c) + y_c = y_o f + y_c(1 - f).$$

The geometry of Figure 8.30 justifies these formulas.

The transformation control pattern of a rotation in the image plane specifies the center of the rotation (x_c, y_c) and its magnitude T. Under such a transformation, the destination location for the surface patch held in the spatial location at (x_o, y_o) is (x, y), where

$$x = (x_o - x_c) \cos\Theta - (y_o - y_c) \sin\Theta + x_c, \text{ and}$$
$$y = (x_o - x_c) \sin\Theta - (y_o - y_c) \cos\Theta + y_c.$$

In this case, the components of both the visual flow vector **F** and the surface orientation vector **O** which lie in the image plane must undergo a similar

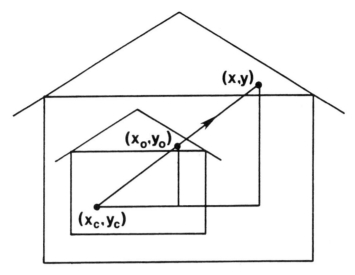

Figure 8.30. The geometry of a scaling transformation. As the image expands (or contracts) by a factor of f around the surface patch at spatial location (x_c, y_c), the surface patch at location (x_0, y_0) moves to location (x, y). Thus $(x - x_c) = f \times (x_0 - x_c)$ and $(y - y_c) = f \times (y_0 - y_c)$. (Reproduced, with permission, from B. A. Julstrom & R. J. Baron, A model of mental imagery. *International Journal of Man-Machine Studies*, 23, 1985, 313-334.)

transformation. Figure 8.31 shows the result of applying a shift pattern for a uniform rotation to the representation of a car in spatial memory. (Figure 8.20 shows a shift pattern for a uniform rotation in the opposite direction.)

REPRESENTING THREE-DIMENSIONAL ROTATIONS

Rotations in three dimensions can be computed in several ways. Many texts describe the use of three-by-three matrices to represent rotations (e.g., Minsky, 1955). When homogeneous coordinates consisting of four components each describe locations in three-space, four-by-four matrices represent both rotations and translations (Newman & Sproull, 1973; Paul, 1981). However, quaternions (Hamilton, 1866; Pervin & Webb, 1982) provide a more efficient representation of rotations and will be used here.

Quaternions are expressions of the form $\mathbf{q} = (a, b, c, d)$, where a, b, c, and d are real numbers. The sum of two quaternions is computed component by component: if $\mathbf{q_1} = (a_1, b_1, c_1, d_1)$ and $\mathbf{q_2} = (a_2, b_2, c_2, d_2)$, then $\mathbf{q_1} + \mathbf{q_2} = (a_1 + a_2, b_1 + b_2, c_1 + c_2, d_1 + d_2)$. If we let $\mathbf{q} = (a, b, c, d) = a + bi + cj + dk$ and define multiplication by

$$i^2 = j^2 = k^2 = ijk = -1$$

225

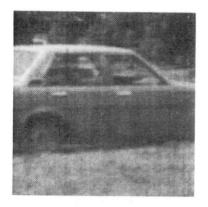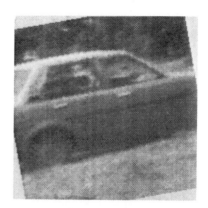

Figure 8.31. A two-dimensional rotation which rotates the image in the image plane about its center. (Reproduced, with permission, from B. A. Julstrom & R. J. Baron, A model of mental imagery. *International Journal of Man-Machine Studies*, 23, 1985, 313-334.)

then quaternions can be multiplied as polynomials in $\mathbf{i}$, $\mathbf{j}$, and $\mathbf{k}$: $q_1q_2 = (r,s,t,u)$, where

$$r = a_1a_2 - b_1b_2 - c_1c_2 - d_1d_2$$
$$s = a_1b_2 + b_1a_2 + c_1d_2 - d_1c_2$$
$$t = a_1c_2 - b_1d_2 + c_1a_2 + d_1b_2$$
$$u = a_1d_2 + b_1c_2 - c_1b_2 + d_1a_2$$

With the operations of addition and multiplication, the quaternions form a four-dimensional system which preserves all the familiar arithmetical properties of the real and complex numbers except multiplicative commutativity.

A quaternion whose real (first) term is zero can represent a three-dimensional vector under the usual identification of $\mathbf{i}$, $\mathbf{j}$, and $\mathbf{k}$ with the unit vectors along the three coordinate axes. With this association, a rotation through an angle θ about an axis a (through the origin) is represented by the quaternion R, where

$$R = \cos(\theta/2) + \sin(\theta/2)\ \mathbf{a}.$$

A location vector $\mathbf{v}$ rotates to $R\mathbf{v}R^{-1}$, where R^{-1} is the inverse of R under quaternion multiplication. If the axis a passes through a point $\mathbf{p}$, not necessarily the origin, $\mathbf{v}$ rotates to $R(\mathbf{v} - \mathbf{p})R^{-1} + \mathbf{p}$. The last section of this appendix gives a fuller discussion of quaternions and rotation.

Each spatial location holds the two-dimensional coordinates and the relative depth values of its current surface patch. Thus spatial memory holds a 2½-D representation of the image's visible surfaces. Upon receiving the **Compute displacements** command from the control system, each spatial location employs quaternion operations to compute the 2½-D position in spatial memory which will encode the same surface patch after rotation. The first two coordinates of this position indicate the spatial location which is the destination of the surface patch. Since each spatial location knows its own coordinates, it can subtract them from the coordinates of the destination location to obtain the displacement over which it must send its image information, its surface patch, according to the rotation. This displacement is identical to the visual flow of the represented surface, assuming the object were actually rotating in space.

For example, suppose the surface patch held in the the spatial location at (100,100) has relative depth value 300; its 2½-D coordinates are then (100,100,300). The image of which this patch is a part will undergo a rotation through five degrees about the axis (1,1,1), which passes through the point (200,200,250). The quaternion R represents the rotation, where

$$R = \cos (5/2)^0 + \sin (5/2)^0 (0,1,1,1)$$
$$= (0.999,0.044,0.044,0.044).$$

The inverse of R under quaternion multiplication is

$$R^{-1} = (0.995,-0.044,-0.044,-0.044),$$

so the surface patch at (100,100,300) must move under the rotation to the 2½-D coordinates (113.6,87.6,289.9):

$$R((0,100,100,300) - (0,200,200,250))R^{-1} + (0,200,200,250)$$
$$= (0,113.6,87.6,298,9).$$

The relative displacement in spatial memory over which the surface patch must be transmitted is then

$$(113.6-100,87.6-100) = (13.6,-12.4)$$

This last pair is broadcast by the spatial location at (100,100) in response to the **broadcast displacements** control signal.

VISUAL FLOW IN SPATIAL MEMORY

Each surface patch held in spatial memory includes a vector **F** which represents the visual flow—the apparent movement—of the corresponding visible surface in the original scene. To transform the image according to this visual flow pattern, the spatial locations compute the destination addresses based on their own addresses and the component of the visual flow lying in the image plane.

The supervisor transmits no transformation control pattern for the visual flow transformation; none is needed. Spatial memory implements visual flow by responding to the control system's **compute displacement** control signal by applying the visual flow vectors of its current surface patches.

The model does not describe how spatial memory transforms the surface patches of an image during the visual flow transformation. In contrast to the other transformations described here in which each spatial location can appropriately transform its surface patch by applying only the information in the transformation's transformation control pattern, in the visual flow transformation, the spatial locations must also have more global information to transform their surface patches correctly. Each spatial location might need to know the visual flow being imposed by its neighbors or even something of the object whose image is being transformed; consider the difference between a blimp inflating and an object exploding.

QUATERNIONS AND ROTATION

Quaternions, invented and described by Hamilton before the turn of the century, form a four-dimensional algebraic system with addition and multiplication. This system preserves all the properties of the real and complex numbers except the commutativity of multiplication.

A quaternion can be represented as

$$a + bi + cj + dk$$

where a, b, c, and d are real numbers. Quaternion addition proceeds in the obvious way, term by term, while the following relations govern quaternion multiplication:

$$i^2 = j^2 = k^2 = ijk = -1.$$

As consequences of these relations, $ij = k$, $ji = -k$, $jk = i$, $kj = -i$, $ki = j$, and $ik = -j$. With these rules, we can multiply quaternions as polynomials in i, j, and k. For example,

$$
\begin{aligned}
(2 + 3i - k)(2i + j) &= 4i + 2j + 6i2 + 3ij - 2ki - kj \\
&= 4i + 2j - 6 + 3k + 2j + i \\
&= -6 + 5i + 3k
\end{aligned}
$$

Quaternion multiplication does not commute, but quaternions preserve the other arithmetical properties of real and complex numbers. Indeed, the set of quaternions for which the coefficients of i, j, and k are zero is isomorphic to the reals, and the set of quaternions formed of a real term and just one of i, j, or k, for example [a + cj : a, c real], is isomorphic to the complex numbers.

The identity element of quaternion multiplication is $1 + 0i + 0j + 0k$, and every nonzero quaternion q has a multiplicative inverse q^{-1} such that qq^{-1} and $q^{-1}q$ both equal the identity. The magnitude $|q|$ of a quaternion q is, analogously to vectors, the square root of the sum of the squares of the four real coefficients in q:

$$|a + bi + cj + dk| = SQRT(a^2 + b^2 + c^2 + d^2),$$

and the inverse q^{-1} of a quaternion $q = a + bi + cj + dk$ is given by this relation:

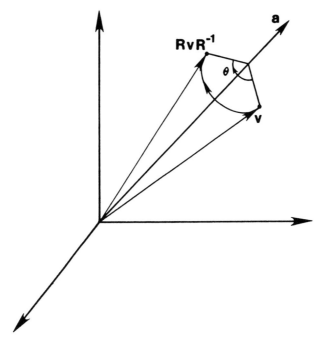

Figure 8.32. Quaternion computation for rotating **v** about axis **a** by θ degrees, when **a** passes through the origin. (Reproduced, with permission, from B. A. Julstrom & R. J. Baron, A model of mental imagery. *International Journal of Man-Machine Studies*, 23, 1985, 313-334.)

$$q^{-1} = (1/|q|)(a - bi - cj - dk)$$

For example, if $q = 2 + i - 2k$, then $|q| = 3$, and

$$q^{-1} = (1/3)(2 - i + 2k) = 2/3 - i/3 + 2k/3$$

A quaternion whose real term is zero can represent a three-dimensional vector, under the usual association of **i**, **j**, and **k** with unit vectors on the three coordinate axes. Interestingly, the quaternion product of two such vectors **q** and **r** is

$$qr = -(q \cdot r) + (q \times r),$$

where q·r and qxr are the usual inner and cross vector products.

As Pervin and Webb (1982) observe, however, "The greatest strength of quaternions is their ability to represent rotations." A rotation through an angle O about an axis a which intersects the coordinate origin, is represented by the quaternion

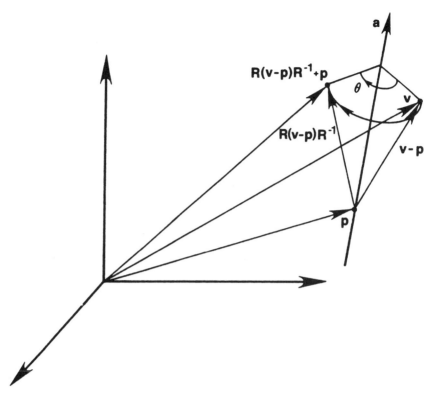

Figure 8.33. Quaternion computation for rotating vector **v** about axis **a** which passes through point **p** by θ degrees. (Reproduced, with permission, from B. A. Julstrom & R. J. Baron, A model of mental imagery. *International Journal of Man-Machine Studies*, 23, 1985, 313-334.)

$$R = \cos (\theta/2) + \sin (\theta/2) \, a.$$

The new location of a vector **v** following the rotation is RvR^{-1}, where R^{-1} is the inverse of R under quaternion multiplication. Figure 8.32 illustrates such a rotation.

Thus, a rotation through 90° bout the z-axis is represented by

$$R = \cos 450 + \sin 450 \, (0 + 0i + 0j + k)$$
$$= 0.707 + 0.707k$$

The inverse of R is $0.707 - 0.707k$, and the new location of the point $(1,1,1)$ under the rotation R represents is

$$RvR^{-1} = (0.707 + 0.707k)(i + j + k)(0.707 - 0.707k)$$
$$= -i + j + ik.$$

For a point **v** to rotate to RvR^{-1}, the axis of the rotation which R represents must pass through the origin of the coordinate frame. If the axis of rotation passes through some point **p** but not through the origin, we must add two simple steps to the process just described to find the new location of **v**. In particular, we move the origin to **p**, rotate, and restore the origin to its initial position, as Figure 8.33 illustrates.

Let **p** indicate a point on the axis **a** of a rotation through an angle θ. The point v will rotate about a. The vector (**v** − **p**) has its tail at **p** and its head at **v**, and so indicates the position of **v** relative to an origin at **p**. The axis a intersects this origin, so the rotated position of **v** relative to **p** is $R(\mathbf{v} - \mathbf{p})R^{-1}$. To restore the origin to its initial location, simply add **p**; **v** rotates to $R(\mathbf{v} - \mathbf{p})R^{-1} + \mathbf{p}$.

REFERENCES

Baron, R. J. (1981). Mechanisms of human facial recognition. *International Journal of Man-Machine Studies, 15*, 137-178.

———— (1985). Visual memories and mental images. *International Journal of Man-Machine Studies, 23*, 275-311.

Hamilton, W. E. (1866). *Elements of quaternions.* London: Longmans, Green.

Hubel, D. H., & Wiesel, T. N. (1977). Ferrier Lecture. Functional architecture of the macaque monkey visual cortex. *Proceedings of the Royal Society of London, B., 198*, 1-59.

Julstrom, B. A., & Baron, R. J. (1985). A model of mental imagery. *International Journal of Man-Machine Studies, 23*, 313-334.

Minsky, L. (1955). *An introduction to linear algebra.* Oxford: Clarendon Press.

Newman, W. M., Sproull, R. F. (1973). *Principles of interactive computer graphics.* New York: McGraw-Hill.

Paul, R. P. (1981). *Robot manipulators.* Cambridge, MA: MIT Press.

Pervin, E., & Webb, J. A. (1982). Quaternions in computer vision and robotics. (Tech. Rep. CMU-CS-82-150), Department of Computer Science, Carnegie-Mellon University, Pittsburgh.

9
ACCESSING
VISUAL MEMORIES
AND VISUAL RECOGNITION

INTRODUCTION

The previous two chapters suggested how visual information is encoded for storage, how storage representations are transformed into mental images, and how mental images are manipulated. This chapter suggests how storage representations are organized, how they are analyzed, and how memories are accessed. Both memory scanning and sequential recognition, also called recognition by hypothesis verification, are discussed.

Storage representations, as you may recall, consist of test patterns which describe surface characteristics of objects, control patterns which describe where the objects were located and how they were encoded for storage, and spatial patterns which describe surface extent, surface orientation, depth (position), and movement. These visual representations are the access windows into the past; they enable the storage system to locate and access related stored information based on structure and appearance.

Visual memories can also be accessed by verbal descriptions of the places, events, or objects in them. When verbal descriptions are used to access visual memories, naming stores convert the tokens in the description into visual (spatial or pictorial) representations which are then presented to the visual memory stores for analysis. Thus visual representations are still the access windows into the past, albeit indirectly. Chapter 11 discusses verbally mediated recall.

THE SPATIAL ORGANIZATION OF VISUAL EXPERIENCES

Whenever we visit new places, we glance around and build internal representations or **world models** of the places we visited and objects we saw. Later, we can recall how the places looked, where the objects were located, how they looked, and how they were oriented. The following section describes how and why we are able to interact with our memories in this way.

Spatial Coordinate Systems

First, the brain uses **spatial coordinates** to encode the locations of objects and events in the world. These coordinates are part of the control pattern for the experience. Although we don't know in fact what types of coordinate system the brain uses, one possibility is illustrated in Figure 9.1. Eight coordinate systems are shown: a **local coordinate system** (shown, in the upper right of the figure using cylindrical coordinates) and seven **global coordinate systems** (shown using Cartesian coordinates). Chapter 5 showed how the brain can represent coordinate values, but the details of the specific encoding are not important to this discussion.

Local coordinates are assigned to each object that is perceived. They specify the location of the object relative to the viewer. When a person looks around from a fixed place, his or her head, eyes, and body continually shift. Transformational networks convert vestibular, kinesthetic (muscle sense), and visual signals into local coordinates and send them to the storage system as part of the control pattern for the experience. How the brain does this is not yet known, but one way local coordinates might be specified is by encoding the height of the object relative to eye level, its angular position relative to straight ahead, and its distance away. This was illustrated in Figure 9.1h.

Whereas local coordinates specify the object's location relative to the viewer, global coordinates locate and orient the viewer in the world. Global coordinates consist of several different sets of values, each specifying the location of a particular set of spatial coordinates within a larger framework. For example, one set of coordinates might locate the viewer within a neighborhood, one set might locate the neighborhood within the city, and one set set might locate the city within the world. In Figure 9.1, the seven sets of global coordinates were selected so that each set specifies the position of the next set of coordinates within an area which is an order of magnitude smaller than specified by the previous set of coordinates: country, state, county, city, neighborhood, building, and room.

Assuming three global and one local coordinate system, and further assuming that each global coordinate system uses three values for location and three for orientation, the entire coordinate specification requires 45 values.

Object-Centered Coordinates

In addition to the local and global coordinates which specify the location of an object in the world, the brain imposes an **object-centered coordinate system** on each perceived object. The storage representation of each object is based on its

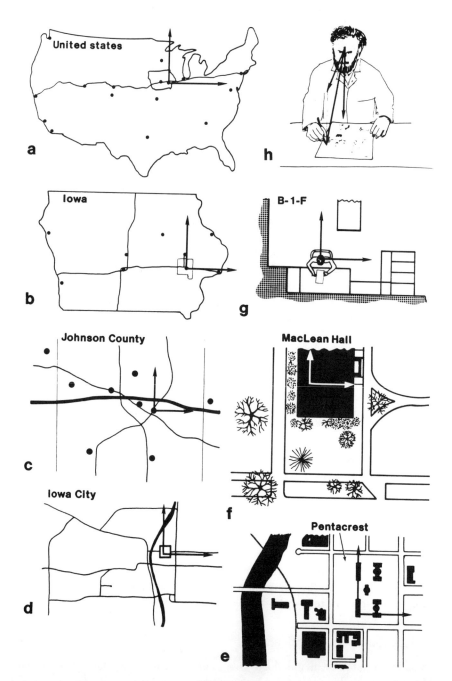

United states

a

Iowa

b

Johnson County

c

Iowa City

d

B-1-F

g

MacLean Hall

f

Pentacrest

e

h

Figure 9.1

own object-centered coordinate system. This happens in some unknown way when an object is selected for the focus of attention and its representation created in an object buffer. Figures 9.2 and 9.3 illustrate several objects and their object-centered coordinate systems. The first frame of Figure 9.2 shows a square and a belt comprised of a sequence of squares while the second frame shows a diamond and a belt comprised of a sequence of diamonds. Figure 9.3 shows a human body with its own coordinate system as well as its right arm, right forearm, and right hand with their own coordinate systems. In each of these figures, the object coordinates are aligned with axes of symmetry of the object. The principal (or Z) coordinate axis is aligned with the object's longitudinal axis. This alignment takes place when the focus of attention (eye fixation point and internal focus) are selected.

How does the brain assign object-centered coordinates? With a newly perceived object, there is no prior identification, so the assignment must be based on naturally occurring visual features of the selected object. These features include symmetry, the ratios of height to length of the object, and so forth. If the object is very long, for example, one axis might be placed along its length or orientation. Each belt in Figure 9.2 is assigned object coordinates based on its orientation, and the assigned object-centered coordinates are then used when scanning the individual components of the object. That is why we perceive squares on one belt and diamonds on the other. The object coordinates are encoded in the way the object enters the focus of attention as described in the previous chapter. For the hand of Figure 9.3, the direction of the fingers establishes the object coordinates. These spatial features require no a priori knowledge of the individual objects, and hence the low-level and intermediate-level visual networks can make the assignment without any high-level control. The result is a canonical representation of each selected object.

Many visual illusions are illusions because the low-level visual networks which assign the object-centered coordinate system find more than one natural way to make the assignment. Each choice results in a different canonical storage representation and hence different perception of the object. When the low-level visual networks switch between these coordinate system assignments, we perceive the object in different ways. Figures 9.4 and 9.5 show examples of visual illusions which illustrate this point. Once the representation of an object activates a permanent memory location, stored knowledge becomes available and can be used both to direct the scan and to specify the object-centered coordinates to use for additional object components. For example, when a hand

---

Figure 9.1. Global and local coordinate systems. Each subfigure, moving from top-left counterclockwise, shows coordinate systems at a scale of reference an order of magnitude smaller than the previous one. These correspond in a natural way to country, state, county, city, neighborhood, immediate neighborhood, local area coordinates, and finally body-centered coordinates.

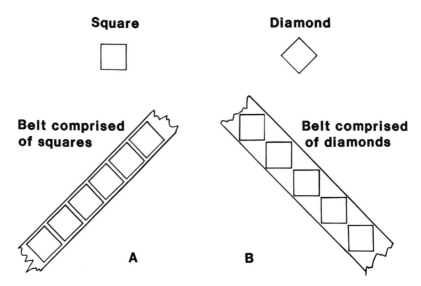

Figure 9.2. Object-centered coordinates. A. A square and a belt composed of squares. B. A diamond and a belt composed of diamonds. (Suggested by G. Hinton at the Third Annual Conference of the Cognitive Science Society, Berkeley, California, 1981.)

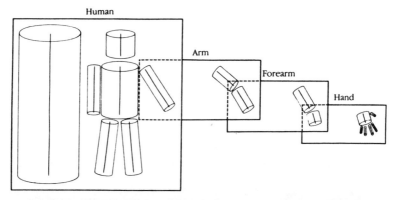

Figure 9.3. Various body components with their own coordinates. (Reproduced, with permission, from D. Marr & H.K. Nishihara, Representation and recognition of the spatial organization of three-dimensional shapes. *Proceedings of the Royal Society of London*, B, 200, 1978, 269-294.)

is recognized, each finger can be processed with its own set of object coordinates.

In summary, the visual control pattern for each storage representation contains the following coordinate information: (1) the location of the viewer in the world, (2) the location of each object relative to the viewer, (3) the object-centered coordinates used while scanning the object, (4) the orientation of the object, and (5) its size.

Reflex actions are not encoded in the visual control pattern. When viewing an object, many small visual reflex actions occur to keep the high-level visual encoding invariant. For example, changes in body attitude and head position mediate small shifts in eye positions; movement of the object in space results in a combination of shifts in eye position, changes in the focal length of the lens, correction in the convergence of the eyes, and selection of an appropriate region of the correlation pattern to occupy the focus of attention. These reflex actions

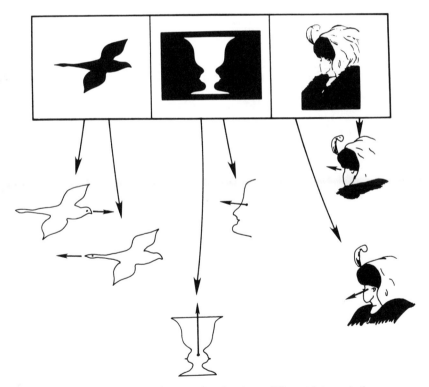

Figure 9.4. Ambiguous figures, showing how different interpretations result when different object-centered coordinates are assigned by the low-level visual networks. (Based on Figure 17, page 19 from J. P. Frisby, *Seeing, Illusion, Brain and Mind*. Copyright © 1979 by Oxford University Press. Used with permission.)

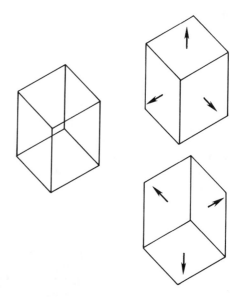

Figure 9.5. Two valid assignments of surface orientations to a wire-frame drawing of a cube.

are the result of a complex sequence of interactions between visual, vestibular, and oculomotor systems and generally take the form of smooth pursuit eye movements.

On the other hand, a change in the point of fixation on the selected object is encoded, as it represents part of the scan path information. Changes in the fixation point, unlike smooth pursuit movements, take the form of saccadic eye movements.

Although the computational details of the visual control pattern are currently not known, they are not necessary for an understanding of how we interact with stored visual experiences.

TEMPORAL ORGANIZATION OF VISUAL EXPERIENCES

Encodings of visual experience appear to be organized within memory according to their time of occurrence. That is, the permanent stores of visual experience appear to be temporal analyzers. All of today's visual experiences are, according to this assumption, stored in physically nearby memory locations. Because people move about rather slowly, events which occur close together in time also take place at nearby places. Thus within the storage system, memories which are stored near one another have identical high-level coordinates, almost

238

identical lower level coordinates, and so forth. The local and object-centered coordinates will, of course, be different for each object attended. These facts, as you will soon see, are important for controlling access to the memories of past events.

Chapter 6 described in considerable detail the nature of stored visual experiences. The spatial components resemble, to a great extent, the images on a strip of motion-picture film: They vary in time exactly as the experiences did during storage. The control pattern is part of each experience and is somewhat like the sound track on the film. When a surgeon stimulates the brain of a patient and causes one of his or her memories to unfold, the patient is always aware of the spatial organization of the objects perceived. Each object is reported just as it was seen, and the patient gives a composite view of all items which once occupied the focus of visual attention. "Oh, a familiar memory—in an office somewhere. I was there and someone was calling to me—a man leaning on a desk with a pencil in his hand" (Penfield & Roberts, 1959, p. 45). The patient did not simply describe a sequence of objects (a desk, a man, a pencil) but rather he described the scene as if he were right there looking around the room. Spatial information, encoded in the control pattern, is always preserved along with pictorial information.

Spatial information is part of each of our records of experience. When asked to describe a particular object, for example the sofa in our home, we normally select from memory a particular set of features and then describe the sofa one feature at a time. The recalled sequence consists of encodings of prior selected features, their spatial relationship to one another, their orientation, and their size. The control information, clearly present in the storage representation, is used when describing the object from memory. During an experience the storage system receives and stores the control pattern and during recall it regenerates it. See Figure 9.6.

CANONICAL STORAGE REPRESENTATIONS

What information can the visual control system use for generating a canonical storage representation of an unknown object? One answer should be clear. The control system can use stored control and test patterns which were used to guide the analysis of similar objects in the past. By using a prior scan path,[1] the current object will be scanned in exactly the same way as before and the resulting high-level visual representation will be the same now as before. It will be a canonical storage representation.

---

[1] Noton and Stark (1971a, 1971b) originally studied the relationships between scan paths of individual subjects, and visual recognition. Baron (1970) incorporated scan path information in a model for the elementary visual networks of the human brain.

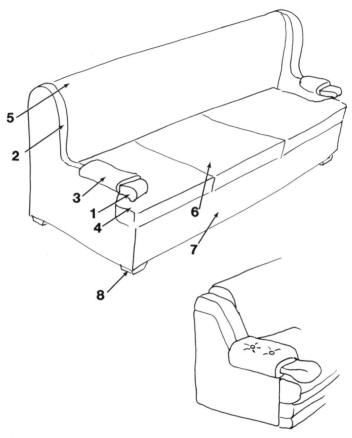

Figure 9.6. Recall of various parts of the sofa in my living room. The upper figure was redrawn from a quickly-drawn sketch (about 30 seconds) made before I paid attention to the details of the sofa. Numbers indicate the order that features came to mind. The inset shows a sketch of the sofa drawn while looking at it and drawn after the original sketch was made.

Canonical storage representations can be formed using previously stored control patterns provided that at least one feature of the current object activates a storage location. In that case, the corresponding stored control pattern can be recalled and used to direct further visual processing. Immediate recognition of the category of object is generally all that is required to activate a storage location. When a face is seen, for example, stored control patterns are used to direct the gaze, and when an automobile is seen, an entirely different scan pattern is used. Different characteristics distinguish objects in different categories and with experience we learn how to "look at" objects in those categories. What we learn, in fact, is to access control patterns that enable a systematic comparison of the distinctive features of the individual objects in each category. Since objects in the same category share the same control patterns, the permanent storage system automatically performs the comparison.

We not only learn how to scan objects in different categories, we learn which low-level encoding to focus on. Rivers, creeks, and streams all share properties of visual flow; buildings share the properties of flat surface boundaries, regularity in surface features (bricks, shingles, siding, etc.), and certain symmetries.

The need for canonical storage representations becomes particularly evident when studying moving objects such as a man walking. The ability to recognize the parts of a moving body requires knowledge of their connectedness, and this knowledge is encoded in the internal representation of the body by the object-centered coordinates imposed on each body component. Although the details of the computations that enable real-time recognition of moving bodies are not yet known, the utility and need for a canonical internal representation should be clear.

At the present time these ideas have only been simulated for faces (see the appendix to this chapter), and even then, the only measure of similarity is pictorial similarity of the image components. Surface orientation, visual flow, surface quality (texture and color) and other attributes such as symmetry have not been incorporated. This is clearly an area for future investigation.

ACTIVATING, RECALLING VISUAL EXPERIENCES

The permanent memory store for visual experience is an associative memory store as described in Chapter 3 and hence analyzes visual experiences as it stores them. The result of the analysis is the activation of selected memory locations. Access to stored experiences is associative: *A pattern must be presented to the storage system which will activate a memory location before recall from that location is possible.* This is, of course, true for all associative stores of all modalities.

Template matching in associative memory stores underlies all visual recognition, but the notion of template matching must properly be understood to include all features that are made explicit by the low-level and intermediate-level visual encoding networks: size, shape, color, surface texture, movement patterns, surface orientations, and so forth. Spatial similarity, which must be understood in this generalized sense, accounts for much of the power and flexibility of our visual machinery.

Activation of a memory location[2] occurs when current information is similar to prior stored information. Within the visual system, stored information that

---

[2]Activation is necessary before recall can take place. However, activation does not imply recall. The access control network must decide what to recall based on which memory locations are activated.

caused a memory location to become activated must be similar to the current high-level visual encodings in at least one of three ways: (1) spatial similarity (surface extent, surface orientation, depth, visual flow), (2) test pattern similarity (surface characteristics), or (3) control pattern similarity (size, location). I will analyze these three possibilities separately.

Before I begin, however, I must point out that none of the details of any of the following coding techniques are yet understood. We do not know how texture is encoded. We do not know how surface orientation or visual flow are encoded. We do not know how the scan path is encoded. As a consequence, we do not know how similarity is measured on any of these characteristics. This is true not only for unchanging patterns but for time-varying patterns as well. Thus considerable effort and modeling will be required before the ideas presented in the following sections can be evaluated.

Spatial Similarity

Storage representations are time-varying patterns. The spatial components, in particular, change when the gaze shifts (thereby changing the retinal image), when the control pattern selects a different portion of the correlation pattern (corresponding to zooming or rotating the eye), or when the test pattern changes (resulting in the encoding of a different object or feature in the scene). In order for two spatial patterns to generate strong similarity signals, they must be similar during the time interval of comparison. Similarity means that each input cell must now fire at the same rate it did during storage. Thus, in order for the current input pattern to be spatially similar to a stored pattern, both must vary both in time and in space in the same way.

There are several examples of spatial and temporal similarity. The simplest example is when neither the current input pattern nor the prior stored pattern vary at all. This happens when the focus of visual attention is constant during the entire time interval of comparison. An example is the pattern formed during a single eye fixation. A second example is when an object is initially studied in an arbitrary way and the resulting high-level encodings stored. If the same object is later studied in exactly the same way, from the same point of view, and using the same scan path and focus of attention, the resulting high-level encodings, including spatial components, will be the same. Even though the spatial patterns vary as a function of time, both the stored pattern and the current pattern vary in exactly the same way. The memory location holding the stored pattern will therefore generate a high (strong) similarity signal during the presentation of the input pattern, and the memory location will consequently become activated. A third example is when a subject looks at the objects in a given scene in one way and later views the same scene in exactly the same way. Another example is when a subject looks at one of a given set of similar types of objects (for example, faces) and scans them all in a regular and systematic way. When objects are similar, and when the same scan path and control patterns can be utilized, the low-level and intermediate-level visual networks generate similar storage representations—ones with the same temporal and spatial characteristics. Human facial recognition is an example and will be described in detail in the appendix to this chapter.

The situation becomes somewhat more complex when the subject is viewing a scene from a different place than before. Now, the scan path must be systematically modified from the original scan path in order to generate a similar storage representation. However, the geometry of three-dimensional space is well known. Thus the computations necessary to modify the control patterns are easily performed once the relationship is determined between the current and prior points of view. The relationship is determined when an object (such as a building) is recognized, its stored spatial coordinates are recalled, and a comparison is made between its stored and current coordinates.

Spatial similarity refers to the geometry of the selected visual components. When the selected component is brightness, spatial similarity implies that the input and stored patterns are similar in the sense that two photographic prints from the same negative are similar. (In the appendix I will show that spatial similarity is all that is required for human facial recognition.) When either the visual flow pattern or the surface orientation pattern is selected, spatial similarity deals with entirely different aspects of the visual world. As a specific example, consider the class of chairs comprised of a seat, a seat back, and four legs. The seat and seat back can be characterized as square, planar surfaces intersecting perpendicularly at an edge. The legs are attached to the corners of the seat on the side opposite the seat back. When looking at a chair, one possible scan path is to look first at the seat, then at the seat back, and finally at the legs. The resulting storage representation would consist of the encoding of an approximately flat surface (as encoded in its surface orientation pattern), a second flat surface perpendicular to the first, and legs which are perpendicular to the first surface. The control pattern encodes the scan path used when inspecting the chair, and if all chairs are analyzed using the same control patterns, and if similarity is based on surface orientation, then differences in color, specific shapes of surfaces, and styles are disregarded.

Now suppose that an object is seen that has a flat surface of about two square feet. Suppose, also, that a memory location containing the representation of a chair is activated. If the control pattern in the activated memory location is used to control the gaze, the current object, which has not yet been identified, will be scanned as if it were a chair. If it happens to be a chair, the new storage representation will be recognized by other memory locations holding chair representations. Consequently, the representation of the current chair will not only be recognized but will automatically be added to the class of chairs in memory.

In contrast, if one wants to recognize a particular chair, then one must select for the focus of attention particular "distinguishing features," such as color, shape, or style; unusual markings, blemishes, and so forth.

Test Pattern Similarity

Now consider the significance of test pattern similarity for visual recognition. The test pattern is a pattern of small dimensionality that describes a surface characteristic, such as color or texture. These surface characteristics are independent of surface shape. When a test pattern is selected, for example the color yellow, the resulting surface extent pattern describes the shape of all yellow surfaces in the visual field. The entries in the surface extent patterns do not encode the color yellow: Only the test pattern does that.

Test patterns are stored in the storage system and are compared in exactly the same way that spatial patterns are compared. However, activation of a memory location based on test pattern similarity is independent of surface shape. We recognize many things by their color (the orange roof of Howard Johnsons, the pink of Pepto-Bismol), or texture (the fuzziness of a peach, the mottled surface of an orange), or visual flow (the water in a river, the undulant movement of a snake). When the test pattern is derived from within the visual field, it is immediately compared with prior test patterns. Comparison results in the activation of memory locations containing similar stored test patterns. Their activation enables access to the representations of objects having the same surface characteristics regardless of their shape. When combined with shape similarity from the spatial encodings, access to specific associated experiences is rapid and accurate. Unfortunately, the details of the encodings and the measures of similarity are currently unknown. Considerable research is needed, therefore, before these ideas can be incorporated into a detailed model for human visual recognition.

Control Pattern Similarity

Finally, associative access can be gained to experiences which have similar control patterns. Since the size and location of an object selected for the focus of attention is encoded in the control pattern, the selection of a memory based on its spatial location is mediated by the control pattern. Memory scanning is an example which will be discussed in detail shortly. Similarly, while recalling a specific control pattern to use in guiding the current visual field analysis, all prior objects that share that control pattern may be made available for recall. Attributes such as size, general shape (broad, tall, slender), and location (high up, on the ground) are encoded in the control pattern and therefore contribute to recognition of visual patterns. Control patterns can also be used to activate memory locations and therefore access specific memories (e.g., objects that are on the floor or objects attached to the wall).

Verbally Mediated Recall of Visual Exerience

When we want to access a particular visual memory, the verbal system must send appropriate associated patterns to the visual system for analysis. (This chapter will not address the question of how the verbal system gets the patterns in the first place.) The associated patterns may be spatial patterns, control patterns, or test patterns, depending on the nature of the request. The patterns arriving from the verbal system may activate none, a few, or many visual memory locations, and the first goal of the visual memory store's access control system is to isolate those memory locations that are most likely to contain the desired information. The access control system may deactivate unlikely memory locations, but it cannot activate any inactive ones: Activation can only be done associatively.

There are several ways the access control system may select active memory locations as relevant for recall. One way is by the time of occurrence of the associated event. Keep in mind the fact that the time of occurrence of an event determines the approximate position within the memory store of the memories of that event. Based on the time of occurrence of the desired event, the access control network can deactivate all memory locations which are not located in the appropriate part of the memory store. Recall can then be initiated, in sequence, from each of the remaining activated memory locations until the desired information is found.

The time of occurrence of each event is unique. However, since time is encoded by the position of the memory location in the memory store, time alone cannot be used to activate storage locations. A verbal specification, such as "what did you see on your way to work today?" isolates a specific set of memory locations, those with today's memories, but unless one has already been activated by association, information is not available for recall. A specification such as, "did you see the accident on the way to work today?", in contrast, suggests a specific event (an accident) which can be used to activate specific memory locations. In this case, once again, time restricts access to memory locations which are not relevant to the request; association, on the other hand, activates specific memory locations.

The access control system can bias the way that memory locations can be activated. Once an interval of time is specified, the access control system can facilitate access to the memory locations that hold memories which occurred during that time interval. Once facilitated, a memory location can be activated by presenting information which is less similar than usually required. Specifying a time interval for recall establishes a **context** so that the records of experience with that context are more available. When talking about last summer's vacation, for example, many events come to mind which would not otherwise come to mind. They are made easier to recall. The particular memories which are recalled are activated by an association, but the time of occurrence—last summer—delimits the context.

The coordinates of an experience in memory are unique only if the place was visited exactly one time. Thus it is often necessary to constrain verbal specification in other ways than by specifying a time alone: "the blue house *which we saw yesterday while on the bus*," or "the red building **two blocks east of the White House**." In summary, the verbal system must send to the visual system an adequate set of patterns to establish a context, and it must also send patterns which activate specific memory locations. After that, the access control system can initiate recall of specific memories from within the activated set.

Memory Scanning

Once a context is established for recall, local coordinates can be used as an input pattern to activate particular memory locations. This is the basis of **memory scanning**, the process of accessing memories by using local coordinates to activate memory locations.

One question immediately comes to mind: What operations are needed for scanning the memories of an experience? Conceptually, memory scanning takes place when we mentally put ourselves in the place we wish to see—"imagine standing in front of the Washington Monument looking east"—and then looking around (in the mind's eye). Two mental processes are involved: (1) putting ourselves in the place we want to be, and (2) looking around. Putting ourselves in the place we want to be means generating its spatial coordinates and using them to establish a context in memory. Generating spatial coordinates means recalling memories containing those spatial coordinates. That is, the term "Washington Monument" would be delivered to a naming store from which images of the monument would be recalled. Those images, in turn, would be sent to the stores of visual experience where they would activate memory locations containing representations of the monument. Since those memories contain the spatial coordinates of their occurrence, recall of those memories generates the required spatial coordinates. Establishing a context in memory means facilitating access to storage locations within that context—in this case, those memory locations holding memories having the desired global coordinates. Mentally looking around is done by generating the control patterns for moving the eyes, head, and body for looking around, but not actually sending them to the motor system for orchestration. They are only used to generate the local coordinates which would be part of the storage representation if we were to look around. The resulting local coordinates are sent to the storage system for analysis. During analysis, they activate storage locations having the same local coordinates. If any memory locations are activated, then the corresponding stored information has the same set of local coordinates that were just generated and therefore comes from the place where we would be looking. On the other hand, if coordinates are generated which do not activate any memory locations, stored information cannot be recalled and we are unable to remember what would be present if we were actually looking rather than mentally looking. In summary, we are able to "look around" in the mind's eye, but we are only able to see things we noticed before.

The representations of many stored objects share the same set of local coordinates. Thus local coordinates alone do not adequately select a memory location for access. However, when the global coordinates are used to specify a context in memory, local coordinates may be used to select among the memories in that context. Part of memory scanning, therefore, consists of using global coordinates to establish the desired context.

It is sometimes impossible, when mentally scanning a scene, to access memories of an object in a specific location. Either the specified location was not attended during the experience, or current access parameters to the desired memories make recall impossible. In the second case we say the desired information is forgotten. Occasionally, it is possible to switch contexts and gain access to the desired information from a different set of memories of the same place. If contexts are switched and different memories are used, incorrect information is sometimes recalled: "My wallet was on the dresser, but I don't remember if it was there this morning or yesterday morning."

A considerable amount of time is required for memory scanning. First, the context must be established. Next, the local coordinates must be generated and sent to the storage system for analysis, and finally, if a memory location is activated, recall must be initiated. If no memory locations are activated, context switching may take place, adding a considerable amount of time to the process.

GESTALT VERSUS SEQUENTIAL RECOGNITION

Gestalt recognition is a passive instantaneous process. Whenever the storage representation of an object is sent to a storage system, the storage system compares it with all stored representations and generates similarity information. Storage locations may be activated during this analysis, and when the similarity signals that caused activation are high enough, a positive identification of the object may occur. Positive identification, **recognition**, is the decision made by the high-level control networks that the current object is known and needs no further processing. Recall is not part of recognition.

Not all visual recognition is immediate, however. A careful analysis of the current object may be required before positive identification can occur and hence before the object can be recognized. This is particularly true when the object is camouflaged, partly hidden from view, seen from an unusual perspective, or seen out of context.

Consider the processes of recognizing the object in Figure 9.7 which is partly hidden from view by a piece of cardboard that has holes in it. In order to recognize the object, both the individual features must be recognized and their relationships to one another must be determined. A representation is created in spatial memory and a hypothesis made as to what the hidden object is. A guess means that a memory location has been activated which may contain a stored representation (or perhaps characterization[3]) of the hidden object. This is the hypothesis that must be verified. The control information from the memory location holding the hypothesized representation is used to control the visual scan, and if, using that control pattern, there is recognition of each feature that is viewed, the hidden object is recognized. (See Noton & Stark, 1971a, 1971b; or Farley, 1974.) Recognition is the high-level decision that the hypothesis has been verified. Figures 9.8 and 9.9 differ from Figure 9.7 in that Figure 9.8 has an invalid feature and therefore can not represent the same object while Figure 9.9 has all of the correct features but they are located in the wrong places. In these cases, the hypothesis is contradicted.

Spatial memory can be used for hypothesis verification even when one of the images is not represented in permanent memory. When asked to find occurrences of a given face among a collection of alternatives, as in Figure 9.10, the usual procedure is hypothesis verification. One of the known faces is selected (the hypothesis). The selected face is generally one which is similar in the gestalt sense to the unknown face. The selected face is scanned. This creates a representation in spatial memory (as well as permanent memory). The other face is then scanned in the same way, by using the same control pattern, and the representations compared. The comparison may take place in temporary memory, permanent memory, spatial memory, or all of them. Several scans of each face may be required, each scan focusing on a different feature for comparison. If enough selected features are similar, the hypothesis is verified; otherwise an alternate hypothesis is made. (The high-level control networks make these decisions.) Note that identification of the given face does not require that all features match. Features such as hairdos and facial expressions change from time to time. What is required is a match between essential features such as the shape of the face, the shape of the lips and nose, and the color of the hair and eyes. It is not known how the mind determines which features are essential.

Identification of objects that have been spatially rotated can also be done by hypothesis verification. When comparing pictures of such objects (See Figure 8.2), immediate identification of one object as the other is not possible. In order to determine if the pictures represent the same object, they must be scanned and a hypothesis made as to the point of view which will make one of the pictures appear like the other. If both pictures represent the same object, a single

---

[3]Entrance stairs can be characterized as a series of steps leading up to a landing. Each of the steps in the series is similar; the number of steps differs from one set of entrance stairs to another. How an individual step is encoded in memory is not known.

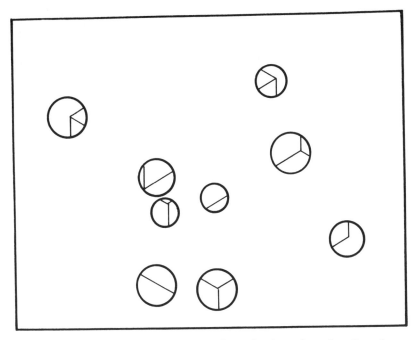

Figure 9.7. An object partially hidden from view by a piece of cardboard with holes in it.

perspective transformation applied to the storage representation of one of the pictures will produce a storage representation that is similar to the other. The hypothesis for this problem is the choice of perspective transformation. Once a transformation is selected, the same testing process is used that was described earlier, and the hypothesis is either verified or contradicted. If contradicted, either another transformation must be selected or a decision must be made that the two objects are not one in the same. The latter decision is usually nonvisual and based on counting the number of cubes in each object, discovering the handedness of the objects, and so forth.

Local features of the two objects are used for selecting a candidate transformation. If, for example, a guess is made that a particular edge of one object corresponds to a particular edge of the other, a family of perspective transformations is indicated. After the selected edge of one of the objects is mentally rotated to align with the corresponding edge of the other, there is still a possible rotation in space about the selected edge to bring the two objects into registration. The mental apparatus, however, cannot process an entire image; it is too complicated. Only one feature at a time can be processed, and the feature that is selected occupies the focus of attention. The mental rotation of one object into the other requires that each selected feature be placed in spatial memory at a position determined by transforming the control pattern to

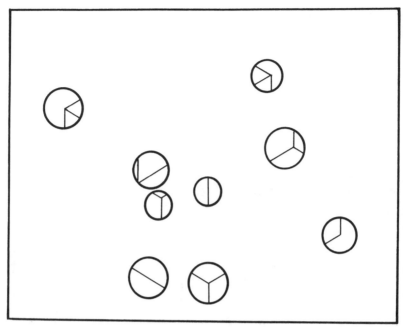

Figure 9.8. The same illustration as in Figure 9.7 only one feature is incorrect. Compare this with a misspilled word.

correspond to the selected point of view. Once the location for the feature is determined, the spatial image must be transformed and stored there. Each selected feature must be properly placed in spatial memory, and during this process, each feature is compared with the corresponding visual representation of the second object. If all features are similar, the hypothesis is verified, but if features are significantly different either the hypothesis must be rejected or the objects found to be different.

There are similarities and differences between gestalt recognition and hypothesis verification. Both types of recognition require the analysis of time-varying patterns, and both types of recognition require a sequence of comparisons. Both types of recognition use storage representations to control the gaze. They differ in several respects also. Gestalt recognition is a passive process while hypothesis testing is an active process. For hypothesis verification, a single storage representation is reconstructed and the comparisons usually take place in spatial memory. For gestalt recognition, all memory locations partici- pate, all comparisons are simultaneous, they all take place in permanent memory, and the results are immediate. Gestalt recognition is clearly the faster process, but it is also less sensitive to details.

As with all mental activity, hypothesis verification is controlled by a mental procedure. (I will describe mental procedures in Chapter 11.) The mental apparatus controls all computational operations, including the routing of information to spatial memory, specifying criteria for storage, specifying transfer conditions, routing control patterns to direct the gaze, modifying them appropriately, and so forth. The procedures which control hypothesis verification must be invoked when needed, and although we cannot say when they will be invoked, certainly the lack of a suitably high similarity signal in response to a memory search seems to invoke hypothesis testing.

SUMMARY

Visual experiences appear to be organized in memory according to their time of occurrence: Events which occurred close together in time are stored in nearby memory locations.

Visual memories not only contain the pictorial data but also the spatial coordinates of where the events took place. The coordinates, which are part of the control pattern, also specify the relative location of each object in the scene and the object-centered coordinates used while attending the objects.

The access control system enables access to selected fragments of an

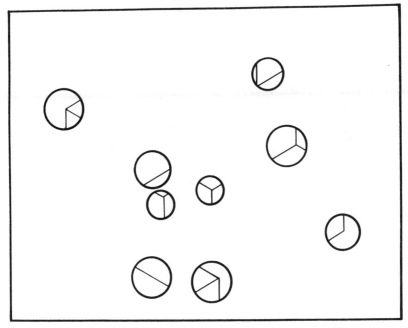

Figure 9.9. The same features shown in Figure 9.7. only several of them are out of place. Compare words sentence this with order out a of whose are.

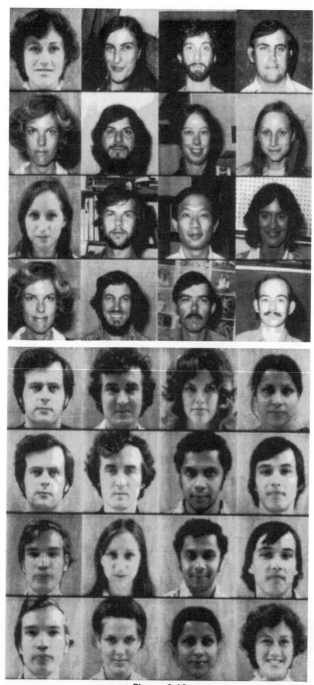

Figure 9.10

experience based either on spatial similarity, test pattern similarity, or control pattern similarity. Experiences can be mentally scanned by establishing the context of an event (either by its time or location of occurrence) and then using local coordinates to select specific memories within that context. The local coordinates are the access keys for the desired representations.

Gestalt recognition is an instantaneous passive recognition process. Gestalt recognition occurs when patterns presented to a permanent storage system are so similar to stored patterns that the resulting similarity signals are accepted by the high-level control system as positive indications that the current object is a known object. Sequential recognition, in contrast, is an active process. One or more memory locations are activated by the initial presentation of the unknown object. The control system guesses that one of the activated memory locations holds a representation of the unknown object. This is the hypothesis. The stored information is recalled and the control pattern used to direct the gaze and focus the attention. At the same time, the stored patterns are reconstructed and compared with the current encodings of the unknown object. If the comparisons are successful, the hypothesis is verified and the high-level control system accepts the result as a positive identification. Otherwise the hypothesis is contradicted.

REFERENCES

Baron, R. J. (1970). A model for the elementary visual networks of the human brain. *International Journal of Man-Machine Studies, 2,* 267-290.

Farley, A. M. (1974). VIPS: A visual imagery and perception system; the result of a protocol analysis. Vols. 1, 2. Technical Reports of the Computer Science Department, Carnegie-Mellon University, Pittsburgh.

Noton, D., & Stark, L. (1971a). Scanpaths in eye movements during pattern perception. *Science, 171,* 308-311.

_____ (1971b). Scanpaths in saccadic eye movements while viewing and recognizing patterns. *Vision Research, 11,* 929-942.

SUGGESTED READINGS

There are many excellent books on vision and memory, particularly those suggested in previous chapters. You might also find the following references interesting and relevant.

Beck, J. (1982). *Organization and representation in perception.* Hillsdale, NJ: Lawrence Erlbaum Associates.

Figure 9.10. Part of the image file used in the computer face recognition studies described here. Can you identify the face that appears four times?

Neisser, U. (1976). *Cognition and reality. Principles and implications of cognitive psychology.* San Francisco: W. H. Freeman.

———— (1967). *Cognitive psychology.* New York: Appleton-Century-Crofts.

Pick, H. L. Jr., & Saltzman, E. (Eds.). (1978). *Modes of perceiving and processing information.* Hillsdale, NJ: Lawrence Erlbaum Associates.

Ullman, S. (1980). Against direct perception. *The Behavioral and Brain Sciences, 3,* 373-415.

Vernon, M. D. (Ed.). (1966). *Experiments in visual perception.* Baltimore, MD: Penguin Books.

APPENDIX 4: SIMULATING HUMAN FACIAL RECOGNITION

In order to understand the nature of the storage representation better, the ideas were incorporated in a benchmark computer program[4] for human facial recognition. A brief overview of that program will be presented, insofar as it relates to human memory and recognition. Additional details can be found in Baron (1981).

THE INITIAL DATA

The data used for these studies consisted of more than 150 digitized images of faces. See Figures 9.10, 9.11, and 9.12 for examples. These images were generated from a collection of black-and-white Polaroid snapshots of students and staff at the University of Iowa. The snapshots were full face pictures taken with the subject looking directly toward the camera. Some snapshots were taken indoors with flash while others were taken outdoors without flash. No attempt was made to control the background, what the subjects wore, hairdo's, and so forth.

The snapshots were then digitized using a Spatial Data 806 Computer Eye and TM11/TU10 magnetic tape system. The digitizing equipment was located at the University of Missouri in the Biomedical and Automation Laboratory of the Department of Engineering. Attempts were made to ensure that the eyes were horizontal in the digitized image, and contrast and intensity were adjusted to be uniform. We have already described the ways the human visual system compensates for changes in brightness, size of object, and its orientation. The resulting digitized images were 512-by-480 pixels (picture elements) on a gray scale of 64. These images were then reduced to 128-by-120 pixels by averaging the values in 4-by-4 squares in the original images. The resulting digitized images were used as input for the face recognition system, and roughly correspond to the low-level visual encodings produced by the retina.

---

[4]This work was done by Ralph James Dawe while working toward a Ph.D. degree at the University of Iowa. All programs were coded in PL/I and run on an IBM system 360 model 65 computer.

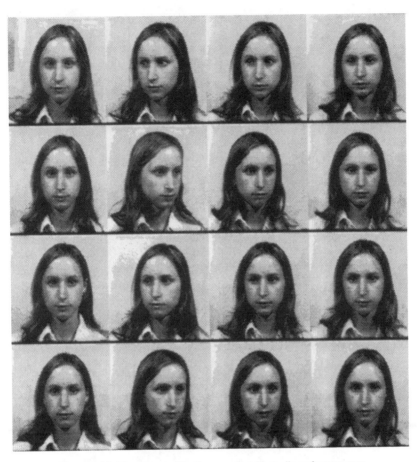

Figure 9.11. Figures used in the parametric studies of computer face recognition showing different orientations and directions of gaze.

LOCATING EYES IN A DIGITIZED IMAGE

In order to reduce the size of the initial 128-by-120 image for storage, the first step was to standardize the size of each face. This was done automatically by the program by locating the eyes in the input image and then reducing or enlarging the size of the input image if necessary so that the distance between the eyes was the same for all faces. The corresponding size standardization in the brain is done by selecting the appropriate fixation point upon which to focus the attention, and then selecting the proper part of the correlation. Specific environmental cues are probably used by biological visual systems for this process, including dark-light-dark surrounds (iris—white of the eye—eyebrow) detected by retinal cells and movements.

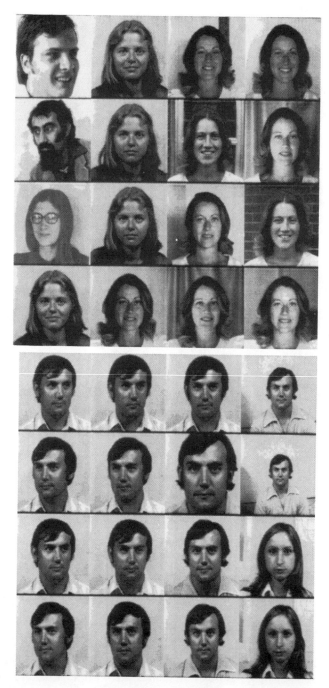

Figure 9.12

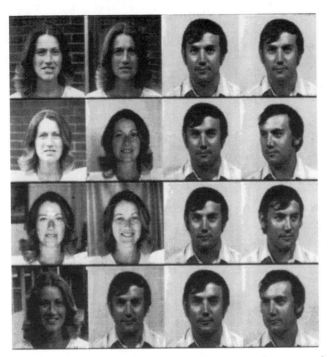

Figure 9.12. Figures used in the parametric studies of computer face recognition showing different backgrounds, lighting conditions, and sizes.

The actual procedure used for locating the eyes in the 128-by-120 input images consisted of correlating up to sixteen 20-by-23 "eye templates" against each 20-by-23 subimage of the input image. See Figure 9.13. These eye templates were obtained by an adaptive procedure that incorporates the features of specific eyes into templates which match a large class of eye images. The process is similar to the feature combination process I will describe shortly. A correlation value greater than .8 for any eye template indicated that an eye was located. The results compared within one row and column of the eye location determined by students when looking at prints of the digitized images.

THE DATA BASE

The data base has provisions for storing the memory representations of up to 75 different faces. The memory representation for each face contains up to five facial features, and each facial feature contains up to four distinctly different

1. **Select the next region from the input image. If the input image is completely processed, then no eyes are found. Quit with failure.**
2. **Extract the selected sub - image from the input image.**
3. **Normalize the extracted subimage.**
4. **Correlate the normalized subimage with each mask. If any correlation exceeds .8, an eye is located. Otherwise, go to step 1.**

Input image

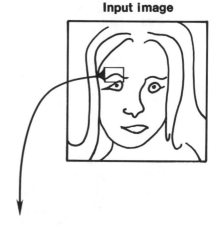

Eye templates

Figure 9.13. Locating eyes in a digitized image by comparing each 20-by-23 pixel subimage with a set of 20-by-23 pixel eye templates. (Slightly modified, with permission, from R. J. Baron, Mechanisms of human facial recognition. *International Journal of Man-Machine Studies*, 15, 1981, 137-178.)

templates for that feature. (In these simulations, a feature is simply a selected part of the face.) Thus each face is represented by up to 20 pictorial templates. Each pictorial template in the data base has 15 by 16 pixels obtained from the input images by reducing selected areas to 15 by 16 points, and then possibly combining (to be described) the resulting image with an image already in memory.[5]

Associated with each pictorial feature in the data base is a control pattern that specifies the size and location of the corresponding feature in the input image. Also stored with each template is the number of input images that have been combined to create it, and also some additional information that reduces the computation time for subsequent processing. See Figure 9.14.

The computer cannot store time-varying patterns. Thus the sequence of stored images for a given face is used to simulate time-varying patterns com-

---

[5]Each storage representation requires at most 20 templates of size 15-by-16 or 4800 data points, but for a single image, only five templates or 1200 data points are used. Each input image is 128-by-120 or 15,360 data points. The storage representation therefore represents a reduction in the amount of information by a minimum factor of 12.8 to 1.0. As a general rule, a much greater reduction factor is evident. If six input images result in the formation of 10 templates, which is typical, the reduction factor is 38.3.

prised of several different points of fixation. The control information, likewise, corresponds to the control pattern stored along with the pictorial pattern; it specifies the focus of attention of the computer.

The storage representation for each different face is derived from one or more input images of that person by a combination of user-supplied data and computer-generated data. For each face, the user supplies a list of features of interest. Thus by giving its coordinates and size in the input image, and possibly its name (nose, chin, etc.) for bookkeeping purposes. The coordinates of a feature are the row and column numbers of its upper-left corner in the input image, and its size is the number of rows and columns it takes in the input image. The selected area containing the feature is reduced to the standard 15 by 16 size for storage. The corresponding process in the brain is controlled by the networks that determine the focus of visual attention and corresponding scan path.

I must emphasize that a "facial feature" is simply an image derived by selecting a particular area in the input image for further processing. There is no other significance attached to the concept. A facial image can lead to a gestalt or immediate recognition of a face in just the same way that a stored face feature can lead to a gestalt recognition of a similar feature.

The only process that was not automatic was the selection of features to be used while creating the storage representation. The experimenter took the digitized images and selected features which to him were interesting, such as the eyes, nose, chin and so forth. These features were then used during subsequent processing. Personal experience certainly plays an important role in a human's choice of features, but there is no corresponding automatic mechanism for selection built into the computer programs.

When the first picture of a person is processed, the computer locates the eyes and standardizes the size of the picture as described earlier. The entire face image is then reduced to 15-by-16 pixels for storage. This 15-by-16 **full face image** or **gestalt image** becomes the first feature image in the face representation. It is the computer's "initial impression" of the face and corresponds exactly to using a uniform intensity test pattern to produce the correlation pattern. The remaining features specified by the user are then obtained and stored, and the appropriate control information automatically added to the storage representation.

If a second image of the same person is incorporated in the data base, processing is somewhat different. After the face is standardized, the full face image is reduced to 15-by-16 and correlated with the stored full face representation. If the correlation value is above a constant called the **recognition threshold** the data base is not modified at all. One might say that if a face is already sufficiently familiar, the program pays no particular attention to it. If the correlation value is between a constant called the **combine threshold** and the recognition threshold, the current 15-by-16 image is combined with the corresponding stored image. In this case, the novelty of the image is high, so

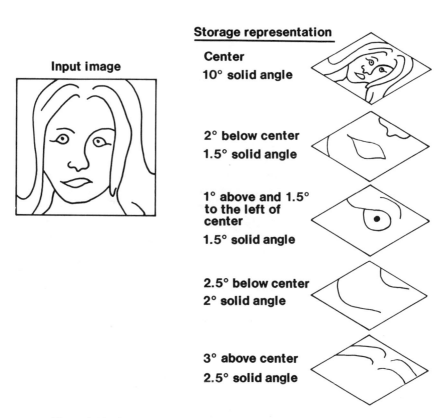

Input image

Storage representation

Center
10° solid angle

2° below center
1.5° solid angle

1° above and 1.5°
to the left of
center
1.5° solid angle

2.5° below center
2° solid angle

3° above center
2.5° solid angle

Figure 9.14. The storage representation of a face. (Slightly modified, with permission, from R. J. Baron, Mechanisms of human facial recognition. *International Journal of Man-Machine Studies*, 15, 1981, 137-178.)

that the program does pay attention to it. The combination is obtained by replacing each stored pixel in the template by the weighted average of the stored pixel value and the new pixel value. The weight is determined by the number of images that have already been combined, and that number is then incremented.[6] If, however, the correlation is below the combine threshold, the entire image is added to the file as an alternate full face image. This leads to an alternate gestalt image for the same person.

After the full face image is processed, the remaining features are processed in

---

[6]The process of template combination corresponds to the modification (adaptation) of memory traces. If there is an analogous network in the human brain, then it should have adaptive memory traces. Since it is our belief that the memory traces of experience are not adaptive, this suggests the possibility that the storage system that holds the storage representations of faces is different from the experiential storage system.

the same way. However, the features are now determined from the control vectors in the stored representation rather than from user-supplied data. That is, the incorporation of subsequent images of a person is fully automatic.[7] Said another way, the storage representation of the prior scan path is used to control the current scan path. Thus the current analysis is directed by past experience.

When the data base was completed, it represented 42 different people and was created by processing 89 different 128-by-120 pixel input images. The recognition threshold was set at .8 and the combine threshold was set at .7 when the data base was created.

FACE RECOGNITION

An input image is **recognized** by the face recognition system if it is correctly identified as one of the people in the data base. An input image is **mistakenly recognized** if it is incorrectly identified as one of the people represented by the data base, and a face is **missed** if it is an image of a person in the data base, but it is not identified as such.

In order to identify an unknown face, the eyes are located and the face standardized as described earlier. The full face image is then extracted and reduced to 15-by-16 for comparison with the data base. The resulting 15-by-16 full face image is correlated with every full face image in the data base. This corresponds exactly, we believe, to the first step in human face recognition. Corresponding to each storage representation are two values, a high value called the **threshold of recognition**, and a lower value called the **threshold of recall**. If the correlation value between the input pattern and the full face template in one of the storage representations exceeds its threshold of recognition, the system responds immediately with a statement of **recognition**, and the name associated with the responding storage representation is given as the name of the input. Otherwise each storage representation for which the correlation value exceeds the threshold of recall is said to **respond** to the input pattern, and the set of all such responding representations is the **conflict set**.[8] If recognition does not occur, the system attempts to verify that the input image corresponds to the one of the images in the conflict set. That representation in the conflict set with the highest correlation value is checked first.

Verification is the process of determining if the input face is the same face

---

[7]In the computer programs, the representations consist of a linked collection of images. Since we assume for human storage that each memory location holds a sequence of images but not a structure, the corresponding neural representation for a face would consist of a set of sequences of images, one sequence in each memory location.

[8]The term "conflict set" is borrowed from production system terminology because of the close correspondence between these two systems (Newell, 1973). In this model, the full face image is the entry condition and the verification procedure described shortly is the corresponding action.

that is in the storage representation, and proceeds as follows. The stored control information for each feature in the storage representation is recalled and used to select the same feature from the input image. Once again, the scan path is controlled by experience. Each feature is correlated against the corresponding stored feature template. This corresponds to comparing time-varying patterns in memory; an automatic process in the brain. If for at least three out of four of the features one of the resulting correlation values exceeds the threshold of recall, the face is identified and the process terminated. Otherwise, verification is attempted for the next face in the conflict set.

There is a direct correspondence between recognition by this system and recognition in the brain. Here, each representation in the conflict set is used to guide the search of the input image, and during the search, correlations are performed only on the images stored in that representation. In the brain, the processing of sequences of images is a consequence of the structure of the storage network. Furthermore, incoming images are correlated against all stored images that correspond to the same relative time of input. Thus the human process is much faster. Since, in the brain, the new incoming images may be stored in memory at the same time or immediately following presentation, a face that was not seen before will get a storage representation created immediately following an unsuccessful verification. As a result, many facial representations share the same control patterns, and during verification, many faces are verified simultaneously.

COMPUTER FACE RECOGNITION EXPERIMENTS

Experiments were conducted to determine the performance of this system. The following tests were included:

- Effect of size of template on recognition accuracy,
- Effect of changing the recognition and combine thresholds on the storage representation,
- Effect of changing the lighting on recognition and storage representation,
- Effect of face rotation on recognition,
- Effect of changing the size of an input image on recognition.

Among the notable results were the following: A recognition accuracy of 100% was achieved for a data base consisting of 42 faces which was created with a recognition threshold of .8 and a combine threshold of .7. More than 150 different faces were then presented to the system, including the faces used to create the data base. All of the original faces were recognized, and faces not in the data base were rejected. The recognition accuracy was not enhanced by using templates larger than 15 by 16. In fact, the 15-by-16 size seemed to contain the essential gestalt information for recognition, and increasing the size substantially increased the execution time with no particular qualitative advantage. Changing the values of the recognition and combine thresholds changed the storage representation as follows. When the combine threshold was decreased, fewer new images were created since more images were combined into a single template, but this resulted in lower correlation values when the same input images were later used as an input. The system therefore became less discriminatory. When the recognition threshold was decreased, fewer images were incorporated in the templates. The result was that different pictures of the same face resulted in lower correlation values and were missed during recognition.

Different lighting conditions have a notable effect on the size of the storage representation for a given person. Pictures taken with flash tend to be recognized by templates that were made from other pictures taken with flash whereas pictures taken without flash tended to correlate below the combine threshold and therefore resulted in new storage representations. Said another way, if the data base is created only with pictures taken with flash, then it does not recognize the same faces when taken without flash, and vice versa. Face rotations of up to 20 degrees did not affect recognition while rotations beyond 20 degrees were not recognized. By creating a new face representation with the face viewed at a 20-degree rotation, the system could then recognize all rotations up to 35 degrees. Finally, large changes in the size of the input image could not be adequately processed.

SIGNIFICANCE OF THE SIMULATION RESULTS

I have described various information-processing operations that relate directly to human face recognition. These include location of the face within the visual field, determination of its size, standardization of its size, correlation of the standardized input image with stored pictorial representations of known faces, location of facial features based on information contained in the storage representations of known faces, correlation of features of new faces with corresponding features of stored representations, and threshold analysis of the correlation values for determining whether or not a recognition criterion is satisfied. Each of these operations appears to be performed in the brain.

The first conclusion to be drawn is that the assumed storage operations are sufficient to account for much of our ability to recognize faces. The second and more significant conclusion is that the number of cells involved in the brain's storage representation, its **dimensionality**, need not be very large, and probably isn't. I showed that storage representations having templates whose sizes were 15-by-16 (240 image points) were sufficient for recognition based on correlation, and in fact, earlier experiments indicated that images having larger dimensionality were no better and often not as good. This agrees with estimates on the size of neural patterns in permanent memory based on the architecture and connectivity of the cerebral cortex (Chapter 7). This also agrees with studies by Harmon (1971, 1973) showing how little information is required for people to recognize pictures of faces. In brief, the human storage representation of the pictorial component of permanently stored visual patterns needs to be no larger than a few hundred elements. *The detail in memory derives from having many small patterns together with the appropriate control information; not in having large detailed patterns.*

REFERENCES

Baron, R. J. (1981). Mechanisms of human facial recognition. *International Journal of Man-Machine Studies, 15,* 137-178.

Harmon, L. D. (1971). Some aspects of recognition of human faces. In O.-J. Grüsser, (Ed.), *Pattern recognition in biological and technical systems,* New York: Springer-Verlag, 196-219.

——— (1973). The recognition of faces. *Scientific American, 229,* 70-82.

Newell, A. (1973). Production systems: models of control structures. In W. G. Chase, (Ed.), *Visual information processing.* New York: Academic Press.

Penfield, W. & Roberts, L. (1959). *Speech and Brain Mechanisms.* Princeton, NJ: Princeton University Press.

10
THE
AUDITORY
SYSTEM

INTRODUCTION

This chapter describes the structure and functioning of the human auditory system. The global architecture of the auditory system is first outlined, followed by a description of the anatomy and physiology of the ear. Particular attention is focused on the cochlea, which converts mechanical vibrations into neural impulses. A description of the low-level and intermediate-level auditory networks along the pathway from ear to cortex follows. The final sections describe the high-level encodings of auditory experience, including mechanisms of auditory recognition.

Auditory recognition, like visual recognition, has many facets. From a person's voice we not only recognize what is said, but who the speaker is. Musical compositions are recognized when played in different keys, at different loudness levels, at different speeds, and even from different arrangements. Still, each arrangement retains its uniqueness. Moreover, the auditory system is highly selective: when in a crowded room, a person may select one individual to listen to, even if the individual is far away or barely audible. The location of a sound source is readily determined, and just as the visual world does not appear to move when the head is turned, the world perceived through the ears also remains stable.

People classify sounds on the basis of pitch, timbre, and loudness or intensity, and each of these characteristics appears to be independent of the others. Pitch is related to the fundamental frequency of the sound: the higher the fundamental frequency, the higher the pitch. For a mixture of pure tones, however, the relationship is far from simple. The perceived pitch of a mixture of pure tones at 1000 Hz, 1200 Hz, and 1400 Hz may be 200 Hz! Although the pitch of the mixture may be 200 Hz, the quality of the sound for the mixture is very different from a 200-Hz pure tone.

The quality of a perceived tone is called its timbre. When different musical instruments play the same note, the pitch is the same although the instruments sound different. The difference partly lies in the component waves that each instrument produces.[1] Music synthesizers sound like different instruments by generating the appropriate component waveforms for each instrument. Figure 10.1 shows oscilloscope traces of a pure tone produced by a tuning fork, and the waveforms produced by several sources playing the same note. The horizontal axis of each waveform is time and the vertical axis is air pressure. Figure 10.2 shows the amount of each component waveform for several of the sounds illustrated in Figure 10.1.

Loudness is a measure of the pressure variations of the sound wave. For the faintest perceptible 1000-Hz pure tone, the pressure variations at the ear are about .0002 dyne/cm^2, which corresponds to air movement of about 10^{-9} cm or one-half the diameter of an hydrogen atom! In contrast, the loudest tolerable sound of the same pitch corresponds to a million times the pressure variation: 280 dyne/cm^2 or air movement of 10^{-3} cm. The incredibly sensitive ear is remarkably tolerant as well!

LOW-LEVEL AUDITORY ENCODING MACHINERY

The low-level auditory machinery converts sound waves into neural depolarization patterns which, through successive stages of transformation, are finally sent to the primary auditory cortex for processing. The principal processing stations along the auditory pathway are the ear, auditory nerve, cochlear nucleus, superior olivary complex, inferior colliculus, medial geniculate nuclei, and primary auditory cortex. See Figure 10.3. The ear converts sound waves into the **primary auditory pattern**, which is conveyed by the auditory or cochlear nerve to the cochlear nucleus for further processing. This nucleus transforms the primary auditory pattern and sends its results to the superior olivary complex for further processing. The result of olivary processing is sent to the inferior colliculus and medial geniculate nucleus. The medial geniculate nucleus is the final processing station before the auditory encoding reaches the primary auditory cortex. The ear has three anatomical divisions: the external or outer ear, the middle ear, and the inner ear. See Figure 10.4.

The outer ear, which consists of the ear lobe or pinna, external ear canal, and ear drum or tympanic membrane, serves as a pressure amplifier for frequencies in the speech range[2] and also helps to maintain a constant temperature and

---

[1] Other factors also contribute to the distinctive sound of each musical instrument, including attack time, decay time, sustain level, sustain time, release time, vibrato, and tremolo of each note, to name a few, but these factors will not be considered here.

[2] The frequencies of most speech sounds range between 100 Hz and 8000 Hz, the majority falling below about 1000 Hz. For reference, the average male voice has a fundamental frequency of 130 Hz and the average female voice has a fundamental frequency of 230 Hz.

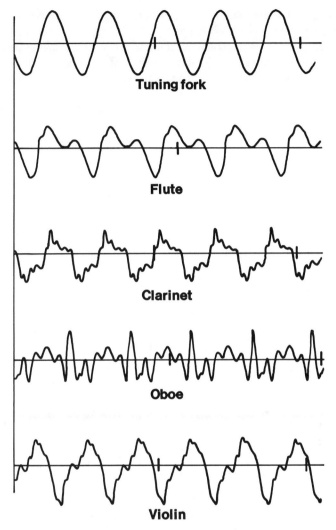

Figure 10.1. Waveform patterns of a tuning fork and various musical instruments. All instruments were sounding middle C or 256 vibrations per second. (Redrawn, with permission of Macmillan Publishing Company, from Dayton C. Miller. *Sound Waves—Their Shape and Speed.* Copyright 1937 by Macmillan Publishing Company, renewed 1965 by The Clarence Trust Company.)

humidity at the ear drum. This is important since the elastic properties of the ear drum depend on temperature and pressure.

The middle ear is a mechanical transformer which matches the sonic properties of the air with the hydraulic properties of the inner ear. It consists of the tympanic cavity, auditory or eustachian tube, and three tiny bones called ossicles. The ossicles are the hammer or malleus, the anvil or incus, and the stirrup or stapes. See Figures 10.4 and 10.5. The middle ear is separated from the outer ear by the ear drum and from the inner ear by two additional membranes called the oval window and the round window. The ossicles form a system of

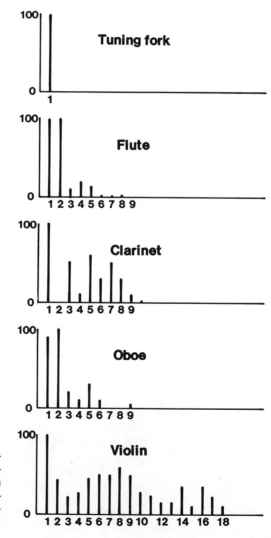

Figure 10.2. Frequency spectra of steady tones of some musical instruments. (Data from D. C. Miller. *The Science of Musical Sounds*. Macmillan Publishing Company, 1916.)

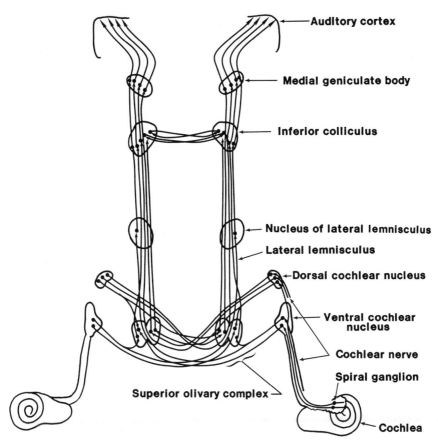

Figure 10.3. The principal auditory processing stations along the ascending auditory pathway.

levers which convert the inward and outward movements of the ear drum caused by sound waves into much smaller movements of the oval window. Not only are the movements of the oval window smaller, but the ratio of the area of the ear drum to the area of the oval window is about 14:1. As a result, the forces exerted on the oval window are about 20 times greater than on the ear drum. Two tiny muscles, the stapedius and the tensor tympani muscles shown in Figure 10.5 help prevent ruptures of the ear drum and oval window caused by extreme movements of the ossicles. Finally, the eustachian tube equalizes the pressure between the outside world and the tympanic cavity, leaving the ear drum unflexed in the absence of noise.

Compared with the outer ear and middle ear, the inner ear is far more complex. It consists of the cochlea and vestibular apparatus. Since the vestibular apparatus is not part of the auditory system, it will not be discussed here. The

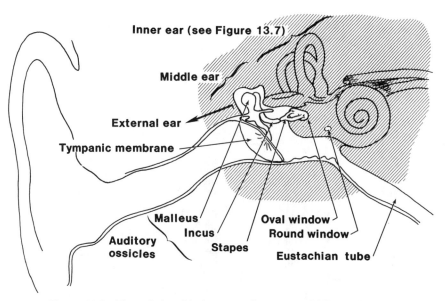

Figure 10.4. The relationship between the outer, middle, and inner ear.

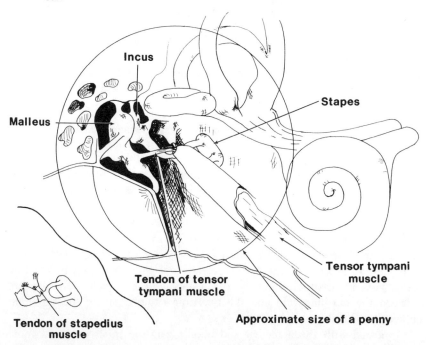

Figure 10.5. The middle ear, showing the stapedius and tensor tympanic muscles.

270

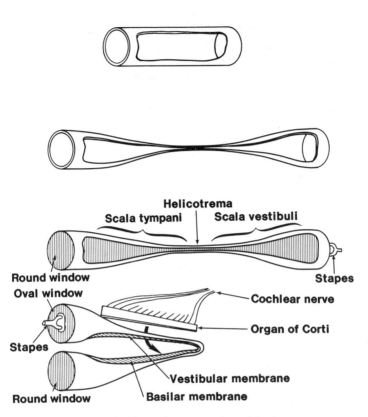

Figure 10.6. A schematic construction of the inner ear.

cochlea analyzes sound frequencies and converts them into a two-dimensional pattern, the **primary auditory pattern**, where sound frequency is related to spatial position in the cochlear nerve. This will be described shortly. The cochlea, coiled like the shell (and hence its name), is a tube whose diameter decreases toward its apex. The tube is divided lengthwise into three chambers: the scala vestibuli, the scala tympani, and the scala media or cochlear duct. The helicotrema is a small passage at the apex of the cochlea between the scala vestibula and the scala tympani.

One way of forming the inner ear in principle is shown in Figure 10.6. When unwound and split apart, the cochlea may be pictured as a half-tube which has been stretched to form a narrow channel. Two membranes are stretched across the tube, and the ends of the tube are capped with the oval window and round window. The stapes ossicle is attached to the oval window. The membrane closest to the oval window, the vestibular or Reissner's membrane, encloses the scala vestibula; the membrane closest to the round window, the basilar membrane, encloses the scala tympani. The small passage at the narrowest part

271

of the tube is the helicotrema. Finally, the tube is filled with an incompressible liquid called perilymph fluid.

The next step in this imaginary formation of the cochlea is the folding of the cochlear tube at its narrowest part as shown in Figure 10.6. During the folding process, the receptor hardware, the organ of Corti, is inserted between the vestibular and basilar membranes. The receptors or hair cells end up within the cochlear tube so the neural filaments, the auditory nerve, must pass through the wall of the cochlear tube. When the cochlear tube is folded upon itself, the space between the scala vestibula and the scala tympani becomes the scala media or cochlear duct. The cochlear duct is filled with endolymph, another incompressible fluid, and the resulting three-chambered structure is coiled into its final form. The cochlea fits snugly within the skull except for the oval and round windows which open into the inner ear.

Mechanical motion is converted into neural activity in the cochlear duct. A cross section of the cochlear duct, including hair cells and related cells, is shown in Figure 10.7. The hair cells are the receptor cells, and as can be seen, the cochlear duct is somewhat more complex than just described. There are roughly 25,000 hair cells divided into two groups: inner cells, and outer cells. See Figure 10.7. An approximately triangular support bridge composed of pillar cells separates the two groups. There is always one row of outer cells but there are from three to five rows of inner cells. The number of rows of inner cells increases toward the apex of the cochlea. Fine hairs emerge from the hair cells in a definite pattern. There are more than 100 of these fine hairs per outer hair cell, and from 40 to 60 hairs per inner hair cell. The hairs touch the tectorial plate, so that any movement of the tectorial plate relative to the basilar membrane causes the hairs to move. The hair cells sense the movements of the hairs and depolarize by an amount that depends on the severity and direction of the movement. This is the final stage in the conversion of sound to neural activity.

The inner and outer hair cells respond to different types of movements and connect differently to the auditory nerve. Thus they appear to encode different stimulus information.

Outer hair cells respond when their hairs are bent perpendicular to the long dimension of the basilar membrane, and in the direction away from the arch of Corti. This particular bending motion occurs when the basilar membrane moves upward due to increased pressure in the scala tympani. Upward motion of the basilar membrane displaces the tectorial plate in the transverse direction as shown in Figure 10.8. In contrast, inner hair cells respond when the hairs are bent parallel to the long dimension of the basilar membrane. Thus inner hair cells respond to the longitudinal gradient of the basilar membrane's displacement. Said another way, the inner hair cells measure how quickly the basilar membrane bends as a function of position in the direction toward the apex. See Figure 10.9.

Outer and inner hair cells have different patterns of connections with the auditory nerve. The auditory nerve consists of the myelinated axons of the spiral

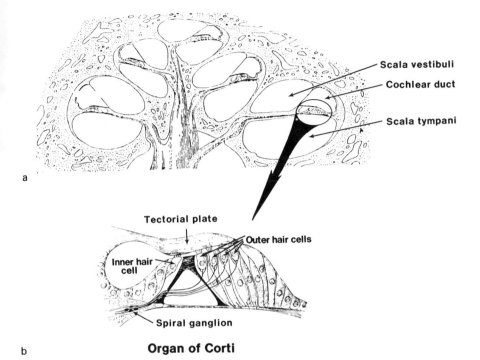

Scala vestibuli

Cochlear duct

Scala tympani

a

Tectorial plate

Outer hair cells

Inner hair cell

Spiral ganglion

b

Organ of Corti

Figure 10.7.   a. A cross section of the cochlear duct. (Reproduced, from Georg von Békésy, The Ear. Copyright © 1957 by Scientific American, Inc. All rights reserved.) b. An enlarged diagram of the organ of Corti. (Reproduced, with permission, from Derek A. Sanders. *The Auditory Perception of Speech. An Introduction to Principles and Problems*, p. 57. Copyright © 1977 by Prentice-Hall, Inc.)

ganglion cells. The spiral ganglion cells are bipolar: Their axons form the auditory nerve; each dendrite consists of a single filament which passes through the cochlear wall, extends toward the hair cells, and branches near the hair cells that innervate it. One collection of spiral ganglion cells, the inner radial bundle, only contacts inner hair cells. Each ganglion cell of the inner bundle contacts one or two inner hair cells, and each inner hair cell contacts one or two of these spiral ganglia. A similar group of spiral ganglion cells, the outer radial bundle, connects in a similar manner to outer hair cells. This group tends to be somewhat less orderly and less frequent than the inner radial ganglia. The majority of the spiral ganglion cells that connect to outer hair cells form the external spiral fibers. The dendrite branches of these cells cross the tunnel of Corti and then run parallel to the tunnel usually toward the base of the cochlea. They often run as far as a third of a turn of the cochlea, and they contact many outer hair cells. In addition, they often change from inner to outer rows as they progress along the organ of Corti. The final set of fibers, the internal spiral fibers, convey information to the hair cells from outside the cochlea. It is not yet understood how these efferent fibers regulate the hair cells.

How are sound waves converted into neural patterns? Sound waves move the ear drum which, through the ossicles, move the oval window in a similar manner. Since the oval window directly contacts the perilymph fluid of the scala vestibula, the mechanical movement creates pressure in the fluid. Because the fluid is incompressible and the cochlea is encased by the skull, the only place for the perilymph fluid to expand is at the round window. Either the fluid moves along the scala vestibula, through the helicotrema, and down the scala tympani, or the cochlear duct must give way as shown in Figure 10.8.

Both types of movement occur. If the oval window is held flexed due to a constant pressure difference between outer and inner ears, the perilymph fluid moves through the helicotrema to normalize the pressure in the scala vestibula and scala tympani. In contrast, ordinary sound moves the oval window so rapidly that the perilymph fluid has no time to travel the long path through the helicotrema. In this case the cochlear duct flexes. The higher the sound frequency, the faster the movement of the oval window and the less time the perilymph fluid has to move. The cochlear membrane bulges near the oval window, and the bulge propagates as a traveling wave along the cochlear duct.

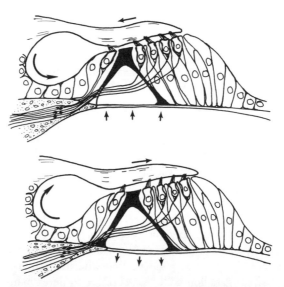

Figure 10.8. One mechanism of sound transduction in the inner ear. Flexion of the basilar membrane is caused by changes in fluid pressure in the inner ear. The resulting movement of the hair cells relative to the tectorial plate are converted by the hair cells into neural impulses.

Figure 10.9. a. Mechanical generation of neural impulses by the hair cells. When the sensory hairs are inclined toward and away from the kinocilium, depolarization and hyperpolarization, respectively, stimulate and inhibit the associated afferent neurons. Motion, direction of motion of stereocilia; pot, potential changes inside the hair cell in response to motion; nap, nerve action potential changes in response to pot. b. Diagram showing why the frequency of the microphonic potential is the same as the stimulus frequency if the hair cells are oriented in one direction. c. Diagram showing why paired hair cells with opposite orientation produce a response at double the stimulus frequency. (Reproduced, by permission, from Yasuji Katsuki. *Receptive Mechanisms of Sound in the Ear.* Copyright © 1982 by Cambridge University Press.)

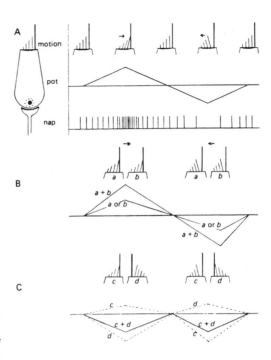

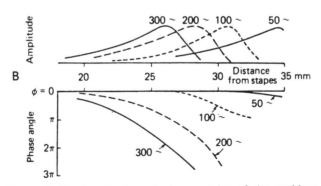

Figure 10.10. Amplitude and phase angles of the cochlear partition at various distances from stapes. (Reproduced, with permission, from G. von Békésy, *Experiments in Hearing.* Copyright © 1960 by McGraw-Hill Book Company.)

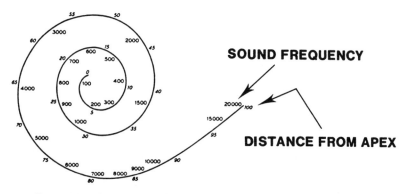

Figure 10.11. Positions in the cochlea for maximum responses to pure tones. (Reproduced from Francis Weston Sears, *Mechanics, Heat, and Sound*, Figure 28-6, page 529. Copyright © 1950 by Addison-Wesley Publishing Company, Reading, Massachusetts. Courtesy of Dr. Harvey Fletcher.)

See Figure 10.10. The amplitude and shape of the wave depends on its position and on the sound frequency and intensity that caused it. For a given sound intensity, lower frequencies produce waves of higher amplitude. The basilar membrane, very rigid near the base of the cochlea, gets broader and less rigid toward the apex. As a result, each traveling wave reaches a maximum amplitude some distance from the base and then dies away. The position of maximum amplitude depends on the amount of energy absorbed and, as measured from the apex, is linearly related to the logarithm of the sound frequency which produced it. See Figure 10.11. The speed of the wave, on the other hand, is independent of its size or shape but depends only on the tensile properties of the basilar membrane.

You may better understand how the organ of Corti works by considering the vibrations of piano strings. If a person hums a tone into a piano, the strings corresponding to that tone will continue to resonate even after the person stops humming. Each string absorbs energy, with maximum energy absorption taking place for the string's natural or fundamental frequency. The lowest frequency that a given piano string will continue to vibrate without external stimulation is its fundamental frequency, also called its first harmonic. The same string can also be set into motion at exactly twice its fundamental frequency, which is called its first overtone or second harmonic. A given string can be set into motion at any integral multiple of its fundamental frequency, and for integer N, the frequency is the Nth harmonic. See Figure 10.12. The sound of a given piano string is always a combination of its harmonic frequencies, and because these are its natural frequencies of vibration, the string more efficiently absorbs energy at these frequencies.

Although the analogy is far from exact, the basilar membrane can be pictured

276

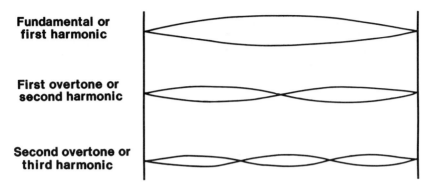

Fundamental or first harmonic

First overtone or second harmonic

Second overtone or third harmonic

Figure 10.12. Standing waves in a stretched string, showing the relationships between the fundamental frequency, its harmonics, and its overtones.

as a collection of parallel strings which are tuned, as are the strings of a piano, to a sequence of specific frequencies. For a piano, the strings are arranged linearly, and since the frequencies of the notes of one octave are double the frequencies of the corresponding notes of the next lower octave, the logarithm of frequency is linearly related to position.[3] The organ of Corti uses this same arrangement. In the piano, high-note strings are thinner and stretched more tightly than low-note strings; in the organ of Corti, high frequencies are sensed most strongly near the base where the basilar membrane is narrower and more tense. This is also analogous to the arrangement of a piano. Figure 10.13 shows how the positions of maximum response along the organ of Corti are related to the sounds of a piano's notes.

If, as is currently believed, the basilar membrane is positionally tuned to different sound frequencies like a piano, then one would expect maximum energy absorption to take place not only at the location tuned to the sound's fundamental frequency, but also at each location tuned to an harmonic of the fundamental. Figure 10.14, based on a theoretical model of the basilar membrane and cochlear duct, shows that this is the case.

Although the analogy between piano and cochlea is close, it is not perfect. Unlike a piano, the basilar membrane is not comprised of strings. And unlike a piano, where sound arrives independently at all strings, each wave traveling along the basilar membrane must first propagate past receptors that detect high frequencies and then past receptors that detect lower frequencies, until all energy has been absorbed.

---

[3] As an example, middle C on a piano has a fundamental frequency of 264 Hz. The lowest C on a piano is three octaves lower and has a fundamental frequency of 33 Hz, which is 1/2 x 1/2 x 1/2 x 264. High C on a piano is four octaves above middle C and has a fundamental frequency of 4224 Hz, which is 2 x 2 x 2 x 2 x 264.

For high frequencies, the organ of Corti appears to measure one or more quantities from which energy absorption can be determined as a function of position along the basilar membrane. What properties enable energy absorption to be determined? First, the hair cells might measure the maximum deflection of the basilar membrane. By comparing these measurements, subsequent networks can determine places of local maximum energy absorption and hence places where the basilar membrane is tuned to the stimulating sound. Second, the hair cells might measure acceleration of the basilar membrane. Places where the acceleration has a local maximum are places of local maximum energy absorption. Third, the hair cells might measure the relative local distortion of the basilar membrane. This is a measure of the longitudinal gradient of the traveling wave and is one property that some outer hair cells appear to measure. The variety of cell morphologies and local connections suggests in fact that several of these quantities are measured simultaneously.

The situation is different for very low frequencies. For frequencies below about 100 Hz, the oval window moves so slowly that the entire basilar membrane oscillates. All regions send nerve impulse volleys which are synchronous with the sound frequency. The tuning effect, which is apparent for high

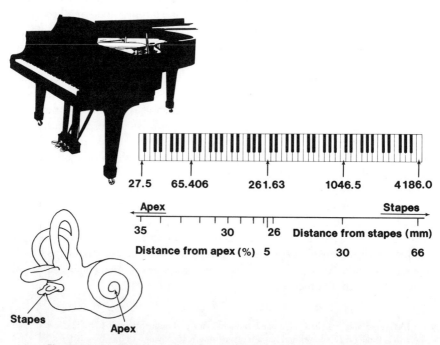

Figure 10.13.   Relationship between position of maximum response of the cochlea and position of a note on a piano.

frequencies, does not occur. It appears, therefore, that for low frequencies the organ of Corti simply responds to upward deflection of the basilar membrane.

The Auditory Pathway

Unlike the visual system, for which years of intensive research have painted a detailed picture of the electrical responses of many different types of cells, the auditory system is less understood. There is some degree of uncertainty and fragmentation in present findings, which will be evident in the following presentation. Nonetheless, the anatomy and physiology of the auditory networks along the pathways from cochlea to cortex provide considerable evidence for several stages of coding and recoding with increasing complexity. The evidence is presented in an attempt to shed insight into the information processing being done.

As with all sensory modalities, the geometrical arrangement of the receptor surface is preserved throughout the system. Within the cochlea and all subsequent processing stations, sound frequency is related to position: High-frequency sounds are encoded at one side of the network and low-frequency sounds are encoded at the other.

The auditory encoding becomes increasingly more complex as it moves from station to station along the auditory pathway. The cochlea contains about 25,000 hair cells and the cochlear nerve has approximately 30,000 elements. The cochlear nucleus contains about 90,000 cells, whereas the inferior colliculus and medial geniculate nucleus contain 400,000 and 360,000 cells. Finally, the auditory cortex contains about 10 million cells.

Auditory Nerve

Each auditory nerve fiber, an axon of a spiral ganglion cell, responds in a characteristic way. First, each cell responds to tones in a limited frequency range, which narrows as the intensity of the sound is reduced. The pattern of responses of a cell is its response curve, and its frequency of maximum response is its characteristic or best frequency. The response curve and best frequency are determined by the mechanical properties of the organ of Corti as described earlier. Second, the rate of firing of a given cell increases monotonically with increasing sound intensity. For a sustained tone, the response adapts over time. As many as 10,000 cells may respond to a single tone, and in the absence of noise, most cells fire spontaneously. For high frequencies, responses of stimulated cells appear to occur at random but with a statistical distribution as described above. Finally, for sharp clicks, cells respond at preferred times after the stimulus. The preferred times show a periodic structure with as many as six peaks for middle frequencies and as few as a single peak for high frequencies.

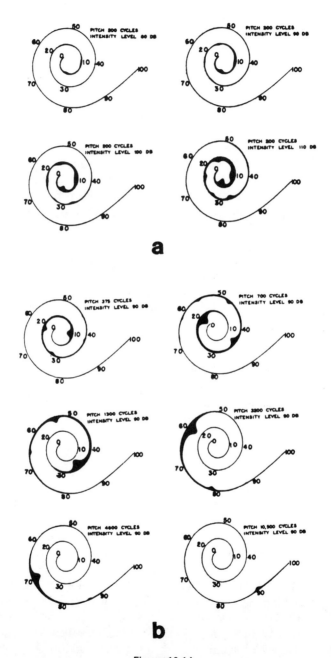

Figure 10.14.

Differences between responses for inner and outer radial fibers and outer spiral fibers have not been characterized.

Cochlear Nucleus

The auditory nerve enters the cochlear nucleus where it divides and terminates in three separate subnuclei: the anteroventral, posteroventral, and dorsal cochlear nuclei. The division is orderly: One branch innervates the anteroventral cochlear nucleus and the other innervates both the dorsal and posteroventral cochlear nuclei. The terminating branches of each cell not only retain their positional relationships, but they spread out into approximately parallel planar surfaces. Within each of the three subnuclei, therefore, the terminating branches form parallel surfaces which have a single best frequency and are arranged tonotopically.

Each of the three subnuclei is composed of numerous types of cells having a variety of synaptic arrangements. A recent review by Brugge and Geisler (1978) describes the morphology and pharmacology of the cells in each part of the cochlear nucleus.

Different discharge patterns have been observed in the cells of the cochlear nuclei. Many cells fire spontaneously. Among the spontaneously active cells, many discharge at random like auditory nerve cells and are called primary-like. Others have a more regular discharge pattern and are therefore not classified as primary-like. One property that differentiates cells in the ventral and dorsal cochlear nuclei is that spontaneous activity of cells in the ventral cochlear nucleus ceases when the auditory nerve is severed; the same is not true for cells in the dorsal cochlear nucleus.

Cells with primary-like responses have been found throughout the cochlear nucleus. Primary-like cells of the anteroventral cochlear nucleus accurately relay the primary auditory pattern to the superior olivary complex as described shortly. The primary-like discharge patterns of these cells are distinguished from the discharge patterns of auditory nerve cells by a short delay in the response time to a click stimulus. Like auditory nerve cells, these cells also have a best-frequency response. Although primary-like cells have been seen in the posteroventral and dorsal cochlear nuclei as well, cells of these nuclei often pause briefly after stimulus onset, and many are inhibited by frequencies near their best frequency. Auditory nerve cells show no such inhibition.

Cells with complex response patterns to simple stimuli are found mostly in

Figure 10.14.   Auditory patterns in the cochlear duct produced by a) a 200 Hz pure tone at various intensity levels, b) 375 Hz, 700 Hz, 1300 Hz, 3200 Hz, 4600 Hz, and 10,500 Hz tones at 90 db. (Reproduced from Francis Weston Sears. *Mechanics, Heat, and Sound*, Figure 28-6, page 528. Copyright © 1950 by Addison-Wesley Publishing Company, Reading, Massachusetts. Courtesy of Dr. Harvey Fletcher.)

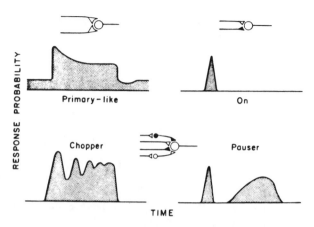

Figure 10.15. Schematic diagram of poststimulus time histograms showing four categories of temporal discharge patterns that can be recorded from cells in the cochlear nucleus. Each inset indicates a model of spatial arrangements of excitatory synapses (open symbols) and inhibitory synapses (shaded symbols) due to primary afferent inputs that could produce that response. (Reproduced, with permission, from J. F. Brugge & C. D. Geisler, Auditory mechanisms of the lower brainstem. *Annual Review of Neuroscience*, 1, 363-394. Copyright © 1978 by Annual Reviews Inc.)

the posteroventral and dorsal cochlear nuclei. Complex response patterns fall into five categories: on-type I, on-type L, chopper, pauser, and buildup. The chopper and pauser patterns are shown in Figure 10.15.

On-type I and on-type L cells are not spontaneously active but respond actively to the onset of sound at all frequencies within their response area. On-type I cells continue to respond at a low rate to sustained sound; on-type L cells fire only at stimulus onset and then quit firing with sustained sound. Both on-type I and on-type L cells will again show their initially strong onset activity after a brief silence, which for some cells is as short as 1.5 milliseconds. Most respond actively to a click stimulus.

The remaining response patterns are less regular and may vary with changing stimulus. The chopper pattern, which lasts for 25 to 50 seconds after stimulus onset, shows a probability of discharge related to the stimulus frequency. The pauser pattern shows an initial burst of activity resembling the on-type response, a subsequent pause in activity, and finally a resumption of activity. The buildup response is characterized by slowly increasing activity which begins shortly after stimulus onset. Cells of the dorsal cochlear nucleus have many inhibitory influences, some from other cells of the same structure and some from external structures. Evans and Nelson (1973) suggest that the complex response patterns are part of a continuum of responses which result from all excitatory and inhibitory influences affecting the cell.

Some cells of the dorsal cochlear nucleus are either excited or inhibited by inputs from the opposite ear. The pathway giving rise to this contralateral influence is not known.

Superior Olivary Complex

Most outputs from the dorsal and ventral cochlear nuclei terminate in the superior olivary complex, although some outputs pass the contralateral olivary complex and continue directly to the inferior colliculus. The superior olivary complex is therefore the first network receiving binaural inputs. The superior olivary complex, like the cochlear nucleus, comprises several subnuclei including the lateral superior olive and the medial superior olive.

The lateral superior olive, also known as the S-shaped segment because of its appearance, is a highly specialized network designed, it appears, to compare information arriving from each ear. The encodings for each best frequency are compared separately as follows. Half the inputs for a given best frequency arrive from one cochlear nucleus and spread out along one edge of a plane surface. The remaining inputs for the same best frequency arrive from the other cochlear nucleus and spread out along the opposite edge of the same plane. Inputs from the same side originate in the front part of the anteroventral cochlear nucleus and are almost exclusively excitatory; inputs from the opposite side arrive both from the back part of the anteroventral cochlear nucleus and from the front part of the posteroventral cochlear nucleus and are almost exclusively inhibitory. Neurons of the lateral superior olive each have two dendrite trees. One spreads out and is innervated by the excitatory inputs; the other spreads out and is innervated by inhibitory inputs. The dendrite trees for a given cell remain approximately within the best frequency plane of its two principal inputs as shown in Figure 10.16. Planes of different best frequency are stacked orderly according to best frequency, with a large percentage devoted to the highest frequencies. When both ears are simultaneously stimulated with a click, the initial spike responses are inhibited, indicating that the time it takes nerve impulses to arrive from the same and opposite ears is the same. In general, the outputs respond to the difference between contributions from the two ears. The responses are regular and demonstrate the chopper pattern.

The structure of the medial superior olive or accessory nucleus is similar to that of the lateral superior olive, though smaller. The inputs come from the anteroventral cochlear nucleus of each side of the brain, and although most cells are excited from both sets of inputs, a few are inhibited by inputs from opposite sides. The output responses of the accessory nucleus are irregular and resemble the primary-like responses of the cells of the anteroventral cochlear nucleus. The responses of most binaurally excited cells are relatively insensitive to

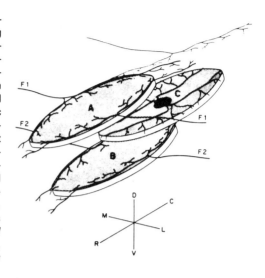

Figure 10.16. Schematic diagram of three (A-C) interleaving disc-shaped neurons in the lateral superior olive (LSO) or medial superior olive (MSO). Dendritic organization is shown only in neuron C. The flattened neuropil between dendritic fields is shown as it would appear from two cells of the left and right cochlear nuclei, respectively, which have two different best frequencies (F1 and F2). (Reproduced, with permission, from J. F. Brugge & C. D. Geisler, Auditory mechanisms of the lower brainstem. *Annual Review of Neuroscience*, 1, 363-394. Copyright © 1978 by Annual Reviews Inc.)

changes in sound levels at the two ears as long as the average sound level remains constant. When both ears are stimulated by a click, the probability of an initial response is maximum for simultaneous stimulus presentation. The probability of an initial response decreases rapidly as the difference between the stimulus times increases, dropping from about .6 for simultaneous presentations to .1 when the presentation times differ by .5 milliseconds. By comparison, the absolute latency of firing after stimulus presentation is about 5 milliseconds.

Although the remaining subnuclei of the superior olivary complex have been studied by several researchers, the studies have not given a clear characterization of the cell types and responses. The reader is directed to the review by Brugge and Geisler (1978) for further details.

Inferior Colliculus and Medial Geniculate Body

The auditory encodings produced by the superior olivary complex are sent to the inferior colliculus via the lemniscal pathway. Cells of the inferior colliculus have many discharge patterns. Some cells respond to clicks but not to any tones; others respond to tones as well. Of the cells responding to tones, there are representatives from all of the complex cell categories described for the cochlear nucleus, with variations which depend on sound frequency and stimulated ear.

Outputs from the inferior colliculus terminate in the medial geniculate nucleus as shown in Figure 10.3. The pathway from inferior colliculus to medial geniculate nucleus conveys the bulk of inputs to the medial geniculate nucleus. Of all auditory processing stations along the auditory pathway, the medial geniculate nucleus has been the least studied, and the few studies which were undertaken show cells with responses similar to the inferior colliculus. Perhaps the biggest distinction is the lack of evidence for a tonotopical organization that is so evident in the other auditory stations.

The Auditory Cortex

The auditory cortex is the final station on the ascending pathway from the ears and also the first station for high-level analysis of sound. Even though the auditory cortex plays a crucial role in auditory encoding, our knowledge of its functioning is severely lacking. This brief section summarizes some of its better-known properties.

The auditory cortex, not nearly as well delimited as the primary visual cortex, receives the bulk of its sensory inputs from the medial geniculate nucleus through the auditory radiations. The cochlea projects to at least two distinct areas of the cerebral cortex which are called areas AI and AII. Since area AI gives rise to projections to area AII, AI is called primary and AII secondary. Nevertheless, area AII appears to receive direct inputs from lower auditory nuclei as well, and most parts of the cortex respond to nonauditory stimulation in addition to auditory stimulation.

Assuming the auditory and visual systems are somewhat similar, the auditory cortex is a sensory buffer which converts the low-level auditory representations it receives into the high-level representations that are stored and analyzed by the auditory memory stores. By analogy with the visual cortex, we might expect to find the auditory cortex tonotopically organized and divided into columns, each column processing the encodings for a particular range of best frequencies. Furthermore, within each column we might expect to find individual cells responding to particular features of the auditory stimulus. The present evidence is suggestive but not overwhelming.

Some evidence indicates a tonotopical organization, although different researchers have arrived at conflicting viewpoints. Cells within any area of the cortex have a variety of best frequencies. Cells on one side of the auditory cortex favor low frequencies and cells on the other side favor high frequencies; still, one cannot state with certainty that there is a continuous progression from low to high frequencies across the cortex. Furthermore, in dogs and cats, which have provided much of the current data, the results differ markedly.

Evidence for columnar organization was gathered by measuring the characteristic frequencies of cells along vertical penetrations of the cortex using microelectrodes.[4] Each set of measurements taken along such a penetration

---

[4]See Chapter 7 for details.

show a small set of values, which may be quite different.[5] If each vertical column processes a single best frequency, the different values might be caused by a slightly nonvertical penetrating microelectrode entering several different adjacent columns.

The assertion that cells of the auditory cortex respond to particular features of the stimulating sound is also supported to some degree by experimental data. Many cells do not respond at all to pure tones but respond either to increasing or decreasing sound frequency. For some cells, when the sound frequency is increased and decreased (modulated) about a particular central frequency, the likelihood of a cell discharging is high only when the frequency increases through a specific value; there is no similar discharge when the frequency decreases through the same value. See Figure 10.17. Other cells respond to decreasing but not increasing sound frequency. In general, cells that respond to increasing or decreasing frequency do so over a broad band of different values, with some cells responding in the opposite way when the central frequency changes from a high to a low value. This evidence suggests that the cells either encode a change in frequency—the frequency gradient, or a change in the frequency gradient—the frequency acceleration. In either case, the evidence supports the hypothesis that cells encode high-level features of the sound stimulus.

HIGH-LEVEL AUDITORY ENCODINGS

There is a remarkable similarity in the way the auditory and visual systems encode information. Both systems construct multiple internal representations of the external world, both systems reduce the information quantity prior to storage and analysis, and both systems form storage representations which enable rapid access to prior related events.

Sensory transducers produce multiple encodings of their stimuli. The eye produces several independent representations of the ocular image which are conveyed by the optic nerve to different layers in the lateral geniculate nucleus. The three cone subsystems encode color in three independent subpatterns, and the rod subsystem encodes the spatial gradient of brightness in another independent subpattern. The cochlea likewise encodes several properties of the sound spectrum. The inner and outer hair cells respond to different movements of the basilar membrane, and the resulting encodings are conveyed by separate nerve bundles to the cochlear nucleus for further processing. Although it is not known whether the different nerve bundles innervate different parts of the cochlear nucleus, it is very likely in view of the fact that the different retinal encodings innervate different layers in the lateral geniculate nucleus.

---

[5]For example, the values along one penetration might be 7, 27, 35, and 25 KHz, or 35, 34, 32, 33, and 5 KHz.

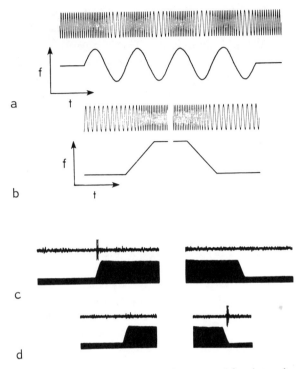

Figure 10.17. a. Auditory waveforms used for determining single cell responses to auditory signals. Top: sinusoidal modulation; bottom: ramp modulation. b. On-cell and off-cell responses to ramp modulation. Top: on-cell; bottom: off-cell. (Reproduced, with permission, from I. C. Whitfield & E. F. Evans, Responses of auditory cortical neurons to stimuli of changing frequency. *Journal of Neurophysiology*, 28, 1965, 655-672.)

The ability of the auditory system to discriminate different tones parallels the ability of the visual system to discriminate different colors. In the visual system, each type of color receptor responds to a broad band of colors. Yet for a given perceived color, the ratios of normalized integrated reflectance values, as measured by the different color receptors, is invariant. In the auditory system, each hair cell responds to a broad band of sound frequencies. Moreover, at a given position along the cochlea, the inner and outer hair cells respond to different components of movement of the basilar membrane and therefore encode different integrated frequency values. Other auditory networks can extract precise frequency information by comparing values in the different encodings. It is still an open question whether the physical correlate of pitch is a ratio of values in these different subpatterns, but the analogy with the visual system is hard to ignore.

The ability of the auditory system to determine the direction and distance of a sound source resembles the ability of the visual system to determine the distance of an object from disparity information. Three properties of sound are fundamental in locating its source: its time of arrival at each ear, the phases of sound waves at each ear, and the relative loudness at each ear. The time it takes a signal to arrive from its source depends on the distance traveled. For an instantaneous noise like a click, the difference in arrival times at the two ears indicates the direction of the source, and as noted earlier, the accessory nucleus of the superior olivary complex accurately determines the difference in arrival times.

For noises which are not instantaneous, phase differences of sound waves arriving at the two ears can be used to determine the direction of the sound source. Since the hair cells are sensitive to the direction of movement of the basilar membrane, the phase differences at each ear can be determined as a function of frequency. It is not yet known if or where phase differences are computed.

Finally, the sound intensity at each ear will differ when the head is turned away from the sound source. As noted before, differences in loudness are determined in the S-shaped segment of the superior olivary complex. The superior olivary complex is clearly implicated in locating the origin of a sound source.

Once the location of a sound source is known, its movement can easily be determined. Changes in loudness and pitch indicate movement: Both the frequency of sound and its intensity increase for a source moving toward a listener and decrease for a source moving away from a listener. Cells have already been observed which respond to changes in pitch, and cells have also been observed which respond to changes in intensity. It therefore appears that both of these attributes are explicitly encoded by the low-level auditory networks.

The Auditory Buffer

The structure of the auditory system was summarized in Figure 10.3. The low-level auditory networks code and recode sound information into multiple representations of high dimensionality which are sent to the auditory cortex for analysis. The low-level encodings include a frequency representation, a frequency gradient representation, an intensity representation, a distance representation, and a movement representation (auditory flow).

By analogy with the visual system, the auditory cortex is assumed to be a sensory buffer which temporarily stores this collection of representations, called the **primal score** by analogy with the visual system's primal sketch. At the same time, the auditory cortex analyzes the primal score and forms the high-level auditory representation. The high-level auditory representation has much smaller size than the primal score and is the canonical representation stored and processed by all other auditory storage systems.

Pursuing the analogy with the visual system a bit further, the auditory buffer is divided into multiple independent storage locations. These storage locations correspond to the cortical hypercolumns. Each storage location receives two distinctly different input patterns. One input pattern is that part of each low-level auditory encoding projected only to that area of the cortex. Whereas each hypercolumn of the visual system processes information originating at a particular neighborhood of the retina, each auditory hypercolumn processes information originating at a particular neighborhood of the cochlea. The second input pattern is an **auditory test pattern**, which is sent to all storage locations of the auditory buffer. Each storage location correlates its sensory input with the test pattern and produces a single output value, the **correlation** between the two input patterns. The **auditory correlation pattern** comprises the set of all correlation outputs generated by the auditory buffer.

The final stage in the formation of the high-level auditory representation is the selection of a particular subpattern of the auditory correlation pattern to occupy the focus of auditory attention. The selected subpattern becomes the **spectral pattern**, which is one of three parts of the high-level auditory representation. The auditory test pattern is the second part, and the **control pattern** used for selecting the spectral pattern from the correlation pattern is the third part. The high-level auditory representation is sent to the memory stores of auditory experience and also to other stores for storage and analysis.

Each subpattern of the high-level auditory encoding conveys different information. The spectral pattern conveys gestalt sound information and corresponds to the visual pictorial pattern. The auditory test pattern reduces the primal score to a size suitable for storage and analysis and corresponds to the visual test pattern. The auditory test pattern conveys the timbre of the selected sound in the same way that the visual test pattern conveys the color and texture of a selected object. Finally, the auditory control pattern indicates the origin of the test pattern as well as the origin of the spectral pattern within the primal score. The control pattern therefore conveys pitch and location and corresponds to the visual control pattern which conveys size and location.

Auditory patterns have both spatial and temporal components, just like their visual counterparts. The auditory pattern has at least one spatial component corresponding to frequency, and hence is at least one-dimensional. It is more than likely, however, that it has two spatial dimensions. One possibility is that harmonic frequencies are encoded in the second spatial direction, as illustrated in Figure 10.18. Encoding harmonic frequencies in this way would greatly simplify the isolation of specific sound sources according to their timbre and would therefore be useful for "listening" to a particular person or to a particular musical instrument in the presence of other sounds. It also offers a natural explanation for the different frequency values found in the same region of the cortex as described earlier.

Some evidence (Edelman & Mountcastle, 1978) suggests that the location of

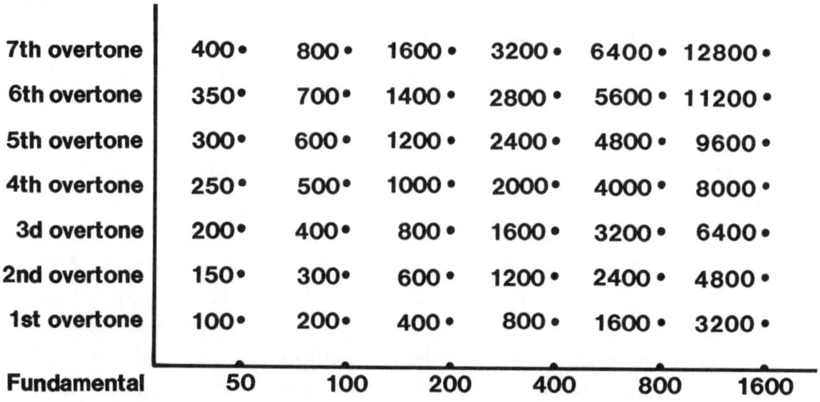

	50	100	200	400	800	1600
7th overtone	400 •	800 •	1600 •	3200 •	6400 •	12800 •
6th overtone	350 •	700 •	1400 •	2800 •	5600 •	11200 •
5th overtone	300 •	600 •	1200 •	2400 •	4800 •	9600 •
4th overtone	250 •	500 •	1000 •	2000 •	4000 •	8000 •
3d overtone	200 •	400 •	800 •	1600 •	3200 •	6400 •
2nd overtone	150 •	300 •	600 •	1200 •	2400 •	4800 •
1st overtone	100 •	200 •	400 •	800 •	1600 •	3200 •
Fundamental	50	100	200	400	800	1600

Figure 10.18. Possible frequency organization of the auditory cortex if the logarithm of the fundamental frequency falls along one direction and the overtone frequency falls along the perpendicular direction.

the sound source is encoded in the second spatial direction. Considerable experimentation is needed before the truth will be known.

The temporal aspects of the auditory encodings are remarkably similar to their visual counterparts. Certainly the auditory encodings vary rapidly as a function of time, but the same is true of the visual encodings, especially when reading is considered. Visual encodings change rapidly, not only because of transients in the receptor systems, but also because of eye movements and changes in the internal focus of attention. Likewise auditory encodings change rapidly not only because sounds change, but also because of head movements and changes in the focus of auditory attention. The auditory and visual systems are extraordinarily similar in view of the incredible differences between the visual and auditory stimuli.

STORAGE OF AUDITORY EXPERIENCE

The differences between the auditory and visual modalities are not in the quantity or quality of stored information, in each case a time-varying neural depolarization pattern, but in the way that the patterns are interpreted.

Auditory experiences, like visual experiences, are stored continuously in time. When a neurosurgeon's electrode chances to activate a past auditory experience (see Chapter 6), the patient reports "hearing" the sounds that were heard once before—sometimes music, sometimes words, but always progressing at time's natural pace. The same is true for visual experiences.

The auditory and visual systems store canonical representations of the stimulus. If one sees an object at two different distances, the images projected on the retina differ in size. Although the retinal images differ, the optic radiations convert them into cortical representations which are size-invariant. Identical high-level encodings are extracted from the cortical representation by selecting the proper subpattern, and the positions of extraction indicate the sizes of the selected objects. For sounds, the cochlea produces a pattern in which the logarithm of sound frequency is linearly related to position. As a result, if one hears the same musical composition in two different keys,[6] the cochlear representations, and presumably the cortical representations, differ only in position. Identical high-level encodings are extracted from the cortical representation by selecting the proper subpattern, and the positions of extraction indicate the keys of the music.

The subpatterns in the high-level auditory and visual representations convey information having conceptually similar interpretations. The test patterns reduce the dimensionality of the encodings for storage. In each case, the test pattern encodes the quality of the stimulus—visual texture versus auditory timbre. The visual pictorial pattern and auditory spectral pattern convey slowly varying information—visual shape versus auditory melody. The control patterns convey scale information—large or small objects versus high- or low-pitched sounds.

Finally, Chapters 6 and 9 have discussed in considerable detail the other types of information that comprise the encodings of experience—the location of an event, the time of its occurrence, and the individual's affect state. These nonauditory components form part of the encodings of auditory experience just as they do for visual experiences. Hence they enable access to associated auditory encodings.

SUMMARY

The auditory system converts sound into auditory storage representations, which enable rapid access to similar stored experiences. The auditory encodings include timbre, pitch, loudness, and location of sound source. The high-level encodings are the only auditory representations available to the high-level systems for analysis, and when stored auditory encodings are reconstructed, they are heard in the mind's ear.

REFERENCES

von Békésy, G. (1957). The ear. *Scientific American*, 197, 66-78.

_____ (1960). *Experiments in hearing*. New York: McGraw-Hill.

Brugge, J. F., & Geisler, C. D. (1978). Auditory mechanisms of the lower brainstem. *Annual Review of Neuroscience*, 1, 363-394.

---

[6]This can easily be visualized by playing a tune on a piano at several different octaves. The keyboard is arranged exactly like the cochlea: The logarithm of frequency is linearly related to keyboard position. Moving one octave to the right therefore doubles all sound frequencies; moving one octave to the left divides them by 2.

Edelman, G. M., & Mountcastle, V. B. (1978). *The mindful brain. Cortical organization and the group-selective theory of higher brain function.* Cambridge, MA: MIT Press.

Evans, E. F., & Nelson, P. G. (1973). On the functional relationship between the dorsal and ventral divisions in the cochlear nucleus of the cat. *Experimental Brain Research, 17,* 428-442.

Katsuki, Y. (1982). *Receptive mechanisms of sound in the ear.* New York: Cambridge University Press.

Miller, D. C. (1937). *Sound waves—Their shape and speed.* New York: Macmillan.

———— (1916). *The science of musical sounds.* New York: Macmillan.

Sanders, D. A. (1977). *Auditory perception of speech. An introduction to principles and problems.* Englewood Cliffs, NJ: Prentice-Hall.

Sears, F. W. (1950). *Mechanics, heat, and sound.* Reading, MA: Addison-Wesley.

Whitfield, I. C., & Evans, E. F. (1965). Responses of auditory cortical neurons to stimuli of changing frequency. *Journal of Neurophysiology, 28,* 655-672.

SUGGESTED READINGS

Hudspeth, A. J. (1983). Mechanoelectrical transduction by hair cells in the acousticolateralis sensory system. *Annual Review of Neuroscience, 6,* 187-215.

Pierce, J. R. (1983). *The science of musical sound.* New York: Scientific American Books, an imprint of W. H. Freeman.

Whitfield, I. C. (1967). *The auditory pathway.* London: Edward Arnold.

11
COGNITION, UNDERSTANDING, AND LANGUAGE

INTRODUCTION

This chapter describes the storage systems required for understanding simple sentences. It also suggests how the brain represents low-level symbolic information. Mental procedures are introduced as parameterized control patterns, while understanding is the process of generating or activating an appropriate mental procedure and its parameters for responding to an utterance, gesture, or situation. Parameters, as you will see, are values held by activated memory locations. A final section suggests some of the processes which underlie a child's ability to learn to understand simple sentences.

The fundamental belief that motivated this work is that our ability to process, understand, and use natural language has nothing whatever to do with grammars studied by most linguists. The fact that grammars can be used to describe natural language (to the extent that they can) is an artifact of the type of computations performed by the networks that process symbolic information. In particular, the meanings of words can only be understood with reference to the internal representations of what they designate in the brain. The significance of most nouns, for example, is that they are symbolic representations that can be used to activate stored representations of the objects they stand for. The stored representations may be pictorial, spatial, olfactory, or whatever. A word such as "yesterday," which is also a noun, has no such pictorial representation; instead, it is associated with appropriate mental procedures for accessing information which took place yesterday. Concepts, ideas, beliefs and other pieces of information can be named and the names are associated with appropriate symbolic representations, often procedural, of the named items. For example, the token "atheism" activates storage locations holding information about a belief system in which there is no god.

Our ability to use language is a consequence of several facts. The memory systems which process different categories of words have different spatial locations in the brain. (Categories are much more restrictive than syntactic classes as you will see later in this chapter.) Because of the spatial distributions, in memory, of words in different categories, the result of processing a sentence is the generation of a unique internal representation, which I call a sentence pattern, for the initial sentence. Sentence patterns can be recognized by associative memory stores. Each sentence pattern is associated with a control pattern that can be used to regulate subsequent computations of the system; the associated control pattern encodes the meaning of the sentence pattern. It is a procedural representation of the meaning of a class of sentences. Moreover, specific words in the sentence are parameters to the encoded procedure. If the control pattern which is activated by a sentence pattern is recalled and used to regulate the computational activity of the brain, the result is a behavior that is consistent with understanding the meaning of the initial sentence.

This chapter describes the neural basis of language and is based on Baron (1974a, 1974b). Recent work by Langacker (1982, 1986) is highly relevant, although he does not attempt to relate his notions to the underlying neural substrate. Also see Chafe (1970), Jackendoff (1983) and Johnson-Laird (1983).

VISUAL AND AUDITORY EXPERIENCES

Chapters 6 through 10 showed, in principle at least, how the brain represents visual and auditory experiences. Each sensory system forms multiple high-resolution representations of its sensory stimulus, which make explicit particular features of the sensory field. These high-resolution representations preserve the essential topologies of the receptor surfaces. High-resolution representations are transformed by the attention networks into low-resolution canonical storage representations, which become part of our memories of experience.

The visual and auditory storage representations are called canonical because all related representations are similar. As a consequence, the memory locations are able to compare current experiences with past experiences and generate strong similarity signals for all related experiences. The access control system can then recall information from an activated memory location, one that contains related information.

SYMBOLIC TOKENS, NAMING, AND IMAGING

Symbolic thought and language require the frequent conversion between sensory and symbolic representations. When we describe a scene with a dog, the token "dog" may come to mind. If the dog is brown, the token "brown" may come to mind. **Naming** is the process of obtaining the symbolic representation of the word or words describing an object or concept (e.g., "dog," "brown") regardless of the modality or submodality of the concept to be named. Naming includes our ability to describe brightness, change in brightness, color, hue, size, shape, texture, movement, spatial location, and surface orientation from their visual representations; pitch, change in pitch, timbre, loudness, change in loudness, and spatial location of sound source from their auditory representations; sharpness, temperature, pressure, shape, surface location, surface orientation, and movement from their tactile and kinesthetic representations; sweetness, happiness, pleasure, hunger, arousal, jealousy, and fear from their affect representations. This partial list is intended to convey the range of objects, characteristics, and sensations that can be named; it is not a comprehensive list.

Naming is the process of accessing a symbolic representation when given a sensory representation. Said another way, naming translates a sensory code into a symbolic code. The first stage of reading or speech understanding is naming: The images and sounds of words are translated into their symbolic codes. I will describe the special storage networks used for these processes later in this chapter.

Imaging is the process of accessing a sensory representation when given a symbolic representation. For example, the token "bell" may bring to mind the image or sound of a bell or an experience in which a bell was heard. The token "up" may bring to mind the necessary control patterns to direct the gaze upward (even if the physical act of looking upward is never performed). In either case, imaging makes available the sensory representation of the corresponding symbolic token.

Neural representations are often translated without utilizing symbolic representations. For example, the sound of rustling leaves may bring to mind the image of an autumn scene without ever bringing up the token "autumn." Direct translation from one neural code to another is neither imaging nor naming.

One question that naturally comes to mind is, what is the modality of symbolic information? There is probably no single answer to this question. For some individuals the symbolic representations appear to be in the modality of premotor patterns, patterns which generate the efferent motor patterns for vocalization. Chapters 12, 14, and 15 will explore motor control in detail. For individuals who mentally hear the sounds of words when reading, the symbolic representations may be in the auditory modality. But regardless of the modality, we can correctly think of symbolic representations as intermediate between sensory and motor encodings.

NAMING STORES

Associative memory stores translate neural patterns from one representation to another and are the fundamental neural subsystems for naming and imaging. The associative stores which perform naming and imaging are **naming stores**.

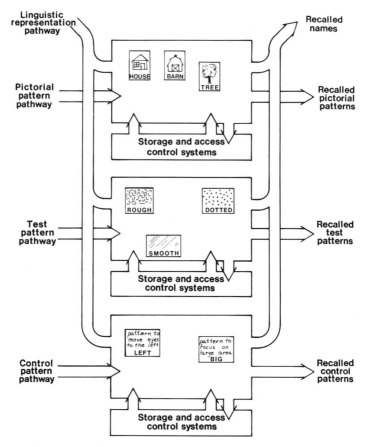

Figure 11.1 A possible structure for the naming stores. Compare with Figure 11.2.

Naming stores have at least two different input and output pathways: those which convey neural representations of symbolic tokens and those which convey neural representations of entities to be named. This is illustrated for three different visual submodalities in Figure 11.1.

In order to name a particular quality such as texture (e.g., glossy, fuzzy, or rough) one or more associative memory stores must be used. When a single associative memory store is used, one input pathway must convey the sensory representation to be named and the other must convey the symbolic representation. When more than one associative memory store is used, the sensory representation must undergo a sequence of translations until the symbolic representation is finally obtained. For example, the assignment of a symbolic code to a printed word may occur by first translating the visual representation of the printed word into a sequence of codes representing the letters and then translating the sequence of letter codes into symbolic codes. Likewise speech may be processed by first translating the auditory representations of speech sounds into a sequence of phoneme representations and then translating the phoneme representations into symbolic codes. On the other hand, intermediate representations are not necessarily used.

Since there are several sensory representations in each sensory modality, there must either be several naming stores within each modality or a single naming store which is functionally divided according to submodality. Figure 11.1 illustrates the possibility that three naming stores are used by the visual system while Figure 11.2 illustrates the possibility that a single naming store is used. As the illustrations show, the principal distinction is whether a single storage control system is used or several.

Within the naming stores, the physical storage sites for the sensory and symbolic representations may be isolated or in registration. The crucial point, which was described at length in Chapter 4, is that a memory location is defined by its control structure and not by its storage structure. Both figures illustrate naming stores where symbolic and sensory engrams are in registration, a situation analogous to the visual cortex where several visual representations are processed by each cortical hypercolumn.

Naming Stores and the Stores of Experience

Experiences are directly encoded by the sensory systems and appear to be stored as they occur. The fact that current experiences may be familiar and remind us of past experiences supports the notion that the stores of experience are

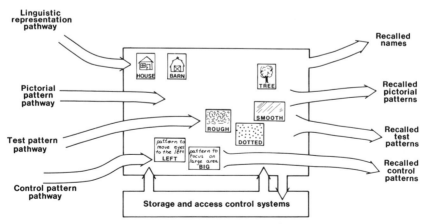

Figure 11.2. A single naming store for visual information. Compare with Figures 11.1 and 11.3.

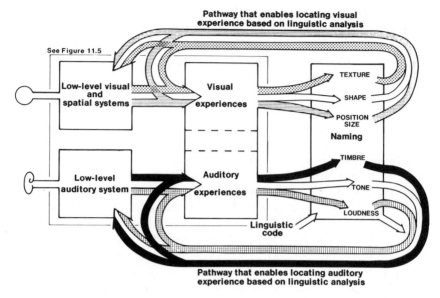

Figure 11.3. Possible relationships between the low-level visual and auditory systems, the permanent stores of experience, and the naming stores. The temporary storage systems are not illustrated. Compare with Figures 11.2, 8.10 and 6.1. Control networks are not shown.

associative. The fact that we can access experiences from their verbal description implies that there are pathways that convey information from the verbal system back to the experiential storage systems. Moreover, these pathways must convey representations which are similar to the ones stored in the stores of experience: They must be sensory representations. It is the naming stores which hold both sensory representations and their symbolic codes and translate between the representations used by these two systems. Figure 11.3 illustrates one possible architecture for the pathways between the visual and symbolic systems, an architecture which will be assumed hereafter.

Organization of the Naming Stores

Our ability to name requires both sensory and symbolic information to be stored in the same memory locations. Because the sensory patterns have different origins and are conveyed by different neural pathways, it is likely that the distribution of memory locations which can be used for naming within a given submodality will depend on where the pathway conveying that representation arrives. That is, the architecture of the brain determines in part its functional organization. The storage control systems, which determine where information is stored within the naming stores, also contribute to the brain's functional organization.

Since the high-level visual encodings comprise a test pattern, a pictorial pattern, and a control pattern, there must either be three naming stores or one functionally divided naming store. Since the visual test pattern encodes surface quality, for example color and texture, the naming store that processes the test pattern must be responsible for naming color and texture.[1]

Our ability to understand and use natural language requires much more than just naming. The following sections will explore the first stages of processing necessary for sentence understanding.

Consider how the naming stores respond during sensory processing. Within each submodality, memory locations that hold patterns which are similar to the current inputs will respond with high similarity signals. If the similarity signals could be used to turn on tiny light bulbs whose brightness indicates similarity, one would see the flickering of those lights as the sensory data are processed by the naming stores. Within the visual system in particular, pictorial patterns would cause flickering in the naming store for pictorial information, color and texture patterns would cause flickering in the naming store for test patterns, and eye movement control patterns would cause flickering in the naming store for spatial relationships. Furthermore, as the focus of visual attention is directed first toward one object and then another, one would see flickering in the naming store for size and spatial relationships (large, small, nearby, far away, to the left, and above). There would, of course, be a similar flickering in the naming stores of each other modality which is actively processing sensory information.

Within a given submodality, the storage control system for that submodality determines where each sensory item is stored and therefore influences the behavior of the system. Before information is stored in a naming store, all memory locations have the same potential for storing information. Once information is stored, however, the placement of additional information can substantially affect the behavior of the system.

There are several storage policies which might be used by the storage control system of a naming store, and each policy will result in a different behavior. Four of them deserve special consideration. First, new patterns can be stored at random. A **random storage policy** would result in a random distribution of information throughout the naming store. Using the previous analogy, during sensory processing the pattern of flickering light bulbs indicating similarity would likewise be random. Second, new patterns can be stored according to their time of arrival. Since sensory items are randomly encountered during one's lifetime, this **temporal storage policy** would also result in random pattern of flickering during sensory processing. A third policy is to store a new pattern in a memory location which is adjacent to memory locations holding similar stored patterns. For this **conceptual storage policy**, although initial data would be

---

[1]Damage to the test pattern pathway would degrade or destroy the ability to name color or texture.

stored at random, subsequent similar items would be stored in nearby storage locations. This would result in clusters of similar information. For pictorial patterns, representations of objects having a similar appearance would be stored nearby, and the pattern of flickering during sensory processing would be organized into clusters based on pictorial similarity. The region containing an active cluster would light up vigorously, and as the focus of attention shifts, other regions would light up. The flickering would no longer be random: It would be conceptually organized.

The fourth and final storage policy places similar names in nearby memory locations. This **similar name storage policy** leads to random flickering during sensory processing but organized flickering during imaging, where access to information is by name rather than by sensory representation. Although at present there is little experimental evidence upon which to base a choice, the organization resulting from the conceptual storage policy appears to be the natural policy and will be assumed hereafter.

UNDERSTANDING

Understanding means knowing what is meant or intended by an utterance, a gesture, or a situation. One understands how a pendulum clock works when one can predict the relationships between the pendulum, escapement mechanism, gears, and mainspring or weight assembly. One understands how checkers or chess is played when one knows which moves are valid and which board configurations result in a win. (This does not imply that one knows how to win the game.) Finally, one understands the meaning of a sentence when one knows how to respond to it. This does not mean that one knows why the sentence was spoken or if there was a hidden meaning intended by it. Understanding always requires the interaction of stored information with sensory information,[2] and understanding generally involves the control of subsequent mental and physical events.

We begin to understand brain function when we can create functional models for its neural circuitry which correctly describe relationships between sensory inputs, storage representations, and responses. The previous chapters have dealt with the conversion of sensory information into storage representations, and so far this chapter has described how sensory representations enable access to symbolic representations. The remainder of this chapter will deal with the far more complicated issue of understanding in general.

We have seen that sensory encodings are converted through a sequence of neural processes into high-level representations which can be recognized by the naming stores. These are by no means simple or well-understood processes.

---

[2]Sensory information includes thought patterns as well as external sensory patterns.

There are two types of outputs from the naming stores. First, during naming or imaging, sensory and symbolic patterns are generated. Second, during sensory analysis, similarity patterns are generated. The similarity patterns correspond to the patterns of flickering lights described earlier. Under the assumption that the engrams in the naming stores are organized by a suitable storage policy, the resulting similarity patterns are highly organized and represent the current situation is a way that will soon become apparent.

Consider what takes place when answering a question such as, "Is there a lamp on the table?" Assume that a subject has understood the question and has decided to respond to it. Further assume he or she is presented with a picture of the scene about which the question was asked. The first thing he or she must do is to look for a lamp and a table. This requires bringing the lamp and table into the focus of visual attention. If either object is missing, a negative response must be generated, but if both a lamp and table are present, the next step is to determine the spatial relationship between them. (If there is more than one lamp or table present, an alternate response will be needed.) If the lamp is on the table, then an affirmative response must be generated; otherwise a negative response must be generated. Understanding implies the ability to carry out such a sequence of mental and physical (eye movement) processes.

Understanding does not mean that the response procedure will be carried out. Rather, understanding means that access is gained to an appropriate response procedure or factual knowledge for carrying out a response. One does not understand a question by answering it.

MENTAL PROCEDURES

Our ability to respond to various situations implies that we can intentionally regulate our physical and mental actions. It is easy to understand what is meant by regulating physical actions. The mental events lead directly to bodily movements which can be readily observed by others. The underlying mental events, however, cannot be seen and are often hidden from introspection by their complexity or subtlety.

Most mental events do not lead to action and cannot be observed at all. One example is directing the focus of visual attention toward a particular object. Focusing the visual attention requires the coordination of body, head, and eye movements (which can be seen) as well as the regulation of internal selection and routing operations (which cannot be seen). As we saw in Chapter 8, directing the focus of visual attention requires selecting an appropriate test pattern for converting the low-level visual representations into a canonical high-level representation (e.g., using an object-centered coordinate system). Once formed, the selected visual representations must be transmitted to the storage systems for analysis. Once the eyes are properly directed and the internal pathways correctly enabled for transmission, the storage systems can finally access related information. Only then can understanding take place.

Our ability to regulate the internal selection and attention processes is a fundamental part of understanding. We learn what to look for; we learn how to look; and we learn how to access related experiences. *It is an inescapable fact that within our brains are memory stores that hold the patterns which control our mental apparatus.*

In order to illustrate what is meant by a mental procedure, 14 questions will be considered. Some deal with the visual system and require specific types of visual analysis; others deal primarily with memories of experience and focus on how access is gained to stored information. Although the particular mental procedures to be considered are only a sampling of the types of thought processes that commonly take place, a sufficient variety will be considered to establish a firm basis for understanding how natural language might be understood. The particular questions to be analyzed are the following:

What is that?
Is that John Smith?
Who is in the car?
What color is the car?
How fast is it moving?
Does the road have a rough surface?
What did you have for dinner yesterday?
Did you ever see the movie, "The Seven Year-Itch?"
Did you enjoy it?
If you could see out the window, what would you see?
How do you get to work from here?
How many people work in your building?
Have you ever felt frustrated?
Are you hungry?

What is that?   In answering this question, attention must either be directed toward the speaker or toward the environment to determine what "that" refers to. If there was a recent loud noise or flash of light, for example, then "that" probably refers to its source. Otherwise, the speaker might be pointing or looking at an object. In either case, once the focus of attention is directed toward the object, it can be recognized and a response generated. If one or more memory locations are activated in the naming store for pictorial information, and if access of the symbolic representation gives a name for the object, then a direct answer can be generated. Otherwise an answer such as, "I don't know" must be given.

The major mental processes for this question are directing the visual apparatus toward the designated object, creating a canonical storage representation so the naming store can recognize it, recalling associated symbolic information from the naming store, and generating a response. Each of the processes—attending the object, forming a canonical representation, recognition, and response generation—is fundamental in answering the original question. Each is a learned high-level procedure, and each is part of thinking and understanding.

Is that John Smith?   The first step in answering this question is attending the person being asked about. Just like the previous example, the encodings must be routed to the naming stores for analysis. Now, however, if an activated memory location holds the name "John Smith," an affirmative answer can be given; if not, a negative answer must be given. The difference between this question and the previous one is not in the selection and encoding processes but in the analysis and response that must be generated. A naming store must contain both the name "John Smith" and pictorial representations which match the current visual encodings before an affirmative answer can be given.

Who is in the car?   Once again the sensory apparatus must be directed, first toward the car and then toward the person in it. If either one is missing, a response such as, "I don't see the car" or "I don't see the person in it" must be generated. If there are several cars present, a request for more information must be generated: "Which car do you mean?" If the car and person are found and the person's name is accessed, then the question can be answered. If the person is not recognized, a negative response must be given.

What color is it?   For this question the reference "it" must be interpreted. If "it" is interpreted as meaning the car, then the car can be selected for the focus of attention. During sensory analysis, the word "color" implies a special type of perceptual analysis. The shape of the car and other pictorial features are not relevant; only the color is. The response must therefore be based on information that is activated by the visual test pattern, not in the naming store for spatial information. Once a name is attached to the neural representation of the color, the question can be answered just as in the previous cases.

How fast is the car moving?   Like the previous question, this one requires that the focus of visual attention be directed toward the car. Now, however, the color is not relevant but its speed is. Since speed is not an attribute of the car but an attribute of the relationship between the car, its background, and the viewer, a special perceptual analysis is required. It is necessary to name an attribute of the visual flow pattern (refer to Chapter 7). Once the visual flow pattern is recognized and a name attached to it, the question can be answered just as in the previous examples.

Does the road have a rough surface?   Once again, the sensory apparatus must be directed. This time the texture of the road must be analyzed, and texture has a different internal representation than color, speed, or shape. Understanding the question means understanding the significance of the word "texture." If the test pattern is recognized and a name accessed (rough, smooth, icy, glassy, etc.), then an answer can be generated.

What did you have for dinner yesterday?   This question differs significantly from the previous ones. It does not require an analysis of the current sensory inputs, but rather, it requires access into the stores of experience. Since the stores of experience are associative, the symbolic apparatus must recall appropriate sensory representations and send them to the stores of experience for analysis. The phrase "what did you have?" implies a memory search, and the term "dinner" specifies what is being sought. However, "dinner" is not a particularly rich clue for setting up an associative search.

It is sometimes possible, by recalling different dinners, to remember what was eaten for dinner yesterday (was it chicken, hot dogs and beans, spaghetti . . . ?), but as often as not this type of exhaustive search doesn't work. When it doesn't, usually the search consists of recalling a particular event that occurred the previous day, and mentally trying to advance forward in time to figure out what dinner was. This is called **temporal chaining** and is an important associative search procedure. Temporal chaining consists of recalling an event from an activated memory location and routing the recalled information back as an associative input to activate additional memory locations. If, by this process, the storage representations of the previous night's dinner are activated, then their representations can be transmitted to the naming stores for analysis. A response can then be generated.

The ability to isolate memories according to their time of occurrence plays a central role in our day-to-day lives. If we could not tell whether a particular event occurred yesterday, last week, or last year, it would be difficult to survive. The mental apparatus was given the power to determine the time of occurrence of an event from its storage representation, and it was also given the power to access information according to its approximate time of occurrence. The question remains, how does verbal information restrict the search to a particular interval of time?

Words and phrases such as "yesterday," "tomorrow," "last year," and "a long time ago" all put restrictions on the memory search. Unlike picture words (nouns) or words describing perceptual features such as color, texture, or speed, words describing the time of an event have no external significance. They do have an internal significance: They help specify information in memory. They must therefore be associated with control patterns which can be used to control the access parameters of the storage networks. If, as suggested in Chapters 6 and 9, the information in the stores of experience is organized according to time of input, then words that describe the time of an event translate into absolute or relative positions in the stores of experience. When asked about yesterday's events, the access control networks can restrict the memory locations from which relevant information might be recalled. (Note that the access control system cannot activate storage locations; it can modify the threshold parameters for access, it can initiate recall from an active memory location, or it can deactivate active memory locations. Activation of memory locations can only be done by association.)

In answering the question "What did you have for dinner yesterday?" the first mental step is to recall the information associated with "dinner" and "yesterday." The pattern associated with "yesterday" is used to restrict access within the stores of experience, and the patterns associated with "dinner" is used both to restrict what is being searched for and to restrict access to specific events in the store—those which occurred at dinner time, hence late in the day. This may, for example, result in modified access parameters to names or experiences related to food. The detailed sequence of analytical processes required to convert from the word "dinner" to the complicated search strategies for this type of search are not yet known.

Did you ever see the movie, "The Seven-Year Itch?"   Like the previous question, this one requires a search of the stores of experience. Unlike the previous question, however, the time is not restricted. The word 'ever' removes any restriction. For this question, the name of the movie is used to access particular experiences, which are then analyzed in attempting to answer the question. If those experiences include one of watching the movie, a positive answer can be given. Sometimes it is not possible to recall specific events that once occurred, in which case an answer like, "I don't know" or "I think so" can be generated. Sometimes the name enables access to specific knowledge about the movie—Marilyn Monroe starred in it—but still not enough information to answer the specific question asked. In any event, answering the question requires activating specific pieces of experiential knowledge, recalling them, and analyzing the recalled representations in an attempt to answer the question.

Did you enjoy it?   Assuming that a positive response was given to the previous question, this question requires a further analysis of the representations which were recalled while answering the previous question. Since the encodings of experience contain an encoding of the time and location of the event as well as the physical and mental state of the individual during the event, this question can be answered by simply recalling the event and sending the recalled affect state encodings to the naming stores for analysis. Words like "happy" and "sad" are associated with specific affect patterns and can therefore be used when responding to the question.

If you could see out the window, what would you see?   This question is significantly different from any of the previous ones. It does not require directing the attention externally, nor does it require a memory search based on time. What is required is a memory search based on the location of the observer. The observer's spatial coordinates, both absolute and relative, are used to access knowledge about the world, and the accesses must be to specific experiences based on their location. Unlike trying to remember what dinner was yesterday, which cannot be accomplished by a simple associative search, access to spatial knowledge is direct and very fast. Fast access implies that part of each experience is an encoding of its spatial location. Moreover, rapid access implies that the mental apparatus is able to translate current coordinate specifications into an appropriate pattern for associative search, which can then access the desired information. How this is done is yet unknown.

How do you get to work from here?   This question, like the previous one, requires access to spatial knowledge. The usual procedure that one follows in answering this question is mentally to follow the same route that is usually driven. Experiences along the route are recalled, and the naming stores are able to analyze and describe them as they are recalled.

Recall of experiences need not take place at the same speed that they were lived. Experiences are organized into packets which can be recalled quite independently, and only the first few moments of a given packet need to be recalled in order to describe its contents. By using spatial coordinates as access keys, and by further restricting access to nearby memory locations, the experiences can be accessed along a spatial path, even one which was never followed. **Spatial chaining** is an associative search technique which resembles both memory scanning (refer to Chapter 9) and temporal chaining. Spatial chaining is also an important memory search technique which consists of recalling an activated event, modifying its spatial coordinates, and transmitting the modified spatial coordinates back to the memory system to activate additional memory locations. By this process, one can mentally retrace one's steps or follow a new path that was never taken before.

How many people work in your building?   This question resembles "What did you have for dinner yesterday?" in that there is not enough information on which to base an associative search. Unlike the dinner question, however, time does not play an important part in accessing the correct information. When answering this question, one technique that is frequently used is mentally to walk around the building, trying to recall the individuals who work in the offices along the corridor that is traveled. Once the memories of an individual are accessed, other unknown computational networks can keep count. The process of mentally walking around the building is another example of spatial chaining. Note that it is not the search process that is important but only its result, the access of specific relevant pieces of knowledge.

Have you ever felt frustrated?   In answering this question, information must be accessed according to the components which encode one's affect state. The word "frustration" has associated with it the affect state patterns of frustration. Answering this question requires routing the recalled encodings of frustration from the naming store into the stores of experience to activate the records of one or more events. Once recalled, the naming stores analyze the events and enable a response to be given to the question.

Are you hungry?   Answering this question requires focusing the attention on one's current physical state. Focusing the attention means sending the physical state encodings to the storage systems for analysis and in particular to the correct naming store. Once the physical state encodings arrive at the naming store, they may activate memory locations containing words such as "hungry," "ravished," or "starving," in which case an affirmative response should be generated; words such as "full," "satiated," or "stuffed" in which case a negative response should be generated; or no hunger-related words at all, in which case a neutral response should be generated. In any case, answering the question requires that the appropriate sensory patterns be sent to the naming stores for analysis.

Parameters to Mental Procedures

Certain mental procedures, or thought processes, are used all the time. Focusing the attention is one example. Within the visual system, focusing the attention requires coordinating body, head, and eye movements, as well as selecting a test pattern and establishing connections to the storage systems. Within the auditory system, focusing the attention requires selecting a particular spatial location upon which to focus and routing the encoded auditory representations to the storage systems for analysis. When focusing the attention on an internal state such as hunger, pain, anger, or fear, the encodings of the selected representation must be routed to the storage systems of that modality for analysis. In general, focusing the attention means selecting a particular modality or submodality and routing its sensory encodings to the appropriate storage systems for analysis.

Naming and imaging are examples of thought processes which require access to particular memory locations. This implies that one or more memory locations must have been recently activated by a process such as attending a sensory event. If, for example, the result of directing the focus of visual attention on a house results in the activation of a memory location containing the token "A-frame," then recall of information from that memory location names the house. If sending the symbolic token "house" to the naming store activates a memory location containing images of the White House, then recall causes imaging of the White House. Both naming and imaging require that information be recalled from an activated memory location.

Temporal and spatial chaining are examples of thought processes which require a sequence of mental actions. In each case, information is recalled from an activated memory location and new information is presented to the storage system for analysis. For temporal chaining the recalled patterns are sent back to the memory store without modification but for spatial chaining the recalled spatial coordinates are generally modified before they are sent back. This enables access to memories which took place in a different nearby spatial location. In each case, the access control system together with the systems which transmit information from one place to another cooperate during chaining.

Terminating Mental Procedures

Most thought processes, including those just mentioned, have some implied termination condition. For example, when naming an object in the visual field, the visual search usually terminates when the object is recognized by the naming store. Naming terminates when the name of the object is recalled from the naming store. When using temporal chaining in an attempt to recall a particular past event, chaining terminates when the event is finally recalled.

Termination conditions are parameters to the procedures: They differ for each invocation of the procedure and they are independent of the action to be carried out. One can look for a house, a car, a person, or a dog, but the process of looking is the same.[3] What differs in each case is the search specification: the desired object and its expected location. Likewise, what differs between one memory search and another are the specifications for a successful search: the conditions under which a search will be terminated. When answering specific questions, the tokens often specify the termination conditions for the mental processes. When attempting to accomplish a specific task, the desired result of the task generally specifies termination conditions.

Termination conditions are partly specified by information contained in activated memory locations in the storage systems. When answering the question "Is that John Doe?" the name "John Doe" activates a set of memory locations in the naming store. Attending the visual field also activates a set of memory locations in the naming store. The search can be terminated if one of the following conditions is satisfied: (1) A memory location activated by "John Doe" generates a high similarity signal when the person in the visual field is attended; (2) The visual representation activates a memory location in the naming store which contains the token "John Doe"; or (3) The visual representation activates a memory location in the naming store which contains a name different from

---

[3]This is not entirely true. When looking for a house, the selected scan path differs than when looking for a dog. We use knowledge associated with the parameters to the procedure (in this case, house and dog) to regulate the scan path. The same parameters which terminate the search may also be used to direct the focus of attention, but different parameters may also be used. Still, it is approximately correct to think of searching the visual field as a single procedure having different parameters for its execution and termination.

"John Doe." In the first two cases the question can be answered affirmatively; in the third case a negative answer must be given. If the visual representation does not activate any memory locations in the naming store, then two more termination conditions may be considered: (4) The person is not recognized at all—either in the naming store or in experiential memory; (5) The person is recognized but a name is not associated with the accessed memories. In the fourth case a response indicating nonrecognition must be given, but in the fifth case a response like, "I can't recall his name," or "I don't know his name," must be given. The important point is that activated memory locations hold some of the information that terminates the search of the visual field.[4]

Activated memory locations, however, do not hold all of the information. The control systems must know which memory stores are involved and which memory location or locations within those stores hold the termination condition. When naming the color of an object, the naming store for color holds the termination condition, when identifying a face, the naming store for pictorial information holds the termination condition, and when attempting to recall a past event, the experiential memory system holds the terminating condition.

UNDERSTANDING SIMPLE SENTENCES

The process of understanding simple sentences consists of translating the sensory inputs (either spoken or written) into the mental procedure for responding (answering questions, storing new factual data, or whatever). In some cases the response sequences are executed but in other cases they are not. The central point is that *sentences activate storage locations holding appropriate response procedures, and at the same time, the tokens in the input sentence establish parameters for those procedures.* In some cases the tokens indicate what to attend; in other cases the tokens restrict a search of memory; in still other cases the tokens indicate which storage system to use.

How do sentences enable access to the appropriate response procedures, that is, how are they understood? Put another way, how are the input sentences recoded into a form which can be recognized by an associative memory store? If the input sentences can be recoded into recognizable patterns, and if the storage representations of the response procedures are associated with those patterns in a storage system, then understanding consists of transmitting their symbolic representations to that storage system to activate the memory locations containing the response procedures. Once the memory locations are activated, then understanding has taken place. If the linguistic input is a question and the response procedure is invoked, then the question will be answered. If the

---

[4]Starting with the networks presented in Chapter 4, it is easy to construct an access control network which delivers a strong similarity signal only when it is generated by an activated memory location. You might like to construct such a network as an exercise.

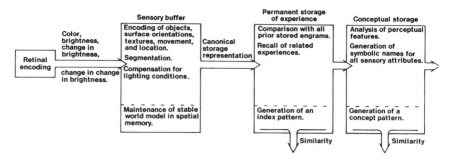

Figure 11.4. The sequence of events that occurs in real time while describing the visual field.

linguistic input is a factual statement and the response procedure is invoked, the result will be the storage of new factual information. The response procedure always determines the nature of the response.

In general, one would not expect an arbitrary sentence to invoke a stored response procedure. Rather, one would expect high-level processing networks to formulate a response procedure based on particular tokens in the sentence, its syntactic form, context, and so forth. In this case, the process that underlies the generation of a response procedure is itself a response. In any event, my intent in this presentation is not to formulate a complete model for how language is processed, but rather, to demonstrate the prelinguistic mechanisms which are necessary for language understanding. Let me proceed with that in mind.

The storage system that associates the encodings for the sentences with response procedures will be called a **concept store**. The brain's representation of language inputs must be recognizable by the concept store, yet the representations must be somewhat independent of the tokens in them. For example, "Is that a house?" should activate the same response procedure as "Is that a cottage?" or "Is that a duplex?" but a different response for "Is that Bo Derek?" or "Is that Marilyn Monroe?" Furthermore, the brain's representation of the language inputs must differ for inputs whose response procedures differ: "Is the car blue?" or "Is the car big?" or "Is the car moving?" Regardless of the representation, the conversion from sensory representation to internal representation must take place in real time, that is, at the same speed that the inputs are read or heard.

Figure 11.4 shows the sequence of events that take place for ordinary sensory inputs. The low-level visual and auditory networks encode the sensory patterns into representations recognizable by the stores of experience and the naming stores. At the same time, the stores of experience record and analyze the current inputs while the naming stores simply analyze them. Words in the input stream activate memory locations both in the naming stores and the stores of experience, while the naming stores generate the similarity representation of the inputs (the pattern of flickering described earlier in this chapter). The similarity representation forms the basis of natural language understanding as I will soon show.

Each word in the naming store has an associated sensory representation. The only difference between two words in the store for pictorial information is the pictorial representations associated with them. The only difference between two words that name color is the specific color pattern associated with them, and the same is true for words that name textures, movements, and spatial relationships. Because there are different naming stores for each modality and submodality, words that name different types of information have distinctly different places of storage. It naturally follows that the similarity patterns generated by the naming stores when analyzing symbolic inputs will differ for sentences which have different meanings but be similar for sentences which have similar meanings. Referring back to the previous examples, "Is that a house?" and "Is that a duplex?" generate similar similarity patterns while "Is the car blue?" and "Is the car moving?" generate different similarity patterns. This follows because "house" and "duplex" would be stored nearby in the naming store whereas "blue" and "moving" would not be stored nearby—they have different sensory submodalities.

The similarity patterns generated by the naming store have high dimensionality and must therefore be reduced for storage. Since there is at least one different memory location for each meaning of each word, and since people have vocabularies of tens of thousands of words, it follows that the similarity pattern has tens of thousands of components. Patterns having that many components are too large for permanent storage, and just like the low-level and intermediate-level visual and auditory representations, they must be reduced prior to storage. The reduced representations, which will be called **sentence patterns**, must differ for sentences having different meanings but be similar for sentences having the same meaning. It follows that words that have a different significance (house, red, fuzzy, moving) must generate different components in the sentence pattern, but words that have the same significance (house, A-frame, cottage, duplex) may generate the same component.

The similarity pattern generated by the naming stores can be reduced into a sentence pattern in exactly the same way that low-level visual information is reduced by the sensory buffer. The similarity signals from different regions of the naming store can be combined (for example, by averaging or by selecting the maximum value) to produce a pattern which has one component for each region in the naming store and therefore each category of item. The generated sentence patterns will differ for sentences having different meanings but be similar for sentences having the same meaning. For example, if the various encodings for different types of chairs reside in nearby locations in the naming stores, then all "chair" words will have identical significance for sentence understanding: They will enable access to the same response procedures. That is not to say that different chair-words are indistinguishable. Different words enable imaging of

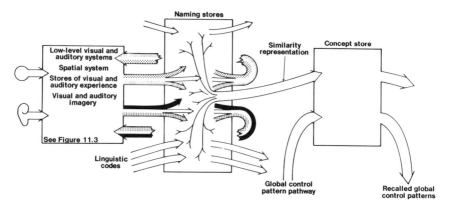

Figure 11.5. Relationships between the low-level visual and auditory subsystems, the naming stores and the concept store.

different objects—a captain's chair, a rocker, or a recliner—so when used for accessing additional information, each word will convey its own unique significance. Since input words activate memory locations in the naming stores, and since activated memory locations act as parameters to the response procedures, the significance of different words is preserved when responding to sentences containing them.

Figure 11.5 illustrates the relationship between the naming stores, the concept store, and networks not yet described which control them. The pathways labeled "global control" convey the brain's representation of various mental procedures to the concept store for storage and analysis and from the concept store for execution. Comparing this figure with Figure 8.9 shows the similarity between the networks for reducing sensory information and those for reducing sentence information. A fundamental principle of brain architecture is: *The similarity signals from one stage of processing form a high-resolution representation for a later stage of processing. The high-resolution representation can be reduced in size by combining nearby elements from the memory store that generates it. The result is a low-resolution, high-level representation of the same sensory event.*

READING AND SPEECH UNDERSTANDING

Reading is a mental procedure which combines several different forms of activity. The visual system must first direct the focus of attention toward the material to be read. For English this requires scanning the page from left to right and from top to bottom. The high-level visual representations must then be translated into symbolic codes before being sent to the naming stores for analysis. Translation requires one or more associative memory stores. The sequence of translations take place in special associative stores which associate symbolic codes with visual codes. Some words, like "STOP," which may be recognized directly from their pictorial presentation may require only one translation. In other cases, the letters may be first translated into an interme- diate code before being translated into their symbolic representation. For example, for a person who reads by sounding out words, the translation is from a visual code to an intermediate auditory code, and then from the auditory code to the symbolic code. Regardless of the number of intermediate codes that are used, when one code is translated into another, the memory location which associates them must be activated and its stored associated pattern recalled. The access control system for the store that does the translation is therefore critically involved with the translation process. Figure 11.6 illustrates the architecture that is assumed if reading takes place with two stores used for translating from visual to symbolic codes.

Speech understanding, like reading, requires that auditory representations be translated into symbolic codes before being presented to the naming stores. Although many speech sounds are translated directly (e.g. one's own name and words such as "stop" and "hot"), others are translated into an intermediate code before being translated into their symbolic codes. Figure 11.6 illustrates the architecture that is assumed if speech understanding takes place with two stores for translating from auditory to symbolic codes. Just like for reading, the access control system for the illustrated store plays a crucial role in the process.

In the simplest cases, Figure 11.6 represents the stages of sensory processing

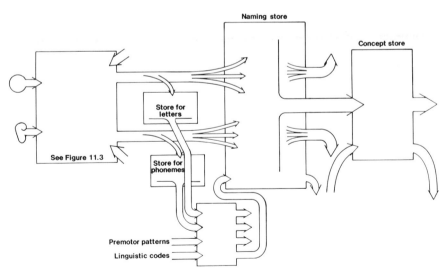

Figure 11.6. An elaboration of Figure 11.5 showing networks for translating phoneme and letter representations into linguistic codes. Control networks are not shown.

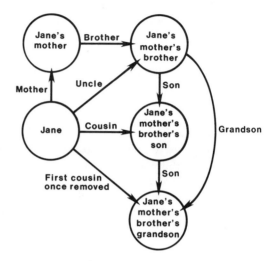

Figure 11.7. A graph showing general relationships (arc labels) and particular people (node labels) mentioned in the phrase "Jane's mother's brother's grandson."

for reading and understanding speech. In general the networks are not as clearly delineated. Some words are understood immediately, which means that response procedures are directly associated with auditory and visual codes. In other cases, understanding requires significantly more processing. For example, understanding the relationship between Jane's mother's brother's grandson and Jane requires a mental procedure which is far more complex than any described previously in this chapter. While attempting to understand the relationship, several presentations of the phrase may be required. If the phrase was written it may be reread and if it was spoken it may be mentally rehearsed. The analysis often requires imaging. When imaging, spatial memory is used to hold tokens for the people described in the phrase. See Figure 11.7. The tokens are placed in spatial memory so they form a family tree, and then the family tree is scanned to determine the relationship between the individuals in question. It is not known how spatial memory is controlled when constructing the mental image of the family tree, nor is it known how the family tree is scanned and the unknown relationship recognized. Regardless of what process is used, the complex mental procedures required for understanding logical relationships are beyond the scope of this book.

THE ONSET OF LANGUAGE

Some insight into the variety of associative stores and procedures which underlie language can be gleaned by considering how children learn language.

One of the first steps is learning to speak. Learning to speak consists (in part) of storing the motor engrams for vocalization and learning how to recall them and play them out over the vocal apparatus.[5] Until the child has stored the motor engrams for vocalization, each attempt at speaking is a conscious effort. At first, the child attempts to duplicate the sounds of his or her parents. It is during this process that the storage system lays down the memory traces for associating the auditory representations of sounds with the motor patterns for their vocalization.

Although I do not know what system initiates storage, the child's effort and concentration appear to be the psychological correlates of the process. The child pays attention to the auditory encodings while consciously controlling the muscles of the vocal tract. The consciously generated motor patterns and the auditory encodings arrive at the storage system together and are therefore stored in the same memory location. They become associated. At first the sounds are random, but as traces are established which associate specific motor patterns with their auditory encodings, the child learns to access the motor encodings and transmit them directly to the vocal apparatus. Some of the earliest sounds are words such as "mama" and "dada," but in time the learned sounds are the phonemes of the language. Thus the child learns to convert intended sounds into vocalizations.

While the child learns to vocalize, he or she also learns to access symbolic representations from the naming stores. Since the symbolic representations are not generally motor patterns, they must be premotor patterns or more specifically, **prevocalization patterns**, patterns which enable access to the motor patterns (which are called **vocalization patterns**). Chapters 14 and 15 describe how premotor patterns are translated into motor patterns by associative memory stores, and the description presented there pertains to speech production as well. Fluent speech consists of translating the symbolic representations, prevocalization patterns, into vocalization patterns, and then transmitting them to the vocal tract for execution. All of this takes place without conscious effort.

As with any associative storage system, access requires that the memory locations containing the desired memory traces be activated. There are two ways that activation can happen. First, the sounds can be heard, in which case the current auditory encodings activate the desired memory locations. This would happen, for example, if the child is imitating its parent's speech. Second, the child can recall information from a storage system which contains memories of speech sounds. When this happens, the child hears the sounds in his mind's ear. The stores of auditory experience are most likely the ones involved. The

---

[5]The process of vocalization is more complicated than simply recalling the vocalization patterns and transmitting them to the vocal tract for execution. For our purposes, however, this simplified description will be sufficient. Chapters 14 and 15 will describe in more detail the mechanisms that are required for converting stored motor patterns into the muscle activity for speech, body movement, and other physical acts.

child recalls a sound he or she wants to make,[6] transmits the recalled sensory encoding to the store, which associates auditory with motor encodings,
and then recalls the vocalization patterns from an activated memory location. If
the vocalization patterns are sent to the vocal apparatus for execution, the
result is the production of the desired sound.[7] If the recalled patterns are not
sent to the vocal apparatus, the result is the mental rehearsal of the speech
sounds.

It is clearly not the case that speech develops first and then other aspects of
language follow. The child learns many different aspects of language at the same
time. Nonetheless, before fluent speech is possible, the child must store a large
number of motor engrams for speech sounds. These engrams can then be
recalled and executed without conscious effort.

Although the motor and premotor encodings for speech sounds are not the
only symbolic codes used, it seems very likely that for the majority of individuals
they are the principal ones. The prevocalization patterns are the tokens of
symbolic thought. Within the naming stores, sensory encodings are associated
with symbolic codes, which I have argued are either prevocalization patterns or
vocalization patterns. Our ability to describe instantaneously what's going on
around us adds strength to this hypothesis.

Learning a language is far more involved than learning to speak. The child
must learn to associate symbolic tokens with various items in the environment:
The child must learn to name. Naming objects is an obvious example, where the
child associates names with pictorial representation. But other aspects of naming
are quickly learned as well. For example, children learn to name physical
sensations (hot, cold, pain, sweet, sour, bright, dim, wet, dry, and so forth),
actions (going potty, eating, bathing), and moods (happy, sad, angry). Once
the child has learned how to name and how to vocalize, the principal
mechanisms for language acquisition are in place.

Consider how a child learns to read. Reading not only requires associating a
symbolic code with a visual representation, but it requires the active control of
the visual apparatus. At first the child learns the names and sounds of the
letters. The machinery for that is already in place: Letters are simply visual
patterns, and learning the sound of a letter means associating a vocalization
pattern with its image. This may take place in a single associative store, or it
may take place in two stages: first by translating a letter into its name, and then
by translating the name of the letter to its vocalization pattern.

The child also learns to control the visual machinery. This entails locating
the words to be read and scanning them in such a way that they can be
recognized. Controlling the visual machinery is a major step in the child's
development. Although, at the start, the letters can only be processed one at a

---

[6]This is the child's intention.

[7]This is the execution of the intention.

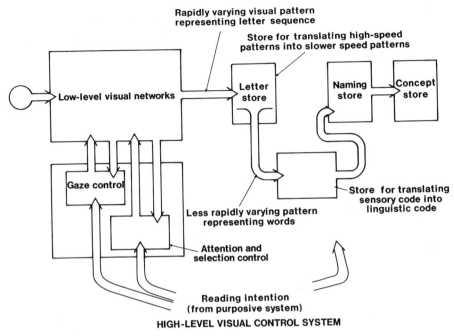

Rapidly varying visual pattern
representing letter sequence

Store for translating high-speed
patterns into slower speed patterns

Low-level visual networks

Letter
store

Naming
store

Concept
store

Gaze control

Store for translating
sensory code into
linguistic code

Less rapidly varying pattern
representing words

Attention and
selection control

Reading intention
(from purposive system)

HIGH-LEVEL VISUAL CONTROL SYSTEM

Figure 11.8. Some of the networks that underlie reading. The "reading intention" establishes the pathway connections and operation modes of the various processing subsystems and enables the gaze control subsystem and visual selection and attention networks to coordinate their activities while generating the sensory sequences representing the written material.

time, reading requires the association of symbolic codes with visual patterns which change very quickly. Not only must the visual machinery scan the page, encode the printed words, and form visual representations for analysis, but the storage system or systems that associate them with symbolic codes must respond and recall the symbolic codes just as quickly as the words are scanned. It seems likely that the associative stores are used as association stores for that purpose. The association store must analyze rapidly varying visual patterns and associate them with their symbolic codes. Figure 11.8 illustrates how the memory stores for reading might be organized.[8]

Reading and speech understanding are examples of high-level mental procedures. Both consist of directing the attention toward a particular stimulus, translating the sensory representation into symbolic form, and analyzing the resulting sentence patterns. Both are learned processes, and hence the patterns

---

[8]This is an area of considerable active research. See, for example, Caramazza (1986).

of neural activity which control the perceptual apparatus and memory stores must themselves be stored in a storage system. When a child learns to use language, he or she not only learns to associate names (prevocalization patterns) with the sensory stimuli, but also how to control the storage systems which do the associations. For example, activated memory locations must be deactivated at the correct times, information from activated memory locations must be recalled, which means selecting the proper storage system and then choosing the correct memory location from which to perform recall, and new information must occasionally be stored. When information is recalled, the recalled information must be transmitted to the correct place for analysis or execution.

What is specified by a mental procedure? First, the submodality and hence the storage system must be specified. This is easy to do since there are a limited number of submodalities to choose from. Within each submodality, however, there are vast amounts of specific knowledge. For example, a huge number of different visual symbols can be named from their pictorial representation alone. It is therefore unlikely that the high-level specification will identify a particular storage location. The high-level specification is probably very general, indicating which storage system to use, which storage operation to perform (analysis, storage, recall), and perhaps restricting somewhat the region of the storage system that is to be used. When information is to be recalled, the high-level specification probably indicates where to transmit the recalled information to, and if information is to be analyzed, the specification indicates the type of analysis that should be performed. Finally, the high-level specification probably indicates what the expected outcome of its execution should be and what to do if the expected does not occur.

Learning language, therefore, includes generating and learning to use these high-level control procedures as well as the low-level procedures, such as naming and speaking.

SUMMARY

In summary, understanding is the process of activating appropriate procedures in response to sensory stimulation while responding is the process of recalling the activated response procedures and transmitting them to the appropriate control networks for activation. Understanding simple sentences consists partly of learning to name, but in addition, it consists of storing the response procedures for responding to sentences along with the sentence patterns that should invoke them. Finally, learning to use language entails learning how to access and execute those response procedures.

This chapter showed the organization of the visual and auditory networks that encode and store experiences, it showed the organization of the naming stores, it showed the organization of the concept stores, and it introduced in detail the notion of a mental procedure or thought process. It described the sequences of translations that take place even during the simplest of mental acts, and it showed how the mental procedures can depend on specific symbolic tokens in the input sentences.

With respect to language understanding in general, the ideas presented here have just scratched the surface. There are many very important aspects of language understanding that were not addressed and for which the neural networks described here are simply inadequate. These include the ability to count, to understand logical relationships, to infer future events, or even to understand complex syntactic forms of almost any type. Understanding the neural mechanisms which underlie these processes awaits future research.

REFERENCES

Baron, R. J. (1974a). A theory for the neural basis of language. P. 1. A neural network model. *International Journal of Man-Machine Studies, 6*, 13-48.

_____ (1974b). A theory for the neural basis of language. P. 2. Simulation studies of the model. *International Journal of Man-Machine Studies, 6*, 155-204.

Caramazza, A. (1986). The role of the (output) phonological buffer in reading, writing, and repetition. *Cognitive Neuropsychology, 3*, 37-76.

Chafe, W. L. (1970). *Meaning and the structure of language.* Chicago: University of Chicago Press.

Jackendoff, R. (1983). *Semantics and cognition.* Cambridge, MA: MIT Press.

Johnson-Laird, P. N. (1983). *Mental models.* Cambridge, MA: Harvard University Press.

Langacker, R. W. (1986). An introduction to cognitive grammar. *Cognitive Science, 10*, 1-40.

_____ (1982). Space grammar, analysability, and the English passive. *Language, 58*, 22-80.

SUGGESTED READINGS

Little has been written on the neural basis of language. Still, there are several references which begin to relate language processing with the neural foundations and with memory representations. I strongly recommend the following material.

Bobrow, D. G., & Collins, A. (Eds.). (1975). *Representation and understanding. Studies in cognitive science.* New York: Academic Press.

Bondarko, L. V., et al. (1970). A model of speech perception by humans. In *Working Papers in Linguistics No. 6* (Tech. Rep. 70-12), Computer and Information Science Research Center, Ohio State University, Columbus, OH.

Caplan, D. (Ed.). (1980). *Biological studies of mental processes.* Cambridge, MA: MIT Press.

Fodor, J. A., Bever, T. G., & Garrett, M. F. (1974). *The psychology of language.* New York: McGraw-Hill.

Geschwind, N. (1974). *Selected papers on language and the brain.* Boston: D. Reidel.

Just, M. A., & Carpenter, P. A. (1977). *Cognitive processes in comprehension.* Hillsdale, NJ: Lawrence Erlbaum Associates.

Lenneberg, E. H. (1967). *Biological foundations of language.* New York: John Wiley & Sons.

Luria, A. R. (1981). *Language and cognition.* New York: John Wiley & Sons.

Rosch, E., & Lloyd, B. B. (Eds.). (1978). *Cognition and categorization.* Hillsdale, NJ: Lawrence Erlbaum Associates.
Schank, R. C. (1975). *Conceptual information processing.* New York: American Elsevier.
Schank, R. C., & Abelson, R. P. (1977). *Scripts, plans, goals, and understanding.* Hillsdale, NJ: Lawrence Erlbaum Associates.
Walker, E. (Ed.). (1978). *Explorations in the biology of language.* Montgomery, VT: Bradford Books.

12

THE ANATOMY
AND PHYSIOLOGY OF
THE SENSORY-MOTOR SYSTEM

INTRODUCTION

This chapter focuses on the anatomy and physiology of the sensory-motor system, which I will take to include muscle tissue, the spinal cord, the cerebellum, the basal ganglia, and the sensory and motor areas of the cerebral cortex. The structure of muscle tissue is first described, followed by a brief description of the spinal cord and reflex arcs. A description of muscle action follows, showing that both the static and dynamic properties are measured by the sensory receptors and controlled by the motor system. The various processing stations along the pathways of motor control are described in the remainder of the chapter.

The sensory-motor system contains four major cortical representations of the entire body: two motor representations which regulate and control voluntary movements, and two sensory representations which hold and process information regarding the state of the body. Different kinesthetic attributes are made explicit within each sensory representation, and different static and dynamic aspects of each movement are regulated from each motor representation. Moreover, just as the topology of the receptor surface is preserved within each processing stage in the visual system, the topology of the body's surface is preserved within each sensory and motor representation. The utility of this organization will be explored in subsequent chapters.

SKELETAL MUSCLE TISSUE

Striated muscles, also called **skeletal** or **voluntary muscles**, are responsible for all body movements, and although there are three types of muscles (striated

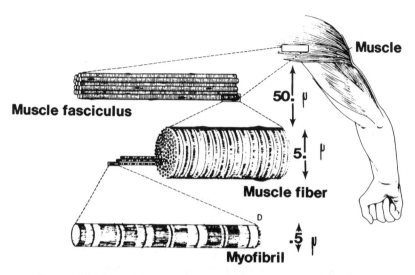

Muscle

Muscle fasciculus

50. µ

5. µ

Muscle fiber

D

-5 µ

Myofibril

Figure 12.1. The architecture of a skeletal muscle. (Modified from W. Bloom & D. W. Fawcett. *A Textbook of Histology. Ninth Edition.* Copyright © 1968 by W. B. Saunders Company. Used with permission.)

smooth, and cardiac),[1] only striated muscles will be described here. Striated muscles are composed of a large number of parallel cylindrical **muscle fibers** which are either extrafusal or intrafusal. **Extrafusal muscle fibers** are the principal contractile elements of the muscle. **Intrafusal muscle fibers** are primarily sensory organs, and although they also have contractile elements, they do not directly add in any significant way to the tension produced by the muscle. However, the outputs from the intrafusal fibers directly or indirectly contact the motor neurons that innervate the muscle and therefore influence the tension produced by the muscle.

Each extrafusal fiber is composed of a large number of tiny cylindrical fibers called **myofibrils** as illustrated in Figure 12.1 The myofibrils are the contractile elements of the muscle. They are encased in the mesh-like **sarcoplasmic reticulum** as shown in Figure 12.2. The sarcoplasmic reticulum initiates their contraction. The entire muscle fiber is encased in the sarcolemma, which is its thin outer membrane. The sarcoplasmic reticulum consists of a lace-like gridwork of sarcotubules which themselves connect larger tubes called terminal cisternae. The terminal cisternae are separated by small tubes called transverse tubules. The sarcoplasmic reticulum is a semipermeable membrane which, like neural tissue, conducts an action potential. When the sarcoplasmic reticulum

---

[1]Smooth muscle occurs in the walls of the uterus, intestine, blood vessels, and so forth, and the heart is composed of cardiac muscle.

depolarizes, the myofibrils contract in an all-or-none fashion. The resulting contraction is a **muscle twitch**. As Figure 12.2 illustrates, the sarcoplasmic reticulum encases many myofibrils, and therefore the resulting twitch is the combined effect of the contraction of all activated myofibrils. Under normal conditions, the action potential is initiated by the discharge of a single **motor neuron**. The motor neuron releases acetylcholine at functional contacts called **motor end plates**, which are illustrated in Figure 12.3. Acetylcholine initiates a spreading action potential in the sarcoplasmic reticulum which propagates throughout the reticulum and quickly reaches all myofibrils in the muscle fiber. As a result, the myofibrils contract. It follows that the muscle fiber is the smallest unit which can be controlled by the nervous system.

The length of a muscle fiber ranges from a few millimeters to about 12 centimeters and attaches to the skeleton either directly to the fascia surrounding the bones or to tendons, which then attach to the skeleton. In long muscles, some muscle fibers attach directly to other muscle fibers. Muscle contraction can shorten a fully extended muscle by up to 40% of its initial length, depending on

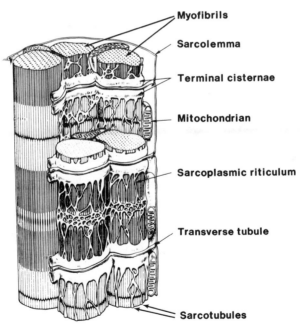

Figure 12.2. The structure of a skeletal muscle showing the relation of endoplasmic reticulum and transverse tubular system to fibrils. (Reproduced, with permission, from Andrew W. Rogers. *Cells and Tissues. An Introduction to Histology and Cell Biology.* Copyright © 1983 by Academic Press, LTD.)

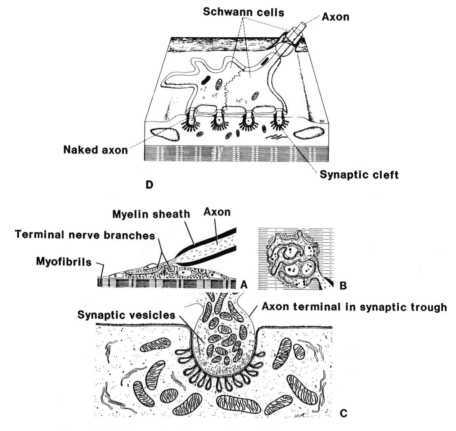

Figure 12.3. Schematic representations of the motor end plate: a. as seen in histological sections, b. as seen in surface view under light microscope, c. terminal branch as seen under an electron microscope, d. and as seen in isometric perspective. (Figures a-c reproduced, with permission, from W. Bloom & D. W. Fawcett. *A Textbook of Histology*. Ninth Edition. Copyright © 1968 by W. B. Saunders Company. Figure d reproduced, with permission, from R. S. Snell, *Clinical Anatomy for Medical Students*. Copyright © 1980 by Little, Brown and Company.)

the particular muscle. Muscles whose contraction tends to extend the attached limb are **extensors** and those which tend to bend it are **flexors**. Different muscles which work to produce the same motion are **synergists**; those which produce opposite motions are **antagonists**. When the constant tension produced by a muscle causes bending or extension of the joint, the contraction is called **isotonic**; when the tension changes but no movement results, the contraction is called **isometric**. Isometric contractions are essential for controlling posture.

Muscles are characterized by the speed at which they can reach peak tension. **Fast muscles** have a contraction time ranging from 7.5 to 40 milliseconds, are pale in color, produce less tension than slow muscle, and are generally adapted for fine control of movements. **Slow muscles**, in contrast, have a contraction rate ranging from 90 to 120 milliseconds. They are often deep red in color, are more resistant to fatigue, are more receptive to reflex inputs, and are adapted to maintain prolonged repetitive discharges for postural control. In addition, the conduction rate of the axons of motor neurons that innervate them are slower than for fast muscles.

The Activation of Muscles

The basic unit of control is the **motor unit**, which consists of a motor neuron together with all muscle fibers it innervates. All movements and all postural adjustments are controlled by motor units. As explained earlier, when the motor neuron discharges, all innervated muscle fibers contract; moreover, except under pathological conditions, a discharging motor neuron is the only cause of a muscle contraction. Small, fine movements are controlled by motor units that have as few as three fibers; coarse movements, such as leg movements, are controlled by motor units that have as many as 200 fibers.

Within a given muscle, motor units are organized into pools according to their physical characteristics. Two characteristics in particular appear to guide the organization: the relative excitability of the particular motor unit within the pool, and its relative size. Larger motor units, which are fed by axons with faster conduction velocities, give rise to contractions having greater force.

The tension in a muscle is the combined force supplied by all twitches of the individual motor units. Tension is increased by recruiting more and more motor units. Recruitment takes place in a systematic and orderly way: Units associated with low twitch amplitudes are the first to be recruited while those with higher twitch amplitudes are recruited later. In general, small motor neurons have the lowest thresholds of excitation, have the smallest twitch amplitudes, and are the first to be recruited. As the size increases, so too does the threshold of activation, the amplitude of the twitch, and the speed of conduction of the axon. Just as recruitment of motor units takes place in increasing order of size and twitch amplitude, the retirement of motor units takes place in decreasing order of size and twitch amplitude: Muscle units having high twitch amplitudes are the first to cease contracting and those with low twitch amplitudes are the last to cease contracting. The orderly sequences of recruitment and retirement are stable and do not seem to depend on the speed of contraction of the muscle.

Motor neurons which innervate extrafusal fibers are **alpha motorneurons**; those which innervate intrafusal muscle fibers are **gamma motorneurons**, and those which innervate both are **beta motorneurons**. Efferent fibers which innervate intrafusal muscle fibers are also called **fusimotor fibers**. The alpha and gamma systems differ substantially both in how they are innervated and on how

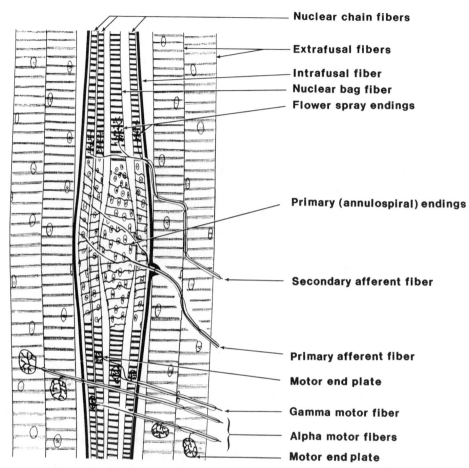

Nuclear chain fibers

Extrafusal fibers

Intrafusal fiber
Nuclear bag fiber
Flower spray endings

Primary (annulospiral) endings

Secondary afferent fiber

Primary afferent fiber

Motor end plate

Gamma motor fiber

Alpha motor fibers

Motor end plate

Figure 12.4. A neuromuscular spindle showing two types of intrafusal fibers: the nuclear bag and nuclear chain fibers.

they control movement. Less is known about the beta system, and little will be said here.

Neuromuscular Sensory Organs. The principal sensory organ in the muscle is the **neuromuscular spindle organ**, which is illustrated in Figure 12.4 There are three types of intrafusal fibers within each spindle organ: **nuclear bag1 fibers**, **nuclear bag2 fibers**, and **nuclear chain fibers**, and there are two classes of receptor endings: **flower spray endings**, and **annulospiral endings**. See Figure 12.4. **Primary afferents** have annulospiral endings. They comprise the **group Ia fibers** and are the largest group of sensory outputs from the muscles. A single primary afferent fiber originates in each spindle organ and is formed from one large myelinated fiber which divides and sends unmyelinated spirals around each of the intrafusal fibers in the spindle. The rate of firing of a type Ia afferent indicates both the length of the muscle (a static property) and the velocity of its stretch (a dynamic property). Sensory fibers with flower spray endings, **group II fibers** or **secondary afferents**, indicate mainly the length of the muscle (a static property). See Figure 12.5.

The **static responsiveness** of an afferent fiber is its rate of firing as a function of muscle length; its **dynamic responsiveness** is its rate of firing as a function of rate of change in muscle length. Both the static and dynamic responsiveness of a primary afferent can be modified by fusimotor inputs whereas only the static responsiveness of a secondary fiber can be modified.

The rate of firing of each sensory fiber depends not only on the length and change in length of the muscle, but also on the fusimotor signals reaching the spindle organ. As mentioned earlier, the gamma efferents only stimulate intrafusal fibers. Stimulation of the intrafusal fibers causes their contraction, which in turn changes the rate of firing of its sensory fibers. Gamma efferents can be subdivided into **static** and **dynamic** fusimotor fibers based on how they modulate afferent activity. As illustrated in Figure 12.5, the primary (type Ia) afferents encode both the instantaneous length of the muscle and the rate of change of the length. The **dynamic index** of an afferent is the decrease in firing rate which occurs during the first half second after the muscle reaches its final extension. A dynamic fusimotor fiber increases the dynamic index of a primary ending whereas a static fusimotor fiber decreases the dynamic index. When the muscle length is unchanging, both static and dynamic fusimotor fibers increase the rate of firing of the primary afferent. The influence that a static or dynamic fusimotor fiber has is always the same, regardless of the length of the muscle or the frequency of stimulation.

In contrast, secondary fibers are only influenced by static fusimotor fibers. Stimulation of a static fiber increases the responsiveness of the secondary fiber to muscle length while leaving its dynamic index unchanged. Stimulation of a dynamic fiber has no effect on the secondary endings, even when stimulation causes a contraction of the intrafusal fiber from which the secondary afferent originates.

The second largest group of afferent fibers, **group Ib fibers**, originate in the Golgi tendon organs. Golgi tendon organs are illustrated in Figure 12.6. Group Ib fibers signal the rate of change in tension in the muscle.

Taken together, the types Ia, Ib, and II afferent fibers convey a relatively complete picture of the body's muscles. It must be understood, however, that the picture can only be interpreted with knowledge of the efferent activity reaching the muscle of origin. The various sensory representations are transmitted to the brain, and like all sensory patterns, the local topology of the receptor surface is preserved.

Fibers in the sensory receptors of the skin and small fibers which detect pain

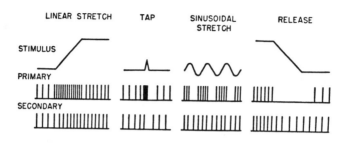

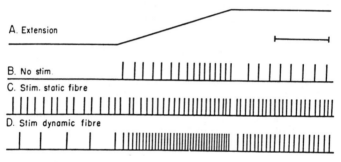

Figure 12.5. a. Comparisons of the responses of "typical" primary and secondary endings to various mechanical stimuli applied to the muscle tendon. The responses are drawn as if the muscle were under moderate initial stretch and as if there were no fusimotor activity. (Reproduced, with permission, from P. B. C. Matthews, Muscle spindles and their motor control. *Physiological Reviews*, 44, 1964, 219-288.) b. Effects of stimulating fusimotor fibers on the response of a primary ending to stretching the muscle 6 mm at 30 mm/sec. A, the mechanical stretch applied to the muscle; B, the discharge of the sensory fiber during stretch. Throughout C (before, during and after stretch) a single static fusimotor fiber was stimulated at 70/sec. Throughout D a single dynamic fusimotor fiber was stimulated at 70/sec. Time marker, 0.1 second. (Reproduced, with permission, from A. Crowe & P.B.C. Matthews, Further studies of static and dynamic fusimotor fibres. *Journal of Physiology*, 174, 1964, 132-151. Copyright © 1964 by Cambridge University Press.)

in the muscle form groups II, III, and IV. Because the skin and muscle pain receptors do not play a crucial role in voluntary movement, their effect will not be further considered.

A Mechanical Analog for the Muscle

Figure 12.7 shows a mechanical muscle, which illustrates the salient features of a biological muscle. The mechanical muscle consists of a closed cylindrical housing which contains a spring, a linear motor, and a tendon, which is attached to the spring. A second tendon is attached directly to the housing at the opposite end of the muscle. The external length of the muscle depends on the internal length, L, and external forces acting on the muscle. In the absence of external forces, a movement of the linear motor by an amount dL changes the external muscle length by the same amount, dL. External forces pulling on the tendons compress the spring and increase the external length of the muscle. The spring is not uniform, so that for a particular setting of its internal length, the forces required to stretch the muscle increase nonlinearly for an increase in the muscle's external length.

The mechanical muscle has the following properties: (1) The maximum tension it can withstand without damage is determined by its physical charac-teristics, (2) For a given external length, the tension in the muscle can be increased by changing its internal length, (3) The same tension can be applied at different external lengths by properly adjusting the internal length.

Figure 12.7 illustrates three sensory organs attached to the mechanical muscle. The sensory organs detect (1) the tension, (2) the internal length

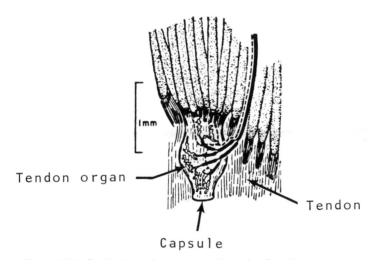

Figure 12.6. Semischematic representation of a Golgi tendon organ. This receptor is innervated by branches of a thick myelinated fiber (1b) and also by some unmyelinated fibers (C fibers) (broken lines). The role of the 1b fibers is to convey tension information to the central nervous system. That of C fibers is less well understood, but it is believed that they may convey painful stimuli to the central nervous system. (Repro-duced, by permission, from C. Eyzaguirre & S. J. Fidone, *Physiology of the Nervous System*, Copyright © 1975 by Year Book Medical Publish-ers Incorporated. Adapted from D. Barker, *Muscle Receptors*, Copyright © 1962 by Hong Kong University Press, p. 227, and used with permission.)

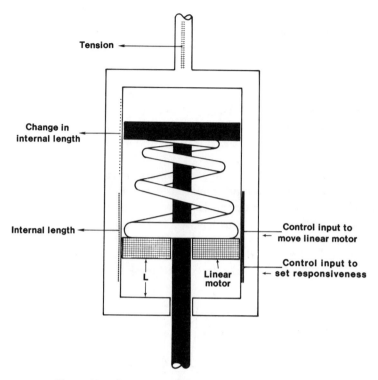

Figure 12.7. A mechanical analog of a skeletal muscle.

expressed as a function of tension, and (3) the change in internal length expressed as a function of tension. Thus the sensory outputs correspond approximately to the outputs of the types Ia and Ib sensory fibers. (Note that the external length is not a measured parameter but can be computed knowing the tension and internal length of the muscle.)

Figure 12.7 also illustrates two control inputs to the muscle. The control inputs specify (1) the internal length of the muscle, and (2) the responsiveness of the muscle to input 1. These inputs only approximately correspond to the control inputs that regulate a biological muscle.

THE SPINAL REFLEX CIRCUITRY

The **spinal cord** connects the muscles and sensory receptors of the body to the brain and consists not only of the afferent pathways (conducting sensory signals toward the brain) and efferent pathways (conducting control signals away from the brain to innervate spinal motor neurons and interneurons), but it also contains the cell bodies and dendrites of the motor neurons and numerous other

330

circuits as well. Among the circuits of the spinal cord are the various reflex pathways. Local pathways that exit and enter the spinal cord are of two types: purely afferent, and purely efferent. This is shown in Figure 12.8. Each efferent pathway is a **motor root**, and each afferent pathway is a **sensory root**. Since the motor roots all exit the spinal cord toward the belly of the animal, they are also called **anterior** or **ventral roots**, and similarly the motor roots are called **posterior** or **dorsal roots**. The ganglion cell bodies of the sensory neurons lie within the posterior roots as shown in the figure, where they cause a swelling called a **spinal ganglion**. Shortly after the sensory and motor roots exit the spinal column they merge into a spinal nerve, and spinal nerves that exit different spinal segments further merge into the spinal plexus as shown in Figure 12.8b. The resulting nerves innervate the muscles and tissues of the body.

Reflex actions result when afferent signals either directly or indirectly activate motor neurons. The sequence of cells that participate in a reflex action

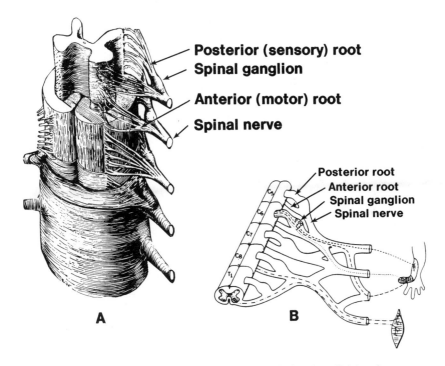

Posterior (sensory) root
Spinal ganglion

Anterior (motor) root
Spinal nerve

Posterior root
Anterior root
Spinal ganglion
Spinal nerve

A   B

Figure 12.8. The structure of the spinal cord showing division into motor and sensory roots. (a. Reproduced, with permission, from W. J. S. Krieg, *Functional Neuroanatomy. Third Edition*. Evanston, IL: Brain Books. Copyright © 1966 by the author. b. Reproduced, with permission, from H. D. Patton, J. W. Sundsten, W. E. Crill & P. D. Swanson, *Introduction to Basic Neurology*. Copyright © 1976 by W. B. Saunders Company.)

is a **reflex arc**. If the afferent signals entering a particular dorsal root activate efferent signals that exit the ventral root of the same spinal segment, the reflex arc is **segmental**. (Figure 12.8b illustrates five spinal segments labeled C5, C6, C7, C8, and T1.) If more than one spinal segment is involved it is **supra-segmental**, and if the brain is involved it is **supraspinal**. The knee jerk is an example of the **stretch reflex**, which is segmental. Limbs are controlled by antagonistic muscle pairs, so that bending a limb requires both contraction of one muscle and relaxation of its antagonist. The **flexion reflex**, which is initiated by painful stimulation to the skin, results in the withdrawal of the limb from the stimulus. It is both segmental and suprasegmental and involves both the excitation of an extensor muscle and the inhibition of its agonist flexor muscle.

A very simplified summary of the major reflex arcs in the spinal columns is as follows. Type Ia fibers make monosynaptic excitatory connections to the motor neurons of the muscle of origin and disynaptic inhibitory connections to the motor neurons of the antagonist muscles. These connections, illustrated in Figure 12.9, are the origin of the stretch reflex. As a result of the cophasic relationship existing for a flexor-extensor pair, a single command which causes a flexor to contract also causes its antagonistic extensor to relax, and vice versa. The group II fibers have only polysynaptic contacts to motor neurons and inhibit extensors and facilitate flexors throughout the limb. Group Ib fibers make only polysynaptic connections to the motor neurons of the muscle of origin. They tend to inhibit the motor neurons of the stimulated extensors and their synergists while facilitating the antagonists. Groups II, III, and IV fibers all inhibit extensors and facilitate flexors throughout the limb, and they have the opposite effect on the opposite limb.

In actuality, the reflex circuitry in the spinal column is significantly more complicated than this simple picture suggests. A given stimulus, such as a prick to the bottom of a foot, may involve only the muscles of the same leg if the subject happens to be seated when the foot is pricked, but the same painful stimulus may involve muscles of the entire body if the subject happens to be walking. In the first case, the leg is simply withdrawn from the painful stimulus; in the second case, the weight of the entire body must be shifted off the violated foot. This involves an extension of the opposite leg as well as a change in the posture of the body. Other reflex actions, such as raising the arms to protect oneself, ducking to avoid a projectile, and rapidly changing one's posture to maintain balance when slipping, are all examples of complex reflexes that are controlled by the spinal circuitry.

It is important to understand that the neural circuitry that serves as the basis for one reflex also participates in numerous other reflexes. In fact, all reflexes as well as all volitional movements are activated by the spinal motor neurons, which serve as the the final common pathway for all actions. It is important to recognize, therefore, that the sensory-motor system must plan and initiate

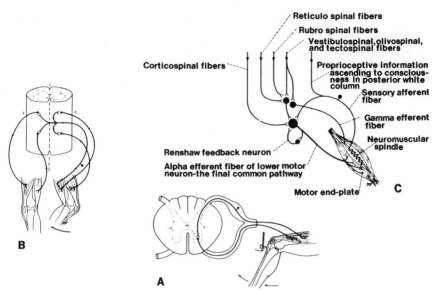

Figure 12.9. Connections of the spinal cord. A, origin of the stretch reflex; b) the law of reciprocal innervation and the crossed extension reflex; and c) the principal connections of the final common pathway. (Reproduced, with permission, from R. S. Snell, *Clinical Neuroanatomy for Medical Students*. Copyright © 1980 by Little, Brown and Company.)

actions with an understanding of how the various reflex arcs modify an intended action.

MUSCLE ACTION

Except under pathological conditions, skeletal muscles are never completely relaxed. The circuits of the cerebellum and spinal column activate some of the muscle fibers to maintain a normal background tension known as **muscle tone**. This corresponds to keeping a slight compression on the spring in the mechanical muscle. Since individual muscle fibers are either fully contracted or fully relaxed, only a small percentage of them are activated at any given time to maintain muscle tone. Movement is accomplished by recruiting more and more muscle fibers into activity and at the same time reducing activity in the antagonistic muscles. By controlling the order of activation of muscle fibers, the sensory-motor system is able to control the speed and force of activation while minimizing the effect of fatigue. The nonlinearity of the spring in the mechanical model is intended to reflect the recruitment of individual muscle fibers thereby nonlinearly increasing the tension in a muscle.

Both alpha motor neurons and gamma motor neurons can initiate muscle action. Alpha motor neurons innervate the extrafusal fibers and therefore activate the main mass of the muscle. The speed of contraction, and the force, are determined by the number of activated alpha motor neurons and the rates of stimulation. Gamma motor neurons can indirectly activate a muscle. The gamma motor neurons actuate the contractile elements in the intrafusal fibers, which in turn causes shortening of those fibers. The primary and secondary endings in the spindle organ are stimulated which, through the stretch reflex arc, innervates the alpha motor neurons. This, then, recruits the extrafusal fibers and activates the main muscle mass.

Movements can be roughly divided into two categories: ballistic and slow. **Ballistic movements** are rapid movements that typically last under 200 milliseconds. They are initiated by a strong impulsive muscle contraction, followed by a relatively passive movement of the body part, and often terminated by a strong impulsive contraction of the antagonist muscle. Moreover, the pattern of stimulation is initiated by the central nervous system and progresses without sensory feedback. **Slow movements** are produced by the relatively continuous action of the muscles involved, and they are often modified as a consequence of sensory processing. Examples of ballistic movements are arm movements for throwing a ball and saccadic eye movements; examples of slow movements are arm movements for drinking a cup of coffee and pursuit eye movements. (It is interesting to note that eye muscles are not represented in the primary motor cortex and pursuit eye movements cannot be initiated voluntarily.)

Alpha and gamma motor neurons are activated together (**alpha gamma coactivation**) to initiate a ballistic movement. When both alpha and gamma motor neurons are coactivated, there is an large signal initially generated in the Ia afferents. This rapidly increases the activity in the alpha motor neurons and brings the bulk of the muscle into activity. The muscle then shortens, which causes a decrease in the activity of the Ia afferents, until a new muscle length is finally reached. Activation then decreases, bringing the movement to an end. In the absence of the gamma system (brought about by drugs that selectively disable gamma activity), subjects are unable to control ballistic movements accurately. Under these conditions, an attempt to move a limb rapidly to a specified position generally results in overshooting the intended position.

The stretch reflex automatically reacts to external forces on a limb. When an external force causes a limb to move, the muscle (and hence intrafusal fibers) stretch slightly. Both the primary and secondary endings are stimulated and the resulting sensory signals reach the alpha-motor neurons through the stretch reflex arc. This causes a contraction in the main mass of the muscle, which opposes the external force and therefore tends to keep the limb from moving. The sensory signals also reach the brain stem and cerebellum, which react by increasing the tension in the muscle thereby opposing the movement. This is a supraspinal reflex.

The fact that gamma efferents play a crucial role in holding a configuration was succinctly summarized by Matthews (1972), as follows (pp. 602-603):

> The stretch reflex has long been recognized as a system for holding the length of a muscle constant in the face of external disturbances. In modern parlance, this is to recognize it as a servomechanism. In the early 1950's the gamma efferents were proved to provide a functionally specific pathway to the muscle spindles. It was then suggested that this enabled them to reset the length of the muscle at which the stretch reflex came into equilibrium. The fusimotor discharge was seen as supplying the command signal for the muscle servo by increasing the Ia firing and producing an excess of alpha motor discharge until the muscle had shortened sufficiently to reduce the Ia discharge back to its original value. The higher centres were thus suggested to be able to produce a movement in either of two rather different ways, that is either "directly" by sending descending activity straight onto the alpha motoneurones themselves, or "indirectly," by sending activity onto the gamma motoneurones in the first place and leaving the servo-loop to produce the desired contraction. The supposed advantage of the indirect gamma route was that it makes use of the valuable servo properties of the stretch reflex and is thereby unaffected by muscle fatigue or the size of the external load.

This original theory, based on a single type of gamma fiber and only the primary sensory ending, has since had to be modified, particularly in light of the differences between the static and dynamic gamma fibers and the added complexity of the secondary afferents. Several suggestions have been made since the earlier one (Matthews, 1972, p. 604):

> On the motor side, however, it can be immediately asked whether one or the other of the two kinds of fusimotor fiber is primarily responsible for injecting the command signal into the servo-loop. The answer appears to be that the static fibers are chiefly if not wholly responsible. This can be said because they alone seem to be able to make the spindle fire faster during shortening of the main muscle, and thereby still allow it to continue to excite the alpha motoneurones reflexively. . . . The dynamic fusimotor fibers may be allocated the role of sensitizing the primary ending and thereby controlling the sensitivity of the stretch reflex. In this respect, equal importance may be attached to their increasing the velocity of responsiveness of the primary ending to large stretches and their parallel action in increasing the absolute value of its sensitivity to small amplitude stretching.

THE ARCHITECTURE OF THE SENSORY-MOTOR SYSTEM

The alpha and gamma motor neurons are the final processing elements along the various pathways of motor control. Moving upward from muscle to brain, one finds the spinal cord which, in addition to the local circuits and reflex pathways, comprises various ascending and descending pathways. Between the spinal cord and higher processing stations of the cerebral cortex are several nuclei, which act as relay stations for various motor control functions. Included is the cerebellum which, although not necessary for motor control, plays a crucial role in the harmonic and fluent execution of virtually all motor acts. At the highest level of control are the cerebral hemispheres, particularly the sensory and motor areas of the cerebral cortex. This section describes the various processing stations between the muscles and the cortical hemispheres.

THE SPINAL PATHWAYS

The spinal pathways, or **spinal tracts** are organized as shown in Figure 12.10, which shows a cross section of the spinal cord. Both ascending (afferent or sensory) and descending (efferent or motor) pathways are duplicated on each side of the spinal cord but only the ascending tracts are labeled on the right in the figure and only the descending tracts are labeled on the left. The sensory functions of the ascending tracts are indicated in Table 12.1.

Figures 12.11 and 12.12 summarize the major ascending and descending spinal tracts, which are described below.

Ascending Pathways

Dorsal Column.   The dorsal column, also called the posterior column, comprises two tracts called the gracile tract (fasciculus gracilis) and the cuneate tract (fasciculus cuneatus). These pathways convey cutaneous (light touch, pressure) and kinesthetic (muscle, joint, and tendon) information to the basal complex of the thalamus. Secondary neurons then project from the thalamus to the cerebral cortex, where the conscious sensations of touch, pressure, and muscle joint

TABLE 12.1
Functions of the Ascending Spinal Tracts

Pathway	Function
Lateral spinothalamic tract	Pain and temperature
Anterior and posterior spinocerebellar tracts	Muscle joint sense to cerebellum
Fasciculus gracilis and fasciculus cuneatus	Discriminative touch, vibratory sense and conscious muscle joint sense
Anterior spinothalamic tract	Light touch and pressure
Spinotectal tract	Afferent information for spinovisual reflexes
Spino-olivary tract	Cutaneous and proprioceptive information to the cerebellum

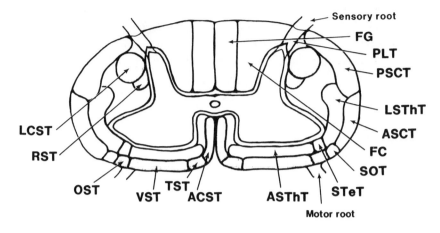

Figure 12.10. A transverse section of the spinal cord showing the general arrangement of the ascending and descending tracts.

Descending tracts (shaded)

LCST	Lateral corticospinal tract
RST	Rubrospinal tract
OST	Olivospinal tract
VST	Vestibulospinal tract
TST	Tectospinal tract
ACST	Anterior corticospinal tract

Ascending tracts (unshaded)

FG	Fasciculus gracilis
PLT	Posterolateral tract
PSCT	Posterior spinocerebellar tract
LSThT	Lateral spinothalamic tract
ASCT	Anterior spinocerebellar tract
FC	Fasciculus cuneatus
SOT	Spino-olivary tract
STeT	Spinotectal tract
ASThT	Anterior spinothalamic tract

sense arise. In addition, some projections terminate in the cerebellum. The dorsal column axons are fast conducting, having a total conduction time ranging between 40 to 110 milliseconds.

Spinothalamic Tracts. There are two separate parts to the spinothalamic tract: the lateral spinothalamic tract, and the ventral or anterior spinothalamic tract. The lateral spinothalamic tract conveys pain (including muscle fatigue), temperature, tickle, itch, and touch to the thalamus and then to the cerebral cortex. The ventral spinothalamic tract conveys mostly kinesthetic information generated by Golgi type Ib tendon organ afferents.

Spinocerebellar Tracts. There are two separate parts to the spinocerebellar tract: the anterior or ventral spinocerebellar tract, and the posterior or dorsal spinocerebellar tract. These pathways convey unconscious muscle, tendon, and joint information to the cerebellum. The receptor afferents terminate in Clark's

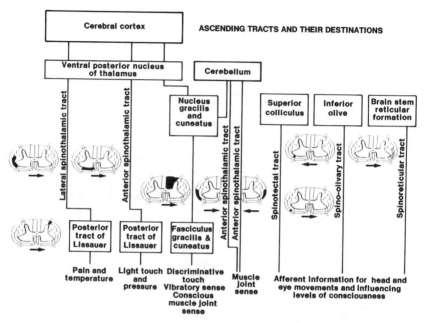

Figure 12.11. Summary of the ascending tracts of the spinal cord.

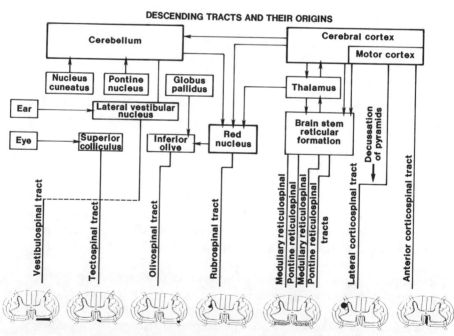

Figure 12.12. Summary of the descending tracts of the spinal cord.

column (the nucleus dorsalis) of the spinal cord, and then secondary neurons project upward to the cerebellum.

Spinotectal Tract. The spinotectal tract consists of second order cells which, after passing through the medulla oblongata and pons terminate in the superior colliculus. Thus this pathway provides information which is related to rotating the head and moving the arms in response to visual stimuli.

Spino-olivary Tract. This pathway consists of second order cells which terminate in the inferior olivary nuclei. Cells of the olivary nuclei send axons to the cerebellum. Both cutaneous and proprioceptive information is relayed through this pathway.

Descending Pathways

Pyramidal Tract. The pyramidal tract consists predominantly of axons of the cerebral cortex. The pyramidal tract splits (decussates), with approximately 80% of the axons descending on the opposite side of the spinal column through the lateral corticospinal tract. The remaining 20% descend uncrossed through the ventral or anterior corticospinal tract. Between 20% and 40% of the axons originate in the motor cortex; the remaining pyramidal efferents, about 60%, originate outside the motor cortex: 40% come from the prefrontal, parietal, temporal, and occipital areas while 20% come from the somatic sensory area. The largest percentage of those which are easily activated by direct electrical stimulation do in fact come from the motor cortex and somatic sensory cortex. About 20% of the pyramidal efferents terminate monosynaptically on the alpha motor neurons; the remaining efferents terminate in the interneurons of the spinal cord. Figure 12.13 illustrates the pyramidal tract and several nearby structures. The corticobulbar fibers, which innervate eye muscles and branchiomeric muscles, are also shown.

Extrapyramidal Tract. The extrapyramidal tract comprises several different pathways which originate in the basal ganglia and various processing stations of the brain stem and cerebellum. The major pathways are the rubrospinal tract, which originates in the red nucleus; the vestibulospinal tract (having both ventral and dorsal pathways), which originates in the vestibular nerve and lateral vestibular nucleus; the reticulospinal tract, which originates in the reticular formation; the tectospinal tract, which originates in the superior colliculus; and the olivospinal tract, which originates in the inferior olivary complex. These pathways convey information which regulates various actions such as visual reflexes (tectospinal tract), orienting reflexes (vestibulospinal tract) and so forth.

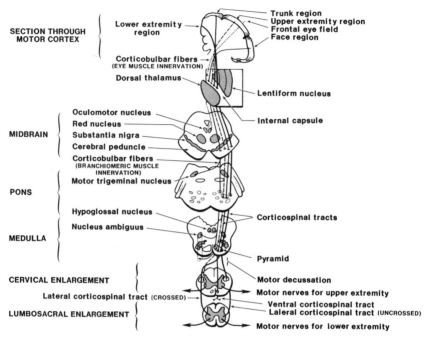

SECTION THROUGH MOTOR CORTEX

Lower extremity region

Trunk region
Upper extremity region
Frontal eye field
Face region

Corticobulbar fibers
(EYE MUSCLE INNERVATION)

Dorsal thalamus

Lentiform nucleus

MIDBRAIN

Oculomotor nucleus
Red nucleus
Substantia nigra
Cerebral peduncle
Corticobulbar fibers
(BRANCHIOMERIC MUSCLE INNERVATION)
Motor trigeminal nucleus

Internal capsule

PONS

MEDULLA

Hypoglossal nucleus
Nucleus ambiguus

Corticospinal tracts

Pyramid

CERVICAL ENLARGEMENT

Motor decussation

Lateral corticospinal tract (CROSSED)

Motor nerves for upper extremity
Ventral corticospinal tract
Lateral corticospinal tract (UNCROSSED)

LUMBOSACRAL ENLARGEMENT

Motor nerves for lower extremity

Figure 12.13. Diagram to illustrate the major components of the pyramidal tract, nearby structures, and the corticobulbar fibers. The corticubulbar fibers innervate eye and branchiomeric muscles. (Figure slightly modified from E. C. Crosby, T. Humphrey, & E. W. Lauer, *Correlative Anatomy of the Nervous System*. Copyright © 1962 by Macmillan Publishing Company. Used with permission.)

The importance of the extrapyramidal pathways to understanding volitional movements derives from two facts: Intentional acts often override reflex actions, and hence a coordination of intention with reflex is mandatory; and second, volitional acts and reflex actions utilize the same circuitry and muscle components, and hence the reflex circuitry must be modulated so as not to oppose a volitional movement. One must understand that the volitional and reflex systems coexist and share, to a greater or lesser degree, the same pathways, sensory receptors, and effectors. This fact was already discussed earlier in this chapter.

THE SENSORY AND MOTOR AREAS OF THE CEREBRAL CORTEX

I have already indicated that the local topology of each receptor surface is preserved by the pathways that conduct afferent information to the cortex. The

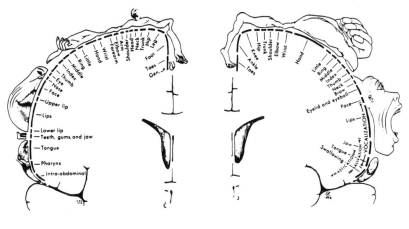

Somatic sensory cortex   **Motor cortex**

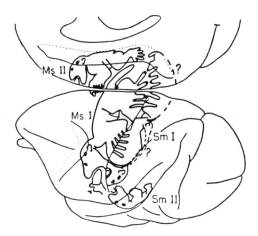

Figure 12.14. a. Relationships between body surface and surface of the cerebral cortex. The figurines are called sensory and motor homunculi. (Reproduced, with permission of Macmillan Publishing Co., from W. Penfield & T. Rasmussen, *The Cerebral Cortex* in Man. Copyright © 1950 by Macmillan Publishing Company. Renewed 1978 by Theodore Rasmussen.) b. A diagram of the monkey cortex showing the two motor (MI and MII) and two sensory (SI and SII) projections. This figure shows topological details not evident in a. (Reproduced, with permission, from G. Schaltenbrand & C. N. Woolsey, *Cerebral Localization and Organization.* Copyright © 1964 by University of Wisconsin Press.)

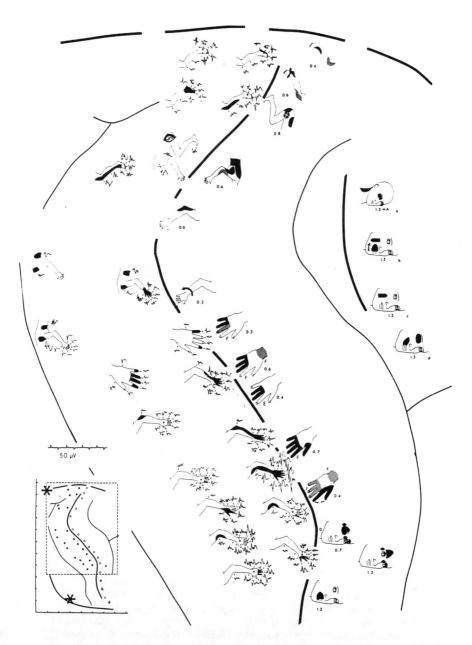

Figure 12.15

local topology of the "motor surface" is also preserved as one backs up along the major efferent pathways. Those cortical areas where the bulk of the motor projections arise are the primary and secondary motor areas, and as one might expect, representations of the entire body's muscles can be found in each area. This is diagrammatically illustrated in Figures 12.14 and 12.15. The figurines in Figure 12.14 are called homunculi. The sensory projections represent all parts of the body as well and they are also shown in Figure 12.14. Figure 12.15 shows in part how the sensory and motor areas of the cortex have been mapped out. The tactile and kinesthetic receptors of the skin, muscles, and tendons not only innervate the various reflex arcs through axon collaterals, but they form the major afferent pathways that project up to the cortex. Tactile and kinesthetic information from a given muscle is analyzed by the control networks which regulate that muscle's activity, and as an apparent consequence of evolution, the sensory and motor projections have similar cortical representations in which both sensory and motor projections from the same muscle are relatively nearby. The importance of this organization will become evident in the following chapters.

The primary motor area, area MI of the cortex, has characteristically large pyramidal cells, Betz cells, whose axons project down into the spinal cord, forming a major portion of the pyramidal tract. Both studies of brain-damaged patients and studies of the effects of electrical stimulation to area MI of the cortex suggest its role in the control of movement. After brain damage, movements lose their finer qualities, skilled movements are performed less smoothly, and movements lose their aim and precision. Although the motor cortex is needed for performing movements skillfully, it is not needed for learning or retaining skilled movements. Strong stimulation may result in organized movements, such as flexing an arm or rotating a wrist, while mild stimulation activates individual muscles. Slightly stronger stimulation is required to activate a flexor than its antagonistic extensor.

The second motor area, MII, also has a complete representation of the body's muscles, and movements can be controlled even after its complete removal. Stimulating the premotor area also results in movements, which are often more complex than elicited by stimulation to areas MI and MII. Still, the fact that complex motor patterns are elicited by area MII does not mean that the motor engrams for those movements are stored there.

Figure 12.15. Evoked potentials at the cerebral cortex caused by stimulating the surface of the body. Positions of stimulation are indicated by the figurines shown at the cortex. Data like these give rise to the homunculus drawings shown in Figures 12.14. (Reproduced, with permission, from C. N. Woolsey, T. C. Erickson & W. E. Gilson, Localization in somatic sensory cortex and motor areas of human cerebral cortex as determined by direct recording of evoked potentials and electrical stimulation. *Journal of Neurosurgery*, 51, 1979, 476-506.)

The two sensory projections correspond approximately to the types of sensory stimuli that are represented. The primary sensory area, SI, receives afferents from the groups Ia and Ib receptors. These are the encodings of tension, velocity, length, and change in length of the various muscles as well as nondamaging stimulation to the skin. The second sensory area, SII, receives inputs from the types II, III, and IV sensory fibers. These are the encodings of temperature, deep pressure, and pain.

There is growing evidence that the sensory and motor cortices are functionally organized into computational hypercolumns much like the primary visual cortex. The sensory cortex is organized so that each segment or small part of a segment of the body is mapped into a narrow strip of cortex running front to back across all of the sensory areas (3a, 3b, 1, and 2). Movement along one such strip of cortex corresponds to movement along the dermatome of the corresponding body segment. (A dermatome is the area of skin supplied by a single segment of the spinal cord.) See Figure 12.16. Moving in the perpendicular direction corresponds to moving between dermatomes in an orderly way. The result is the projection of the body surface as shown in Figures 12.14 and 12.15. Within this mapping, different cortical areas receive and process different sensory representations. Area 3a processes deep afferents, including muscle afferents; area 3b processes slowly adapting cutaneous afferents; area 2 processes deep afferents from joints; and area 1 processes rapidly adapting cutaneous afferents.

The studies which have led to these conclusions are only preliminary, but the evidence is mounting for an orderly cortical representation in which different sensory attributes are processed within cortical columns, and specific sensory attributes are made explicit within the cortical representation. The fact that some neurons of the somatic sensory cortex respond to stimuli moving across the receptive field in a specific direction also suggests a processing structure which resembles that of the primary visual cortex.

Hypercolumns of the motor cortex appear to control individual muscles or localized groups of muscles. Within the primary motor cortex, deep stimulation often produces small movements of single muscles. If stimulation at one point activates a particular muscle, stimulation at a nearby location often results in relaxation of the same muscle. This suggests that the cortex is capable of independently activating individual muscles. The topographical organization of the motor cortex, illustrated in Figure 12.14, showed the similarity in organization between the motor and sensory areas of the cortex. The utility of this organization will be discussed in the next chapter.

I have already described the pyramidal system, which includes the cortical pyramids of both primary and secondary motor areas, and the pyramidal tract which it forms. The extrapyramidal system tends to activate the gamma motor neurons and includes virtually everything else: the cerebellum, basal ganglia, descending reticular formation, and the vestibular system. Figure 12.17 shows part of the extrapyramidal system.

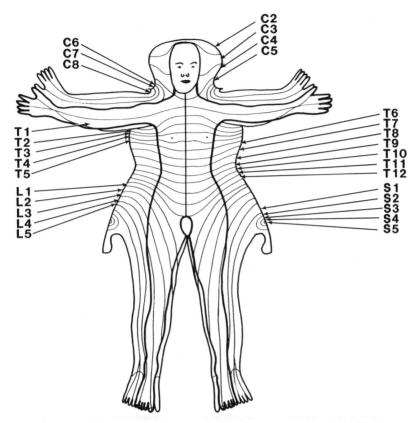

Figure 12.16. Dermatomes of the human body shown as if the back surface was cut along the midline and peeled forward. The labels correspond to the spinal segments of origin: C, cervical; T, thoracic; L, lumbar; and S, sacral.

THE CEREBELLUM

The cerebellum is a major computational network in the sensory-motor system and shares many properties with the cerebral cortex. It consists of two distinct hemispheres which are anatomically corrugated to increase the surface area in a restricted volume. The corrugations or **folia** are separated by numerous transverse fissures. Like the cerebral cortex, the principal processing circuitry of the cerebellum is within a thin sheet at its surface; the interior consists largely of the myelinated afferent and efferent fibers which connect the cerebellum to other processing stations in the brain and spinal cord.

The cerebellum can be anatomically divided into three principal lobes according to evolutionary age and function. The **archicerebellum** comprises the flocculonodular lobe and is the oldest of the three cerebellar lobes. Its primary

345

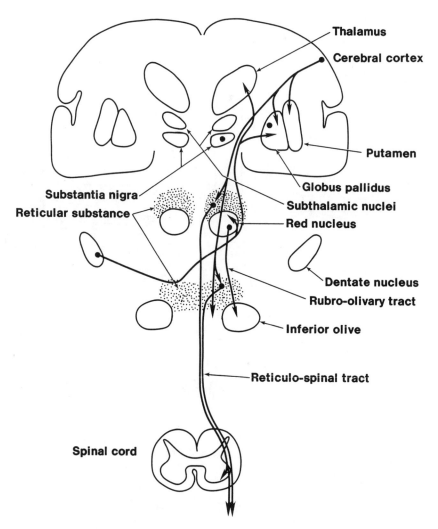

Figure 12.17. A summary of the extrapyramidal system excluding the cerebellum.

inputs come from the vestibular apparatus, and its primary function is to aid in maintaining equilibrium by modifying muscle tone. The **paleocerebellum**, younger than the archicerebellum, comprises the anterior lobe, ulva, and pyramid of the vermis. Its primary inputs come from the sensory endings in muscles and tendons and from touch and pressure receptors, and its primary function is to modify muscle tone for maintaining balance, particularly during voluntary movements. The middle lobe or **neocerebellum** is the newest part. Its primary inputs come from the cerebral cortex of the opposite side of the brain, particularly the sensory and motor areas, and its primary outputs go to the thalamus and motor areas of the cerebral cortex. Its primary function is to coordinate voluntary movements by regulating force, direction, and extent of movement. Figures 12.18 and 12.19 summarize the major pathways connecting the cerebellum to other centers of the brain.

The cortex of the cerebellum has been studied extensively, both anatomically and functionally. Anatomically, it is a highly regular structure comprising only five cell types: **Purkinje, basket, stellate, Golgi,** and **granular cells.** In addition, axon collaterals from external inputs are of two types: **climbing fibers** and **mossy fibers.** See Figure 12.20.

The cerebellar cortex is organized into three layers: the **granular layer,** the **Purkinje cell layer,** and the **molecular layer.** The granular layer comprises the mossy fibers (forming one of the two input systems), the axon collaterals of Golgi cells, some of the dendrites of Golgi cells, and the somas and dendrites of the granule cells. The Purkinje cell layer contains the somas of the Purkinje cells and the axon branches of the basket cells, which engulf the Purkinje cell somas in basket-like structures; hence their name. The molecular layer comprises the dendrite trees of the Purkinje cells, parts of the dendrite trees of Golgi cells, the stellate cells and their processes, the basket cell somas and dendrite trees, and the axon collaterals of the granule cells (called **parallel fibers**).

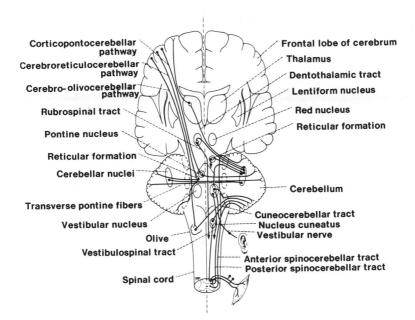

Figure 12.18. Some of the major connections of the cerebellum. The cerebellar peduncles are shown as dashed lines. (Reproduced, with permission, from R. S. Snell, *Clinical Neuroanatomy for Medical Students.* Copyright © 1980 by Little, Brown and Company.)

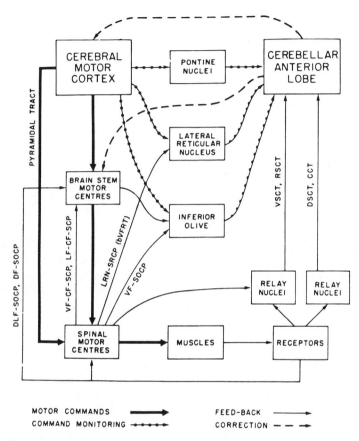

Figure 12.19. Oscarsson's scheme of the cerebellum as a comparator. (Reproduced, with permission, from O. Oscarsson, Functional organization of the spinocerebellar paths. In A. Iggo (Ed.) *Handbook of Sensory Physiology, Vol. II.* Copyright © 1968 by Springer-Verlag New York Inc.)

The Purkinje cells have unique dendritic structures. The dendrites branch many times but extend only vertically into the molecular layer. The branches from a single cell form a fan-like structure which is approximately 250 microns square but only 6 microns thick. Dendrite trees from different cells do not intermingle and they are aligned in a highly regular pattern with all the fan-like trees parallel to one another. See Figure 12.21. A single axon originates at each Purkinje cell and exits the cortex. Purkinje cell axons are the only outputs from the cerebellar cortex, and they always make inhibitory contacts with the cells they stimulate.

Granule cells are the most numerous type in the brain: There are approximately 3×10^{10} of them in the cerebellum. Axons from the granule cells extend up into the molecular layer where they branch once. Each of the two branches goes in the opposite direction, both remaining parallel to the sheet of the cortex and perpendicular to the orientation of the Purkinje cell dendrite trees. Since all granule cell collaterals are parallel, they are called parallel fibers. The parallel fibers are closely packed within the molecular layer, much like pipes stacked up on a truck for delivery. Refer back to Figure 12.21. Each parallel fiber makes a single excitatory synapse with each Purkinje cell whose dendrite tree it passes through. The contacts form only between parallel fibers and dendritic spines, as shown in Figure 12.23. As a result, each Purkinje cell receives inputs from as many as 200,000 different granule cells, one input from each cell. From the other point of view, a three-millimeter long parallel fiber contacts about 300 Purkinje cells. Parallel fibers also contact granule, Golgi, stellate, and basket cells with excitatory synapses.

Within the granular layer, each granule cell has between one and seven dendrite branches which form specialized structures called **cerebellar glomerules** with the mossy fibers and Golgi axons. Cerebellar glomerules comprise axodendritic contacts between the Golgi axons and granule cell dendrites, and axodendritic contacts between mossy fibers and granule cell dendrites. These contacts are illustrated in Figure 12.22. Because of the claw-like structures formed

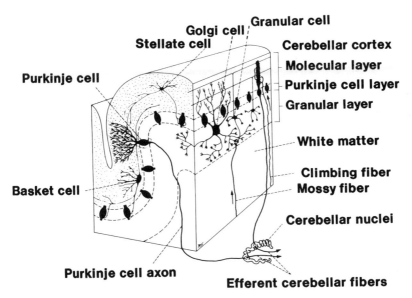

Figure 12.20. Cellular architecture of the cerebellum. (Reproduced, with permission, from R. S. Snell, *Clinical Neuroanatomy for Medical Students*. Copyright © 1980 by Little, Brown and Company.)

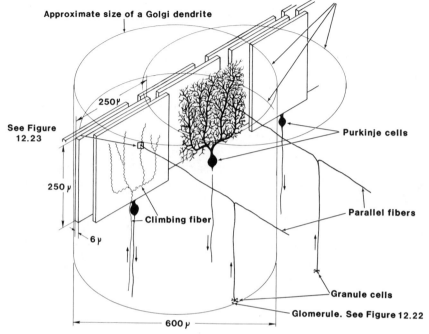

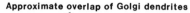

Figure 12.21. The structure of Purkinje cells, parallel fibers, and Golgi cells. Three layers of Purkinje cells are illustrated, showing how their dendrite trees form non-intersecting parallel sheets. The typical branching pattern of the Purkinje dendrite tree is shown only for the middle cell, and the climbing fiber is shown which is associated with the left-front Purkinje cell. Figure 12.23 shows the microstructures of contacts made between Purkinje dendrites, parallel fibers, and climbing fibers. Two granule cells and their parallel fibers are illustrated as are the extent and overlap of three Golgi cells. (Based on Albus, 1972.)

by the granule cells at the glomerules, granule cells are sometimes called **claw cells**.

Golgi cells have large dendrite trees which, as I mentioned before, extend both into the granular layer and molecular layer. These trees are roughly 600 microns in diameter and intermingle with the dendrite trees of about one hundred Purkinje cells. The cylindrical region illustrated in Figure 12.21 indicates the relationship between Purkinje cells and Golgi cells, and the overlap between Golgi cells is indicated by the overlapping ellipses at the top of the figure. There are contacts between parallel fibers to Golgi dendrites and between mossy fibers to Golgi dendrites. Both parallel fibers and mossy fibers contact Golgi dendrites with excitatory synapses.

350

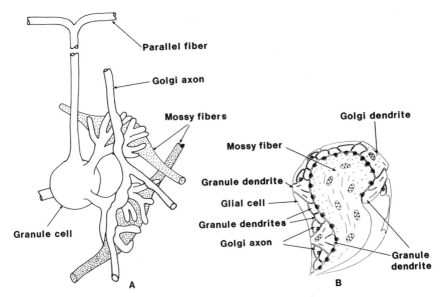

Figure 12.22   The structure of cerebellar gomerules. (a) An isometric sketch showing how the dendrite branches of the granule cells form "claws" around the swellings in the mossy fibers, thereby forming the glomerules. One Golgi axon is shown contacting the granule dendrites; (b) a cross section of a glomerule, showing the synaptic contacts between mossy fibers, granule dentrites, Golgi axons, and golgi dendrites. (Reproduced, with permission, from G. M. Shepherd, *The Synaptic Organization of the Brain: An Introduction.* © 1974 by Oxford University Press. Based on J. C. Eccles, M. Ito, & J. Szentágothai, 1967, *The Cerebellum as a Neuronal Machine.* Berlin: Springer-Verlag.)

Climbing fibers and mossy fibers are the only inputs to the cerebellar cortex.[2] Climbing fibers originate at the inferior olive, divide, and contact about 10 Purkinje cells. However, each Purkinje cell is stimulated by a single climbing fiber. The climbing fiber associated with a Purkinje cell divides and wraps around each dendrite branch of that cell as illustrated in Figure 12.23. Figure 12.21 also illustrates a climbing fiber; the Purkinje branches have been omitted for clarity. Climbing fibers also branch and contact nearby basket cells and stellate cells. Synaptic contacts between climbing fibers and Purkinje dendrites occur only on the dendritic spines as illustrated in the figure.

Basket cells and stellate cells are the remaining cell types in the cerebellar cortex. The dendrite trees of basket cells are similar in size and shape to Purkinje cell dendrite trees, only much less dense. In this respect basket and stellate dendrite trees are similar. Both receive excitatory inputs from parallel fibers.

[2]Recent evidence suggests that additional inputs arise from the locus cereleus; as of yet, however, little is known about them.

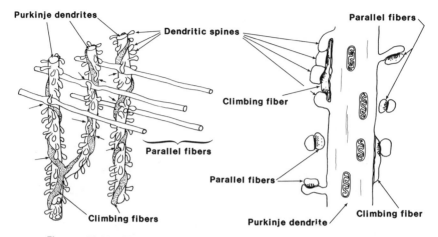

Figure 12.23. The microstructure of contacts between Purkinje dendrites, parallel fibers, and climbing fibers. (Based on illustrations in S. L. Palay & V. Chan-Palay (1974) *Cerebellar Cortex: Cytology and Organization*. New York: Springer-Verlag, and R. R. Llinás (1975) The cortex of the cerebellum. *Scientific American*, 232, 56-71.)

Figure 12.24. The basic neuronal circuitry of the cerebellum. PC, Purkinje cell; PF, parallel fiber; GC, granule cell; MF, mossy fiber; CF, climbing fibers; CNC, cerebellar nucleus cell. Cortical interneurons are omitted. (Reproduced, with permission, from H. D. Patton, J.' W. Sundsten, W. E. Crill & P. D. Swanson, *Introduction to Basic Neurology*. Copyright © 1976 by W. B. Saunders Company.)

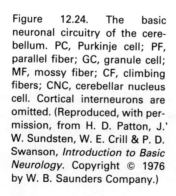

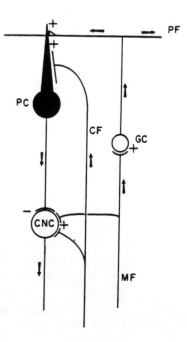

The axons of both types of cells are horizontal to the sheet of the cortex but perpendicular to the parallel fibers. Axons from stellate cells contact and inhibit the dendrites of Purkinje cells; axons from basket cells do the same, in an approximately 1000-by-300 micron elliptical region. However, contacts begin several cells away so the inhibition does not affect adjacent cells. In addition, axons from basket cells engulf and inhibit the preaxon portion of the Purkinje cell in basket-like structures, hence their name.

Figure 12.24 summarizes the basic cerebellar circuitry. Climbing fiber inputs excite Purkinje cells. In fact, because of the large number of contacts, the firing of a climbing fiber always causes its Purkinje cell to fire; the resulting complex spiking pattern is now well understood. Mossy fibers excite Golgi cells, and Golgi cells excite Purkinje cells. Parallel fibers excite granule, Golgi, Purkinje, basket, and stellate cells. Finally, Golgi cells inhibit granule cells. In contrast, Purkinje cells always inhibit the cells they contact.

In addition to the cerebellar cortex, the cerebellum comprises four pairs of internal nuclei: the **fastigial nucleus**, the **globose nucleus**, the **dentate nucleus**, and the **emboliform nucleus**. These nuclei, one of each on each side of the cerebellum, serve as relay stations between the cerebellum and other nuclei of the brain. Their specific functions are not yet understood and they will not be further discussed here.

It is well known that the cerebellum is needed for the smooth execution of ballistic movements. The cerebellum appears to control their timing, predict their outcome, and initiate the intense volleys of impulses (the "step functions") that initiate and terminate them. The cerebellum does not initiate movements, however, and movements can be initiated and performed in its absence. The cerebellum receives and monitors both sensory and motor commands, and it regulates the excitability of various cells in the spinal cord and brain stem during movements. In the absence of voluntary activity, the cerebellum is highly active, but its activity is reduced by inputs from a variety of sources, including the association areas of the cerebral cortex (e.g., visual, auditory, and somatosensory). This makes sense in light of the fact that cerebellar outputs are all inhibitory. Evidently the cerebellum is a special purpose computer, and its complex synaptic organization and specialized architecture have evolved for exactly that purpose.

Damage to the cerebellum decreases muscle tone and disables rapid intentional movements. Force, rate, steadiness, and direction of movements can no longer be accurately controlled. Damage to the flocculondular lobe of the cerebellum causes severe balance disorders corresponding to loss of the vestibular apparatus, while damage to the medial anterior lobe increases the muscle tone in extensors and results in rigidity.

Several detailed theories have been proposed for cerebellar functioning, including the following: Albus, 1971, 1972; Boylls, 1975a, 1975b; Eccles, 1973; Eccles, Ito, and Szentágothai, 1967; Llinás, 1974; Marr, 1969; Pellionisz, 1973;

and Pellionisz and Szentágothai, 1974. Additional references are suggested at the end of this chapter.

MOTOR NUCLEI OF THE BASAL GANGLIA

There are several nuclei of the basal ganglia which are part of the extrapyramidal system and whose functions are not well understood. Among them are the red nucleus, the vestibular nucleus, the caudate nucleus, the putamen, the globus pallidus, the substantia nigra, and the thalamus. The putamen and globus pallidus (or pallidum) comprise the lentiform nucleus. The vestibular nucleus consists of the lateral, superior, inferior, and medial vestibular nuclei. These nuclei receive and relay sensory information regarding gravity and acceleration from the inner ear (semicircular canals, utricle, and saccule) to the cerebellum and spinal reflex centers (via the vestibulospinal tract). These are major sources of information for controlling the gaze (head and eye movements), controlling balance (by adjusting muscle tone of the limbs and trunk) and so forth. The red nucleus acts as a relay station between cortex, cerebellum, and spinal motor neurons (both alpha and gamma), and facilitates flexor muscles and inhibits extensors to compensate for gravity. Damage to the substantia nigra results in Parkinson's syndrome. Although these processing stations are important to motor control, their principal function seems to be to control various motor reflexes and to add smoothness and fluency to volitional motor acts. They will not be further discussed here.

SUMMARY

Motor neurons are the final common pathway for all motor commands, both volitional and reflex. At the highest level, the motor cortex appears to be the source of most motor commands, although other areas of the cortex appear to make demands on the sensory-motor system as well. The patterns of activity which serve to initiate movements are conveyed through various relay stations of the brain and brain stem to the descending pathways of the spinal cord where they actuate the alpha and beta motor neurons and other spinal circuits. In addition, patterns of activity describing intended movements are relayed to the cerebellum and to a lesser extent to other subcortical nuclei. The cerebellum and cortical nuclei integrate the intended movements from the various sources, and taking into account the reflex circuitry and static and dynamic properties of the muscles, determine an optimal control pattern to initiate the action. When the spinal circuits apply the motor commands arising from the cortex, cerebellum, and other motor centers, the result is the smooth performance of the intended movement.

Virtually all senses play a role in the control of movement, particularly because they give rise to various reflexes which may augment or oppose an intended movement. Exceptionally critical are the kinesthetic senses, which tell the higher motor centers the position and change in position of each limb and the tension on each muscle. Since the kinesthetic representation depends on the activity in the gamma efferents, there is an active exchange of information in the spinal column between the afferent and efferent pathways. The brain can only interpret the kinesthetic information if it also knows the current values of the gamma efferents.

Although a general picture of motor control is starting to emerge, detailed explanations of the mechanisms of motor control await further investigation. We do not know what parameters of movement are directly controlled (e.g., muscle length, muscle tension, or both), nor do we know whether groups of muscles which act together to initiate complex movements (synergies) are individually controlled but synchronized by an appropriate motor pattern, or whether they are controlled through a single cortical command system which then, through spinal and cerebellar circuitry, activates the coordinated set of muscles. We do not even know for sure whether the circuits of recruitment of the motor units are spinal or cortical in origin. The answers to these and related questions await further research.

REFERENCES

Albus, J. S. (1971). A theory of cerebellar function. *Mathematical Biosciences, 10,* 25-61.

———— (1972). The cerebellum: a substrate for list-processing in the brain. In H. S. Robinson & D. E. Knight (Eds.), *Cybernetics, artificial intelligence, and ecology.* New York: Spartan Books.

Barker, D. (1962). *Muscle receptors.* Hong Kong: Hong Kong University Press.

Bloom, W., & Fawcett, D. W. (1968). *A textbook of histology. Ninth edition.* Philadelphia: W. B. Saunders.

Boylls, C. C. Jr. (1975a). A theory of cerebellar function with applications to locomotion. I. The physiological role of climbing fiber inputs in anterior lobe operation. (Tech. Rep. 75C–6). Computer and Information Science, University of Massachusetts at Amherst.

———— (1975b). A theory of cerebellar function with applications to locomotion. II. The relation of anterior lobe climbing fiber function to locomotor behavior in the cat. (Tech. Rep. 76–1). Computer and Information Science, University of Massachusetts at Amherst.

Crosby, E. C., Humphrey, T., & Lauer, E. W. (1962). *Correlative anatomy of the nervous system.* New York: Macmillan.

Crowe, A., & Matthews, P. B. C. (1964). Further studies of static and dynamic fusimotor fibres. *Journal of Physiology, 174,* 132-151.

Eccles, J. C. (1973). The cerebellum as a computer: Patterns in space and time. *Journal of Physiology, 229,* 1-32.

Eccles, J. C., Ito, M., & Szentágothai, J. (1967). *The cerebellum as a neuronal machine.* New York: Springer-Verlag.

Eyzaguirre, C., & Fidone, S. J. (1975). *Physiology of the nervous system (2d ed.).* Chicago, IL: Year Book Medical Publishers.

Ho, M. (1985). *The cerebellum and neural control.* New York: Raven Press.

Iggo, A. (Ed.). (1968). *Handbook of sensory physiology, Vol. 2.* New York: Springer-Verlag.

Krieg, W. J. S. (1966). *Functional neuroanatomy (3d ed.).* Evanston, IL: Brain Books.

Llinás, R. R. (1975). The cortex of the cerebellum. *Scientific American, 232,* 56-71.

Marr, D. (1969). A theory of cerebellar cortex. *Journal of Physiology (London), 202,* 437-470.

Matthews, P. B. C. (1972). *Mammalian muscle receptors and their central actions.* London: Edward Arnold.

———— (1964). Muscle spindles and their motor control. *Physiological Reviews, 44,* 219-288.

Palay, S. L., & Chan-Palay, V. (1973). *Cerebellar cortex: Cytology and organization.* Berlin: Springer-Verlag.

Patton, H. D., et al. (1976). *Introduction to basic neurology.* Philadelphia, PA: W. B. Saunders.

Pellionisz, A. (1973). Dynamic single unit stimulation of a realistic cerebellar network model. *Brain Research, 49,* 83-99.

Pellionisz, A., & Szentágothai, J. (1974). Dynamic single unit stimulation of a realistic cerebellar network model. II. Purkinje cell activity within the basic circuit and modified by inhibitory systems. *Brain Research, 68,* 19-40.

Penfield, W., & Rasmussen, T. (1950). *The cerebral cortex in man.* New York: Macmillan.

Rogers, A. W. (1983). *Cells and tissues. An introduction to histology and cell biology.* New York: Academic Press.

Schaltenbrand, G., & Woolsey, C. N. (1964). *Cerebral localization and organization.* Madison, WI: University of Wisconsin Press.

Snell, R. S. (1980). *Clinical anatomy for medical students.* Boston: Little, Brown.

Werner, G., & Whitsel, B. L. (1973). Functional organization of the somatosensory cortex. In I. Ainsley (Ed.), *Handbook of sensory physiology, Vol. 2. Somatosensory system,* 621-700. New York: Springer-Verlag.

Woolsey, C. N., Erickson, T. C., & Gilson, W. E. (1979). Localization in somatic sensory and motor areas of human cerebral cortex as determined by direct recording of evoked potentials and electrical stimulation. *Journal of Neurosurgery, 51,* 476-506.

SUGGESTED READINGS

Asanuma, H. (1975). Recent developments in the study of the columnar arrangement of neurons within the motor cortex. *Physiological Reviews, 55,* 143-156.

Bourne, G. H. (Ed.). (1972, 1973). *The structure and function of muscle (2d ed.). Vol. 1: Structure. Pt. 1, Vol. 2: Structure. Pt. 2, Vol. 3: Physiology and biochemistry. Vol. 4: Pharmacology and disease.* New York: Academic Press.

Brooks, V. B. (Ed.). (1981). *Handbook of physiology, Sec. 1: The Nervous System. Vol. 2: Motor control, Pts. 1, 2.* Baltimore, MD: American Physiological Society.

Carlson, F. D., & Wilkie, D. R. (1974). *Muscle physiology.* Englewood Cliffs, NJ: Prentice-Hall.

Cooke, J. D. (1980). The role of stretch reflexes during active movements. *Brain Research, 181,* 493-497.

Desmedt, J. E. (Ed.). (1980). *Progress in clinical neurophysiology, Vol. 8. Spinal and supraspinal mechanisms of voluntary motor control and locomotion.* New York: Karger.

———— (Ed.). (1981). *Progress in clinical neurophysiology, Vol. 9. Motor unit types, recruitment and plasticity in health and disease.* New York: Karger.

Eaton, T. A. (1972). On the normal use of reflexes. *Scientific American, 60,* 591-599.

Edelman, G. M., & Mountcastle, V. B. (1978). *The mindful brain.* Cambridge, MA: MIT Press.

Evarts, E. V. (1979). Brain mechanisms of movement. *Scientific American, 241,* 164-179.

Evarts, E. V., et al. (1971). Central control of movement. *Neurosciences Research Program Bulletin, 9,* No. 1.

Freund, H.-J. (1983). Motor unit and muscle activity in voluntary motor control. *Physiological Reviews, 63,* 387-436.

Hobson, J. A., & Sheibel, A. B. (Eds.). (1980). The brainstem core: Sensorymotor integration and behavioral state control. *Neurosciences Research Program Bulletin*, *18*, No. 1.

Huxley, A. A. (1979). *Reflections on muscle*. Liverpool, England: Liverpool University Press.

Kaas, J. H., et al. (1979). Multiple representations of the body within the somatosensory cortex of primates. *Science*, *204*, 521-523.

McMahon, T. A. (1984). *Muscles, reflexes, and locomotion*. Princeton, NJ: Princeton University Press.

Merzenich, M. M., & Kaas, J. H. (1980). Principles of organization of sensory-perceptual systems in mammals. In J. M. Sprague, & A. N. Epstein (Eds.). *Progress in psychobiology and physiological psychology*, Vol. 9. New York: Academic Press.

Ochs, S. (1965). *Elements of neurophysiology*. New York: John-Wiley & Sons.

Squire, J. (1981). *The structural basis of muscular contraction*. New York: Plenum Press.

Stein, R. B. (1982). What muscle variable(s) does the nervous system control in limb movements? *The Behavioral and Brain Sciences*, *5*, 535-577.

Stelmach, G. E., & Requin, J. (Eds.). (1980). *Tutorials in motor behavior*. Amsterdam: North-Holland.

Thompson, R. F. (1967). *Foundations of physiological psychology*. New York: Harper & Row.

Wise, S. P. (1985). The primate premotor cortex: Post, present, and preparatory. *Annual Review of Neuroscience*, *8*, 1-19.

13
THE BODY
IN SPACE

INTRODUCTION

Each of us not only maintains a current dynamic representation of our surroundings, our **world model**, but we also maintain a separate current dynamic representation of our body, our **postural model**. We know where our body and limbs are and how to move them to approach and avoid objects. This chapter describes the postural model, its use, and the system used for creating and maintaining it.

Several sensory systems are used for maintaining the postural model. Kinesthetic inputs are crucial and were described in the previous chapter. The cutaneous and vestibular senses are also important. The cutaneous system not only describes the temperature of the environment, it also provides information about the shape and texture of objects that are touched. The vestibular system determines the orientation of the body relative to the direction of gravity, and it determines angular and linear accelerations of the head. Both of these systems will be briefly described in this chapter. Finally, the visual system makes inputs to the postural system, which are used for updating the postural model.

THE POSTURAL BUFFER

Just as the spatial system maintains a current dynamic representation of the world, the **postural system** maintains a current dynamic representation of the body, the **postural model**. This section describes how the postural model is created, how it is maintained, and how it used by the sensory-motor system.

The postural model represents the entire body. Each small part of the body's surface is a **surface patch**. The amount of skin represented by one surface patch depends on its location: The hands have many more surface patches per unit area than other parts of the body. Each surface patch has a position in space, an

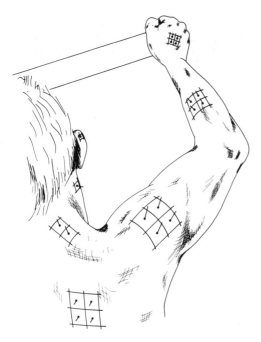

Figure 13.1. The body is conceptually divided into surface patches. Each surface patch has a position in space relative to the body's coordinate system, a surface orientation, and a velocity. The body posture model includes the set of all such surface patch representations. This figure only shows the surface orientation vectors of selected body patches.

orientation, and is moving at some velocity (perhaps zero). Hence a set of three vectors is sufficient for locating each surface patch. The set of all such vectors comprises the postural model. Refer to Figure 13.1. I will assume that the postural system and visual system use the same representations of position, surface orientation, and movement. For example, if spatial memory uses distance, height, and azimuth to specify position, then so does the postural system.

The postural model can be kept current by systematically modifying each of its vectors whenever the body moves. For intentional movements, the motor patterns can be used to calculate the change in each surface patch and update its postural model vectors. The sensory apparatus (cutaneous, kinesthetic, and vestibular) also indicates when a movement takes place and can also be used to update the postural model.

The postural model is maintained in a dynamic, temporary associative storage system called the **postural buffer**. The postural buffer, like spatial memory, is more than a storage device; it contains the computational circuitry needed for updating the postural model whenever a movement takes place. Figure 13.2 illustrates part of the postural buffer. As the figure shows, the postural buffer is distributed across a two-dimensional surface and is divided into computational units called **postural locations**. Each postural location contains the circuitry for updating the postural vectors for the surface patch that it represents and it also contains the circuitry for comparing its postural vectors with an incoming test pattern. The postural buffer preserves the local topology of the receptor surface (e.g., the skin and muscles), so that nearby surface patches on the body are represented by nearby postural locations. Note that unlike the representations held in spatial memory, the representation held in the postural buffer does not shift around; each postural location is dedicated to a particular surface patch of the body. This is important since the transformations that a postural location performs on its surface vectors depend on the body part being represented. A different set of transformations apply to the elbow than to a finger.

Maintaining the Postural Model

Just like motor stores, which you will see are divided into groups according to various body parts, the postural buffer is also functionally divided according to body parts. This organization allows buffer locations to communicate when the postural model is being updated. When an arm is moved at the shoulder, all parts of the postural model for surface patches on the arm must be updated. Moreover, the transformation for each of them is the same, provided no other part of the arm is bending. However, if the elbow is also bending, then the transformations are different for the surface patches below the elbow than above it. Each postural location can transform its part of the postural model provided it knows (1) the transformation that is used for updating the representation of a surface patch between the nearest joint and the trunk of the body, and (2) the way that joint angle is changing. Refer to Fig. 13.3. Moreover, once a postural location determines the transformation it must perform, it can send that information to postural locations representing surface patches farther away from the trunk; they in turn can determine the transformations they must apply and pass that information along to buffer locations which are even farther from the trunk. It follows that if the body is represented as shown in Fig. 13.4, then the information required for updating the postural model can be transmitted between postural locations in an orderly way.

Various information sources are used for maintaining the postural model. When an intentional movement is initiated, the pattern which initiates it is transmitted both to the motor apparatus to control the movement and to the postural system for updating the postural model. The postural system therefore knows what movement is intended and can update the postural model. When looking at a body part, the visual system determines its position. The position vector is sent to the postural buffer and if it does not agree with the current position vector for that body part the postural model can be updated. When one body part touches another, the position vectors for the surfaces of contact are the same. If their position vectors differ in the postural model, the postural model can be corrected. Any movement of the body as a whole also implies a movement of its parts. The vestibular system (described later in this chapter) measures acceleration and orientation (relative to the direction of gravity) and

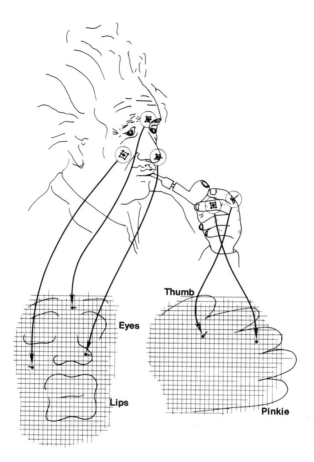

Figure 13.2. A sketch of a person with selected surface patches indicated. Below are parts of the postural buffer showing how specific buffer locations hold surface patch information. Only surface orientation vectors are shown. Compare with Figures 12.14 and 13.4.

therefore provides inertial information for updating the postural model. Finally, muscle and joint receptors continually measure the joint angles and hence provide information for creating and maintaining the postural model.

Although the sources of information required for maintaining the postural model are clear, it is not known how information from different sources is combined to produce and update the postural model. For example, when the visual and kinesthetic senses provide conflicting information, that information must either be combined or one of the sources must be ignored and the postural model made to agree with the other source. Said another way, the ambiguity must be resolved. How that is done is an open question.

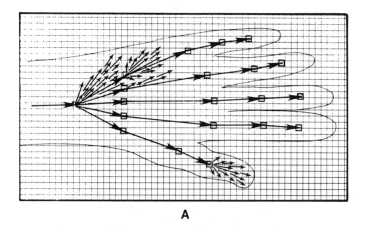

A

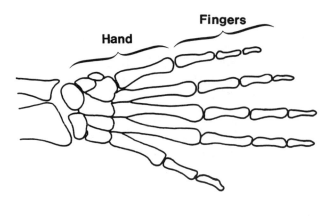

B

Figure 13.3. The structure of the postural buffer. a. Heavy arrows show how information describing movement of one joint can be passed along to buffer locations processing surface patches at subsequent joints along the body; light arrows (only a few are shown) show that identical information can be sent to buffer locations processing surface patches for surfaces between joints. Buffer locations at the tips of the heavy arrows combine movement information from current and previous joints. b. The skeletal structure of the hand.

Extracting Information from Postural Locations.   Position, surface orientation, and movement of any part of the body can be obtained from the postural buffer. To do so only requires that the appropriate postural location be activated: Information can only be extracted from an activated storage location. Postural locations can be activated in several different ways. Cutaneous information, direct stimulation of touch receptors for example, can activate postural locations. Kinesthetic information can also activate postural locations. In addition to the sensory inputs, each part of the postural buffer receives a test pattern which is distributed to all postural locations. The test pattern represents a single position, a single surface orientation, and a single movement. Each postural location compares the test pattern with the corresponding vectors for the surface patch it represents and activates itself if the resulting similarity signal is sufficiently high. Finally, the verbal system associates the name of each body part with a pattern that activates the corresponding postural locations. It is not known how this is done.

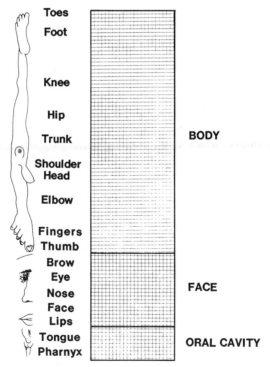

Figure 13.4. The postural buffer is divided into three parts—the body, the face, and the oral cavity. The internal connections reflect the skeletal and muscle structures.

Relating the Body to the Space Around It.   The postural buffer and spatial memory together relate the body to the external world. Whenever part of the body is touched, a particular postural location is activated. The control circuits can then extract its surface patch vectors. This constitutes focusing the attention on the selected body part. Once extracted, the position vector can be used by the high-level control networks to direct the focus of visual attention to the same spatial location. As a result, the visual system and the sensory-motor system can attend the same stimulus. Going the other way, if the visual system is attending a particular spatial location, the position vector of that location is made available. If that vector is sent as a test pattern to the postural buffer, the postural locations which respond, if any, represent the surface patches which currently occupy the selected spatial location. The sensory apparatus can then attend to sensory information from the corresponding surface patch. It follows, therefore, that spatial memory and the postural buffer enable the body to interact with its environment.

The Body Image.   Spatial memory and the postural buffer together create the **body image**, the representation of the body which can be seen in the mind's eye. In order to understand what is meant by the body image, you might like to try the following experiment. Imagine your right arm held out in front of you with clenched fist. Now imagine bending your elbow so your upper and lower arms are perpendicular. Finally, imagine unclenching your fist. Can you see your arm and hand in your mind's eye? Now perform the movements I just described. Is your arm where you imagined it? Is your fist unclenched? The spatial representations of your body which you just imagined are the mind's body image, the dynamic representation which is used while planning a physical action.

The high-level system that receives the body image from the postural buffer is the same system that processes spatial representations from spatial memory; hence the body image can be seen in the mind's eye. It follows that both spatial information and body information can be merged into a single dynamic representation which represents the body in its environment.

PREDICTING THE OUTCOME OF A MOVEMENT

When a pattern that controls a movement is sent to the postural buffer, the postural buffer can compute the postural model that would result if the movement were orchestrated. This is the **anticipated postural model**. The anticipated postural model, rather than the current one, can be sent to the high-level systems for analysis and hence can also be seen in the mind's eye. The resulting representation depicts the outcome of the movement and hence predicts its results. It is precisely because the postural model and spatial representations interact in this way that movements with intended outcomes can be planned.

THE CUTANEOUS SENSES

Skin is a complex tissue comprised not only of the outer layer (epidermis) and inner layer (dermis) but also numerous receptors which describe the state of the environment. Some of the receptors found in the fingertip are illustrated in Figure 13.5; numerous other types are present as well. Skin contains a two-dimensional mosaic of sensory receptors, and the representations generated by the different types of receptors are produced concurrently and transmitted to the brain either in registration or as distinctly separate patterns depending on the type of stimulus being encoded.

Cutaneous receptors can be classified according to function and according to axonal size. When classified according to function, there are three categories: **mechanoreceptors**, which respond to mechanical stimulation; **thermoreceptors**, which respond to heat or cold; and **nociceptors**, which respond to damaging stimulation. When classified according to speed of axonal conduction, there are also three categories: Aα fibers, which are myelinated fibers with a diameter ranging from 6 to 17 microns; Aδ fibers which are myelinated fibers with a diameter ranging from 1 to 5 microns; and C or unmyelinated fibers, with diameters ranging from .3 to 1.5 microns. The largest axons, the Aa axons, are the fastest conducting. There are mechanoreceptors in all three fiber groups, there are nociceptors having Ad and C fibers, while the thermoreceptors have only type C fibers. Within the thermoreceptors are fibers which respond to (1) increasing temperature, (2) decreasing temperature, (3) damaging heat (greater than 50° C), and (4) damaging cold (less than 1° C). Among the mechanoreceptors are fibers which respond to (1) gentle touch, (2) deep touch, (3) position, and (4) movement (Eyzaguirre & Fidone, 1975, p. 73). These categories are not mutually exclusive.

An alternative way to view mechanical stimulation is according to the sensation it produces. When viewed in this way, it is not the particular receptor or its qualities that are important, but the pattern of activity generated in the sensory pathway innervated by the receptors. (If you recall, the sensation of color has its physiological correlate in the ratio of firing rates in three distinct classes of sensory fibers which represent mainly the outputs from three classes (determined by photopigment) of cone cells. Still, each cone received inputs from numerous neighboring rod cells.)

Among the distinguishable cutaneous sensations are touch (pressure), tickle, itch, warm, and cold. The thermal receptors form a single modality where the sensation of warmth indicates increasing temperature and the sensation of coolness indicates decreasing temperature. (This is somewhat like increasing and decreasing brightness, which is signaled by "on" and "off" cells of the retina.) Specific combinations of stimulation result in sensations such as wetness (a combination of coolness and movement) and textures (a combination of light touch, deep touch, and movement). Once again, the origin of the texture

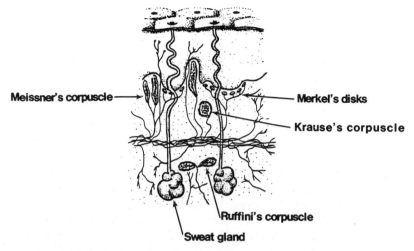

Figure 13.5. Nerve endings found in the epidermis (upper layer) and dermis (lower layers) of the human fingertip. (Reproduced, with permission, from C. Eyzaguirre & S. J. Fidone, *Physiology of the Nervous System. An Introductory Text.* Copyright © 1975 by Year Book Medical Publishers Incorporated. Adapted from V. B. Mountcastle, Physiology of sensory receptors: an introduction to sensory receptors, in V. B. Mountcastle (Ed.) *Medical Physiology, 12th Edition*, Vol. II, 1968, Copyright © 1968 by C.V. Mosby Company, St. Louis, and used with permission.)

sensation is not a single receptor type but the pattern of activity generated by several classes of receptors.

Based on an analogy with the visual system, the sensory cortex probably receives and integrates the patterns from various receptors to make explicit particular features of the stimulating source. The patterns of stimulation are recognizable and are given distinctive names such as "fuzziness." Moreover, one might expect that textures, which can be identified both tactually and visually, have similar tactile and visual representations. Whether or not this is the case is not known.

TACTILE IDENTIFICATION OF OBJECTS

Most of us are able to identify objects by exploring them with our hands. Unlike the visual system, which simultaneously creates a representation of the entire object, the tactile system paints an image of the object by brushing its surfaces with the fingertips. This section describes how this is done.

First, the position and orientation of each surface of the object is determined by touch. Since the postural model gives for each surface patch its position and surface orientation when the fingers pass over a surface, the position and orientation of the surface are immediately available. The tactile receptors of the fingers also encode the texture of the surface. Note that the texture corresponds exactly to the test pattern used by the visual system when scanning the object. Combining tactile representation with information from the posture model—surface orientation, position, and movement—it is clear that the same representations are available that are formed visually. Hence a mental image of the object can be constructed in spatial memory. Once in spatial memory, the representation can be seen in the mind's eye and the object recognized as if the representation were formed by the visual system.

It is interesting to note the parallel between the mechanoreceptors of the fingertips and responses of the X-cells and Y-cells of the retinas. There are two types of mechanoreceptor fibers which will be considered: Type I and Type II. Type I fibers originate in Merkel's disks (see Fig. 13.6); Type II fibers originate in the neighborhood of a Rufini corpuscle. Both are Aα fiber types which are the fastest conducting of the sensory fibers. Both types respond to a tactile stimulus moving across the receptor surface (movement detectors), and both types respond to focal contact (position detectors). Type I fibers respond more vigorously to static contact and less vigorously to movement than Type II fibers, and Type I fibers recover more quickly from fatigue than Type II fibers. Type I fibers have a less regular pattern of discharge than Type II fibers. The similarity between retinal and tactile receptors suggests that the fingers are designed to detect edges and object boundaries and hence perform a low-level encoding for object recognition.

THE VESTIBULAR SYSTEM

I will now change the focus of the discussion from the postural model and its utility to the vestibular system. The vestibular system measures linear and angular accelerations of the head, and it relates the body to the direction of gravity. Vestibular information is therefore crucial to maintaining balance. In general, when the head moves the eyes continue to maintain their direction of gaze by moving in the opposite direction within their orbits. Vestibular information plays a crucial role in initiating the eye movements, which compensate for head movements. This section describes the structure and functioning of the vestibular apparatus.

The vestibular system, part of the inner ear, consists of the vestibular apparatus and the vestibular nerves. The vestibular nerves convey information to and from the vestibular apparatus.

The **vestibular apparatus**, illustrated in Figure 13.7, comprises five receptors: three **semicircular canals**, each with an ampulla that houses the receptor cells; a **utricle**, and a **saccule**. The receptor organs of the semicircular canals are

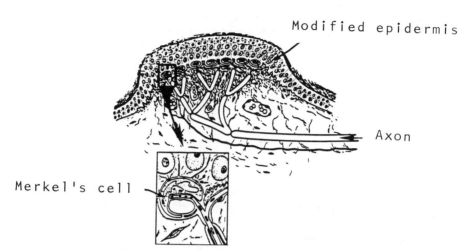

Modified epidermis

Axon

Merkel's cell

Figure 13.6. Diagram of Iggo's type-I "dome receptor." Top, a thick-
ened, modified epidermis containing, just inside the basement mem-
brane, a layer of nerve endings derived from a single myelinated axon.
Inset, detail of one of the nerve endings, together with the cell that
encloses it. (Reproduced, with permission, from C. Eyzaguirre & S. J.
Fidone, *Physiology of the Nervous System. An Introductory Text.*
Copyright © 1975 by Year Book Medical Publishers Incorporated.
Adapted from A. Iggo, Cutaneous receptors with a high sensitivity to
mechanical displacement, in A. V. S. DeReuck & J. Knight (Eds.) *Touch,
Heat and Pain.* Copyright © 1966 by Little, Brown and Company.)

cristae, while those of the saccule and utricle are **maculae**. Like the cochlea,
described in Chapter 10, the vestibular apparatus is encased in a close-fitting
cavity in the skull. Perilymph fluid fills the gap between the vestibular
membrane and the skull, while endolymph fluid fills the inside of the vestibular
apparatus. These fluids provide the necessary chemical environment for the
receptor cells and the mechanical interface for stimulating them. The
endolymph fluid is free to move between the vestibular organs and the cochlea,
and therefore the vestibular and auditory senses are not independent.

Figures 13.8 and 13.9 illustrate the structure of a crista and a macula. As you
can see, both receptors are somewhat similar to each other and also to the hair
cells of the cochlea (refer to Figure 10.7). The receptor cells function in similar
ways: Movement of the cilia toward the kinocilium increases the rate of
discharge of the receptor; movement of the cilia in the opposite direction
decreases the rate of discharge. Understanding how the receptors encode
orientation, linear acceleration, and angular acceleration can be deduced from
understanding what makes the cilia move.

The three semicircular canals (superior, posterior, and lateral) are almost
circular and oriented at right angles to one another. Within the ampulla of each

368

duct, the cilia project into a gelatinous substance which extends prominently into the endolymph fluid thereby obstructing its movement. Except for the partial obstruction, the endolymph fluid is free to move within each duct. Because of the inertia of the endolymph fluid, when the head rotates, the fluid tends to remain stationary and thus moves relative to the walls of the ducts and receptors. When moving past the obstruction formed by the cilia and encasing jelly, the latter deforms. The bending of the cilia generates signals describing the angular acceleration of the head. Since the three semicircular canals are perpendicular to each other, angular acceleration about any spatial axis can be determined.

The saccule and utricle operate on a somewhat different basis. First, gelatinous substance does not project much beyond the ends of the cilia. Second, numerous small calcareous organs called otoliths, are attached to the covering jelly. The otoliths are heavy enough to respond to the force of gravity. Depending on the orientation of the head, the otoliths distort the jelly and bend the cilia. This generates a signal which describes the orientation of the head relative to gravity. When the head accelerates linearly, the inertia of the otoliths resists movement and results in distortion of the cilia. This generates a signal which describes the acceleration.

The responses of the vestibular receptors (and cochlear receptors as well) are not independent. All of these organs share the same endolymph fluid, and the anterior and posterior semicircular canals share a common segment of duct. Moreover, linear acceleration and gravity are not independent stimuli, particularly when the acceleration is in the vertical direction, and each angular

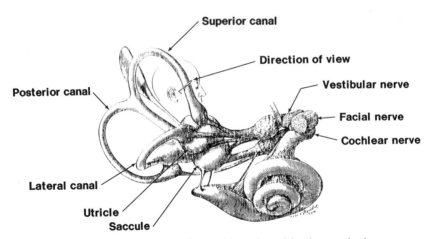

Figure 13.7. Superior, posterior, and lateral semicircular canals shown in relation to their orientation in the human head. (Reproduced, with permission, from M. Hardy, Observations on the innervation of the macula sacculi in man. *Anatomical Record*, 59, 1934, 403-418.)

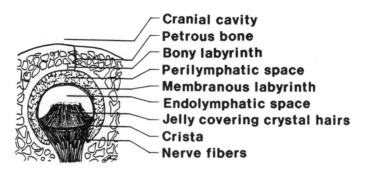

- Cranial cavity
- Petrous bone
- Bony labyrinth
- Perilymphatic space
- Membranous labyrinth
- Endolymphatic space
- Jelly covering crystal hairs
- Crista
- Nerve fibers

a

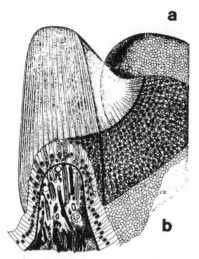

b

Figure 13.8. The structure of an ampulla/crista in a semicircular canal: a. in cross section; and b. an isometric sketch as seen in a longitudinal section of a semicircular canal, passing across a crista. (a. Reproduced, with permission, from W. J. S. Krieg, *Functional Neuroanatomy. Third Edition.* Evanston, IL: Brain Books. Copyright © 1966 by the author. b. Reproduced, with permission, from W. Bloom & D. W. Fawcett, *A Textbook of Histology.* Eighth Edition. Copyright © 1962 by W. B. Saunders Company.)

acceleration has a linear component on at least one side of the head. Even though the responses are not independent, the principles which underlie their functions are sufficiently well understood to recognize that angular acceleration about any axis, linear acceleration in any direction, and orientation relative to gravity can all be detected and encoded.

The vestibular system is often considered as part of the sensory-motor system because of the important role it plays in balance and controlling eye movements. A majority of its function is automatic and will only be mentioned in passing.

The vestibular signals are a major source of input to the visual reflex system.

Whenever the head moves, the eyes must move in the opposite direction if they are to maintain their gaze. The signals which control the movement are of vestibular origin. When the eyes track a moving target, they sometimes move within the orbit and they sometimes remain fixed in the orbit and the head moves. Once again, information from the vestibular apparatus is crucial for controlling the movement.

Vestibular signals are also critical for controlling balance during locomotion and for initiating righting reflexes when the body is off balance or loses balance. The vestibular system makes massive connections with the cerebellum for this purpose.

SUMMARY

The relationship between the body and its surroundings is determined in many different ways. The visual system is a major source of information, and the representation in spatial memory created from visual inputs is one of two representations that are maintained. The other representation is the postural model. The postural model is an up-to-date representation of the body which specifies for each element of the body its position in space, its orientation, and

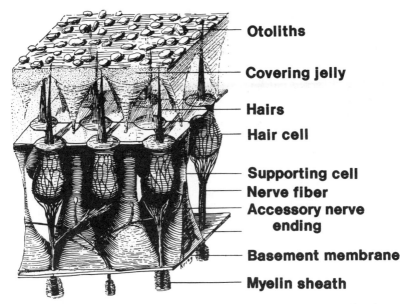

Otoliths

Covering jelly

Hairs

Hair cell

Supporting cell
Nerve fiber
Accessory nerve
    ending

Basement membrane

Myelin sheath

Figure 13.9. Stereogram of epithelium of macula and associated endings of vestibular nerve. (Reproduced, with permission, from W. J.S. Krieg, *Functional Neuroanatomy. Third Edition.* Evanston, IL: Brain Books. Copyright © 1966 by the author.)

its movement. When information describing part of the body is sent to the spatial system, that information can be seen in the mind's eye. When, before a movement, the anticipated body image is sent to the spatial system, the outcome of the intended movement can be determined. This constitutes planning a movement.

The tactile system, postural system, and spatial systems together enable tactile presentations of objects to be converted into mental images. Objects can therefore be recognized as if they were seen directly.

Finally, the orientation of the body relative to gravity, and any accelerations of the body, either linear, or rotational, are encoded by the vestibular apparatus. The vestibular encodings are crucial to maintaining balance, tracking moving objects, and updating the postural model during movements.

Although the general principles of the body profile system have been outlined, there is at present no detailed understanding or model of this system. We do not know, for example, how position, surface orientation, and movement vectors are represented or transformed. We do not know what coordinate systems are used. We do not know how mental images are created from the postural model nor do we know how they are used for planning movements. Thus although general principles have been set forth, details will only come with careful neurophysiological experiments and collaborative theoretical modeling.

REFERENCES

Bloom, W., & Fawcett, D. W. (1962). A textbook of histology(8th ed.). Philadelphia: W. B. Saunders.

DeReuck, A. V. S., Knight, J. (Eds.) (1966). Touch, heat and pain. Boston: Little, Brown.

Eyzaguirre, C., & Fidone, S. J. (1975). Physiology of the nervous system. An introductory text (2d ed.). Chicago, IL: Year Book Medical Publishers.

Hardy, M. (1934). Observations on the innervation of the macula sacculi in man. Anatomical Record, 59, 403-418.

Iggo, A., & Andres, K. H. (1982). Morphology of cutaneous receptors. Annual Review of Neuroscience, 5, 1-31.

Krieg, W. J. S. (1966). Functional neuroanatomy (3d ed.). Evanston, IL: Brain Books.

Mountcastle, V. B. (1968). Medical physiology (12th ed.), Vol. 2. St. Louis: C. V. Mosby.

Precht, W. (1979). Vestibular mechanisms. Annual Review of Neuroscience, 2, 265-289.

SUGGESTED READINGS

Dick, A. O. (1976). Spatial abilities. In H. Whitaker, & H. A. Whitaker (Eds.). Studies in neurolinguistics. New York: Academic Press.

Granit, R. (1977). The purposive brain. Cambridge, MA: MIT Press.

Parker, D. E. (1980). The vestibular apparatus. Scientific American, 243, 118-135.

14

THE CONTROL
OF CONFIGURATION
AND SIMPLE
MOVEMENTS

INTRODUCTION

A **body configuration** is the spatial form of the body and its parts (standing at ease, doubled over, sitting, lying down), while the **configuration system** is the collection of networks which holds and adjusts configurations. The configuration system is subserved by the gamma motor neurons and stretch reflex circuitry. Adjustments to the configuration are movements, and both the static and dynamic properties of a movement are regulated during its orchestration. The **thrust system** accelerates and decelerates body parts during a movement and therefore regulates the velocity of each part along its trajectory. The stretch reflex must be regulated during a movement so as not to oppose it, and hence coactivation of alpha and gamma neurons is implicated for thrust control.

Various storage systems are used when holding or adjusting configurations. Temporary storage systems hold configuration patterns during their application, and temporary storage systems hold sequences of thrust patterns prior to their employment to animate a movement. Permanent storage systems hold configuration patterns, thrust patterns, and control information for skilled movements. The architectures and organizations of these storage systems will be a major focus of this and the next chapter.

MOTOR PATTERNS FOR CONTROL OF MOVEMENT

A **motor pattern** is the final high-level pattern generated by the motor system to control a posture or simple movement, and a **premotor pattern** is any pattern used by the motor system for obtaining a motor pattern. The term **orchestrating a movement** denotes two processes: transforming a premotor pattern into a motor pattern, and applying the motor pattern. **Applying a motor pattern** means transmitting it over the efferent pathways to activate the low-level motor apparatus—the cerebellum, the spinal reflex circuits, the motor neurons, and finally the muscles. Complex movements often consist of sequences of simple movements, and **planning** is the process of recalling or generating premotor patterns for simple movements and **uniting** them into a single premotor pattern for the intended complex movement.

Parameters are values used by the motor system while performing movements, and three parameters of a movement are of particular importance: its intended speed, its intended spatial size, and the expected forces to orchestrate it. The intended speed is a parameter which controls the actual speed of orchestration. Since the motor pattern for a movement depends on the speed of orchestration, the same premotor pattern may be transformed into entirely different motor patterns when orchestrated at different speeds. The intended size of a movement is a parameter which controls the magnitude of each actual movement. When handwriting, for example, the intended size regulates the size of the writing as well as the method of orchestration. Writing small letters is done primarily with finger and hand movements; writing large letters is done with arm movements as well. Intended force is also a parameter to the motor system. When picking up an object, the motor pattern depends on the expected weight of the object. If an object being picked up is much lighter than expected, the result is a sudden, unexpected, overpowered motion which throws the entire body off balance.

There are several different ways that intended force can enter into the control of a movement. First, the motor pattern can be modified as a function of intended force: either each cell that innervates a motor neuron must fire at a faster or slower rate depending on the intended force, or the number of activated efferent fibers must be increased or decreased. In either or both cases, the forces exerted by the muscles will be increased or decreased as specified. A fundamentally different solution is to facilitate or depress the responses of motor neurons to signals arriving along the efferent pathways. In this way, the exact same motor pattern can be used, and the intended force modifies only the animation of the movement. The motor system can be regulated by an independent subsystem, and the pattern of movements is **decoupled** from the intended force.

The motor cortex is a staging area for the control of movement, and viewed in this way, it is tempting to imagine the pyramidal cells as a keyboard on which the score of muscle movements is finally played. In the absence of all other influences this might be so, but we have already seen that there are other influences, including the various reflex arcs, so that this naïve picture of movement control is inadequate. Movements are regulated by a variety of systems, each evaluating a particular aspect of the required movement, and the final efferent pathways simply convey the results of those evaluations to the spinal apparatus. Still, the motor patterns generated by the volitional system determine the essential characteristics of a movement, and this and the next chapters will explore what those patterns do, how they are generated, how they are routed to their correct destinations, and how they are used to control simple movements.

STORAGE SYSTEM FOR MOTOR PATTERNS

One question that naturally arises is, is it possible to use a cortical associative storage system to hold a motor pattern for the entire body? Although it is possible, it is neither likely nor practical. It is not likely because the size of a motor pattern is much larger than can be held by a storage location in a cortical storage system. There are approximately 1.2 million efferent fibers in the pyramidal tract alone, while cortical storage locations are restricted to patterns having a few hundred elements. It is not practical because such motor patterns would have very little utility. The motor system can certainly control the entire body, but to store patterns whose later application is unlikely is simply not an efficient way to do things.

How, then, can a motor pattern for the entire body be stored? The answer is to partition a storage system into independent groups of storage locations, one group for each set of functionally related muscles, and then generate motor patterns for the entire body by recalling subpatterns from each of the independent groups of storage locations.

A **motor store** is a permanent associative memory store for motor patterns. Figure 14.1 illustrates the architecture of a motor store. As with all cortical storage systems, storage locations are locally distributed through the storage medium. Local control circuits, not shown in the figure, control the individual storage locations by specifying when new information will be stored (e.g., during learning) and when stored information will be recalled (e.g., while performing a movement).

Storage locations are partitioned into groups in two different ways, depending on their information input and output pathways. The first partition organizes storage locations into **motor groups**, groups that share the same input and output pathways for motor patterns. Fibers in the input and output pathways control functionally related muscles. As an example, the fibers in one motor group might control all muscles that move a particular joint. These are the smaller of the two types of groups illustrated in Figure 14.1. The second partition organizes storage locations into groups that share the same input and output pathways that convey associated patterns. These are **control groups** and are the larger of the two types of groups illustrated in Figure 14.1. The associated patterns are **premotor patterns**, patterns that enable access to motor patterns. The use of premotor patterns will be discussed in detail later. The sizes of the motor and control groups depend on the body components being controlled and the types of associated patterns.

Motor patterns for the entire body can be generated by simultaneously

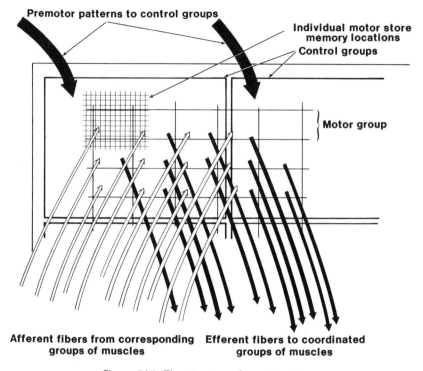

Premotor patterns to control groups

Individual motor store memory locations

Control groups

Motor group

Afferent fibers from corresponding groups of muscles

Efferent fibers to coordinated groups of muscles

Figure 14.1. The structure of a motor store.

recalling motor subpatterns from each of the motor groups in the motor store. Premotor patterns are associated with motor patterns as follows. A set of premotor patterns is selected, one for each control group, and a set of motor subpatterns is selected, one for each motor group. The set of all motor subpatterns comprises a motor pattern for the entire body. Within each control group, the selected premotor pattern is replicated once in every motor group and stored together with the selected motor subpattern for that group. This situation is illustrated in Fig. 14.2. If the given set of premotor patterns is used to activate storage locations, and one motor subpattern is recalled from an activated storage location in each motor group, then the resulting output pattern is a motor pattern for the entire body. In Fig. 14.2, if the premotor pattern 'O' is delivered over the premotor input pathway shown in the lower left, all those motor locations containing the 'O' pattern become activated. When recalled and used to control the hand configuration, the hand will be held in the open configuration shown at the lower right. Similarly, if the fist premotor pattern 'F' is delivered as a premotor input pattern and the resulting activated motor locations used as sources of configuration patterns, the hand will be held in the fist configuration shown at the upper right.

376

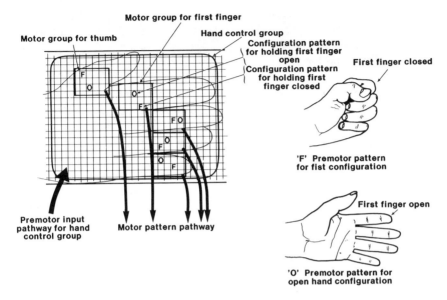

Figure 14.2. The same preconfiguration (premotor) pattern can appear many times in a motor store. As a consequence, one preconfiguration pattern (intention) can specify a complex configuration.

THE CONTROL OF CONFIGURATION

It is well known that a person can intentionally hold his or her body in a specified configuration such as standing at attention.[1] In order to hold such a configuration, each muscle must maintain an appropriate tension. For many muscles, the tension may be very slight, but for others, the tension may be quite large. The control system that keeps the body in a given configuration is the **configuration system**, and the efferent pattern that specifies how the body should be held is a **configuration pattern**. A configuration pattern is one type of motor pattern.

Each configuration pattern comprises two subpatterns. The first subpattern regulates the shape of the body by specifying muscle tension, muscle length, or some other parameter such as ratios of lengths or tensions in agonist-antagonist groups. The second subpattern regulates the responsiveness of the stretch reflex and therefore determines for each muscle how forcefully it will react when stretched from its specified length or tension. If each muscle is commanded to respond vigorously, even to the slightest stretch, the body will not only be held

---

[1] It is interesting to note that direct electrical stimulation to the caudate nucleus of the cat causes an arrest reaction: The entire body is frozen in whatever configuration it happens to be in at the time of stimulation (Thompson, 1967, p. 413).

in a given configuration but it will demonstrate a high degree of rigidity. This chapter will concentrate on the control of shape, not rigidity, but I will use the term "configuration" to designate both shape and rigidity.

A **configuration buffer** is a temporary dynamic storage system that holds a configuration pattern during its application. The output cells of the configuration buffer send signals to the efferent cells that innervate the motor neurons[2] to produce the desired tension and rigidity in each muscle. Each output cell in the configuration buffer is part of a local feedback circuit which keeps it firing at a prescribed rate until instructed to do otherwise. This is how the buffer holds information.

Using the mechanical muscle model introduced in the previous chapter, Figure 14.3a illustrates some of the concepts just described. An arm, with a fixed weight applied, is shown in equilibrium. The configuration pattern required to hold the arm in equilibrium is regulated by the settings on the potentiometers. The potentiometers correspond to the output cells of the configuration buffer and their pattern of settings corresponds to the configuration pattern. Figure 14.3b shows the same arm in equilibrium, only it is now holding a heavier weight. Notice that although the lengths of the muscles are unchanged, the tensions required to hold the heavier object are all different. As a consequence, the internal settings of the muscles are all different.

Also shown in Figure 14.3 are potentiometers which regulate the responsiveness of each muscle to stretch. If the arm is holding a heavy object and the responsiveness is set low, an external impulsive force which moves the arm will be opposed slowly and the arm will move quite far from its initial configuration. If the responsiveness is set high, the arm will be rigid and it will forcefully oppose any externally initiated movements.

Whether or not the configuration pattern changes as weights are applied depends on how configuration is specified by the motor system. If configuration is specified by sending an efferent pattern which regulates muscle tension, then the configuration pattern changes as a function of applied weight. If configuration is specified by sending an efferent pattern which regulates muscle length, then the configuration pattern does not change as a function of applied weight. Figure 14.3 illustrates the situation where the tensions of the muscles are specified, and hence the configuration pattern changes when weights are added to the arm. For purposes of what follows, I will assume that muscle tension is the parameter controlled by the configuration system to specify configuration. Conceptually it makes little difference for the discussion that follows.

Notice that if muscle length is the controlled parameter, then configuration is directly specified whereas if tension is the controlled parameter, then configuration is not directly specified. Moreover, if length is the controlled parameter, then each configuration pattern has a sensory representation since

---

[2]The gamma motor neurons have already been implicated in this function.

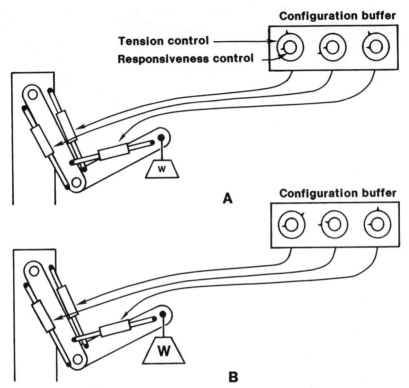

Figure 14.3. The configuration buffer for a robot arm. Notice that although the weight supported by the arm changes from a to b, the arm configuration does not change. Since, in this example, tension is assumed to be the controlled parameter, the configuration pattern changes from a to b.

both types Ia and II sensory fibers indicate the lengths of the muscles. In addition, a configuration pattern can be generated by placing the body in a desired configuration by any means whatever, and then storing the resulting pattern of muscle lengths. Later, during the application of the configuration pattern, the spinal circuits can automatically compare the current pattern of lengths with the desired one and adjust the tensions in the muscles until the desired pattern of lengths—the desired configuration—is achieved. The utility of specifying length is clear, but there are also many difficulties. In the first place, muscles are elastic and hence measuring their lengths is difficult and the measurements are only approximate.

Second, the measurements, obtained by the types Ia and II sensory fibers, depend on fusimotor activity. Hence the muscle lengths can only be determined if the pattern of fusimotor activity is known in advance and its affect on the sensory receptors is also known in advance. There is no evidence that the fusimotor pattern is known in advance. I might point out that tension, like muscle length, has a sensory representation which is directly measured by the Golgi tendon organs of the muscle. Hence if the configuration pattern specifies muscle tension, then it, too, has a sensory representation.

I already showed that when the body is held in a given configuration, any external force that moves the body away from that configuration is countered by an opposite force that attempts to restore the configuration. Forces resulting from the stretch reflex occur first; those initiated by higher brain centers occur later.[3] The opposing forces initiated by the stretch reflex cannot be eliminated by choice; those initiated by the higher brain centers can be.

The motor system holds a configuration by placing a particular pattern of values in the configuration buffer and then applying it by transmitting it over the efferent pathway to activate the spinal cord and muscles. Suppose that a subject is told to hold his or her arm in a horizontal position and maintain that position even while an experimenter places additional weights on it. The moment that an added weight lowers the arm, the stretch reflex circuitry activates muscles which oppose the resulting movement. At the same time, the pattern in the configuration buffer is modified so that the tensions in all stretched muscles are incremented to counteract the additional force. If the modified configuration pattern is incorrect, the subject may intentionally adjust the configuration pattern—raise his or her arm—until the desired configuration is achieved. This voluntary movement is a configurational adjustment and will be described in detail later in this chapter (cf. the section on controlling simple movements).

It is not yet known how the control circuitry analyzes the kinesthetic information and readjusts the configuration pattern, but it is likely that the adjustments are triggered by the primary (type Ia) afferents when they indicate that the arm has started to move. Since the muscles that are stretched as a result of the additional weight are the same ones whose tension parameters have to be increased, the control network may comprise a pathway that connects the spindle afferents of each muscle to the control circuitry in the configuration buffer which regulates that muscle. Moreover, since the acceleration of the limb, as measured by the primary afferents, is proportional to the added weight, and since the required adjustments are also proportional to the added weight, the primary afferent signals originating in the muscle spindles can be used as control signals to adjust the firing rates of the output cells of the configuration buffer. The configuration can therefore be maintained despite changing external forces.

The supraspinal control loop needed for maintaining a configuration is illustrated in Figure 14.4. It is likely that this control loop comprises connections from the primary sensory area of the cerebral cortex to the primary motor area, and

---

[3]The stretch reflex, which is segmental, responds in about 70 milliseconds, while the activity from the higher brain centers, which is supraspinal, responds in about 180-200 milliseconds.

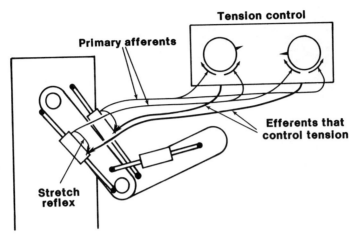

Figure 14.4. Long-loop control of configuration. When an external force tries to alter a configuration, signals from the primary afferents indicate the resulting change in muscle length. Although the stretch reflex opposes the change in configuration, the configuration pattern must also change to compensate for the changed external force. This change occurs when the configuration buffer receives signals from the primary afferents signaling the changing external forces.

if this is so, it is clear why the sensory and motor projections of the cerebral cortex are organized as they are. (Refer to Figure 12.14.) The supraspinal control loop is established by high-level control networks in response to an intention to hold a given configuration. The neural pathway for the control loop already exists; the high-level control networks **carry out the intention** of holding a configuration by gating signals along the pathway and enabling them to modify the firing rates of the output cells of the configuration buffer.

There is some experimental evidence that body configurations can be directly specified by the motor system. Polit and Bizzi (1979) trained normal monkeys in a pointing task and then surgically severed the sensory roots that innervate the arms in the monkey's spinal columns. After recovery from the surgery, the monkeys were still able to perform the arm-positioning task. During experimentation, the monkey's arms were constrained as shown in Figure 14.5, by a device which held the elbow in a fixed position yet enabled the experimenters to control the resistance to movement during testing. The monkeys were prevented from seeing their own arms by an opaque partition placed above the arm. Thus the positioning of the arm was accomplished without any sensory feedback. Polit and Bizzi concluded:

> Clearly this finding indicates that central commands must be able to control final arm position independently of initial position. We believe that, to a first approximation, our seemingly unexpected findings can be explained by postulating

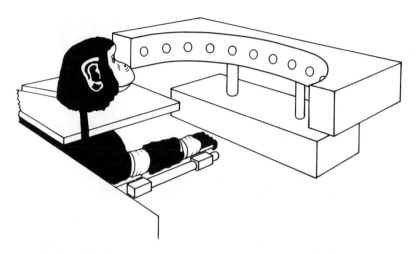

Figure 14.5. The apparatus used by Polit & Bizzi. A monkey was constrained with its arm strapped to a splint. The splint could pivot at the elbow. Target lights were placed at 5-degree intervals in the periphery. During an experimental session, the monkey was not allowed to see its own arm, and the room was darkened. (Redrawn, with permission, from A. Polit & E. Bizzi, Characteristics of motor programs underlying arm movements in monkeys. *Journal of Neurophysiology*, 42, 1979, 183-194.)

that the motor program specifies, through a selection of a set of length-tension properties in agonist and antagonist muscles, an equilibrium point between these two sets of muscles that correctly position the arm in relation to the visual target.

The monkey's arms were later splinted with a new elbow-joint angle and then retested. See Figure 14.6. Only the normal monkeys were able to compensate for the new joint angle after a few movements. This suggests that stored configuration patterns only produce the expected goal configurations when all interacting muscle components of the arm are free to accommodate the movement. Thus it appears that the configuration of the entire arm is one parameter that can be specified.

Preconfiguration Patterns for Controlling Arm Configuration

A **configuration store** is a motor store for holding configuration patterns, and a **preconfiguration pattern** is a premotor pattern which can be used for locating configuration patterns in a configuration store. The configuration store together with its control systems can generate particular configuration patterns when given associated preconfiguration patterns. This section illustrates how the configuration of an arm and hand can be controlled.

For purposes of illustration, assume the configuration store for the arm has three control groups, one for the upper arm, one for the wrist, and one for the hand. See Figure 14.7. Different preconfiguration patterns will be associated with the configuration subpatterns in these three control groups. Simultaneous recall of a configuration pattern from each motor group of each control group specifies a configuration for the entire limb.

The position of an object relative to the body, its surface orientations, its dimensions, and its weight are parameters made available to the motor system by the visual and spatial systems. The first step in grabbing an object is the creation of a representation of the object in spatial memory. For sighted individuals, this is done while the subject looks at the object, but a spatial representation can also be constructed from memory if the individual has prior knowledge of the object and setting, from a description of the object and setting, or by touching it. Refer to Chapters 8 and 13. Once created, the spatial representation indicates the location, orientation, and movement of each surface of the object.

Various parts of the configuration pattern for grabbing an object can be determined independently and then combined to form a single configuration pattern for the entire limb. When grabbing an object, the configuration of the arm (e.g., elbow joint and shoulder joint) depends on the location of the object but not in any major way on its size or orientation. In contrast, the way it is grabbed depends on its size and orientation but not in any major way on its location. It follows that different sensory representations can be used as preconfiguration patterns for locating the configuration patterns for arm, wrist, and hand.

The motor system can control arm configuration by associating the spatial coordinates of points within arm's reach with configuration patterns necessary for holding the arm there. The spatial coordinates, then, are used as

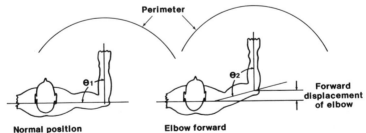

Figure 14.6. Schematic representation of postural manipulation performed by Polit & Bizzi on intact and deafferented monkeys. The normal position of the manipulation is shown at the left. The diagram in the right shows that moving the elbow forward causes the normal relation between joint angles and target light to be changed. (Redrawn, with permission, from A. Polit & E. Bizzi, Characteristics of motor programs underlying arm movements in monkeys. *Journal of Neurophysiology*, 42, 1979, 183-194.)

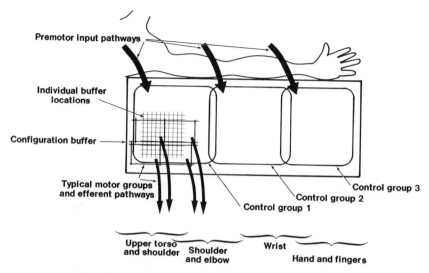

Figure 14.7. The configuration buffer for the arm and hand is divided into three control groups. The first control group specifies the configuration of the arm and hence specifies the position of the hand in space. The second control group specifies the configuration of the wrist and hence the orientation of the hand for grabbing an object. The third control group specifies the configuration of the hand and fingers and therefore determines how an object will be grabbed.

preconfiguration patterns in the control group that holds arm configurations. The area within arm's reach is so limited that it is easy to store for each spatial position the configuration pattern needed to hold the arm there.[4] Moreover, since the spatial system maintains a stable spatial representation of the world in which the position of each object is specified, we may assume that each nearby point has a unique set of spatial coordinates. Since the coordinates of each point (relative to the body) change if the body orientation changes, we may also assume that their encodings within spatial memory change if the body changes orientation. (This is what is meant by a stable representation.) It follows that the configuration pattern for grabbing an object can be orchestrated by extracting the pattern of coordinates of the object from its spatial representation, and using that pattern of coordinates as a preconfiguration pattern, locate and access the desired configuration pattern for the arm. Application of the

---

[4]Since each control group consists of a finite number of storage locations, there is an assumed limit to the accuracy of this type of representation. If, for example, the system stores the configuration patterns for every position on a 2-inch grid, then it would be impossible to position the hand reliably closer than an inch from an arbitrary position. This indeed seems to be the case without using visual or tactile feedback.

desired configuration pattern would hold the arm in approximately the desired position.

The motor system can locate the desired wrist configuration pattern by associating both position and surface orientation patterns with wrist configuration patterns that hold the hand in the orientation that grabs that surface. The position and surface orientation patterns, then, are the preconfiguration patterns in the control group that holds wrist configurations.

The motor system can control the spacing between thumb and fingers by associating patterns representing the object's size with corresponding thumb and finger configuration patterns for grabbing an object of that size. The size patterns, then, are the preconfiguration patterns in the control groups for thumb and finger configurations. Combining arm configuration, wrist configuration, and thumb and finger configuration patterns together, it is easy to see how a configuration pattern can be generated for grabbing any object within arm's reach. See Figure 14.8.

The utility of dividing the configuration store into control groups for body

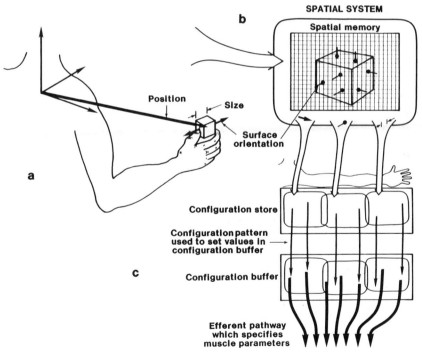

Figure 14.8. Grabbing an object. a. Spatial parameters used by the sensorymotor system. b. Spatial representations of an object used as preconfiguration patterns by the sensory-motor system. c. The configuration store and configuration buffer.

parts and motor groups for functionally related muscles should now be clear. Dividing the configuration store into control groups enables different sensory patterns to serve as preconfiguration patterns for different parts of the body. Dividing the configuration store into motor groups organizes muscles into synergistic units. Rather than having each muscle controlled independently, groups of functionally related muscles are controlled as units. The motor patterns stored in each motor unit organizes the activity of the relevant muscles, and hence the smallest controllable unit of action is an action specified for all muscles in a control group. (Individual muscles can be controlled by storing motor patterns with all entries specifying "no movement" except for the entry controlling the muscle of interest.) The final advantage of organizing the motor store into control groups will be discussed in the following section.

Convergence and Divergence of Information

One fundamental property of cortical storage systems is that individual storage locations can only hold patterns consisting of at most a few hundred elements. This principle applies to all modalities, and we saw for the visual system that low-level sensory patterns, although huge, were processed in small pieces by the visual buffer. Each stage of visual processing resulted in smaller patterns until, at the highest level, visual storage representations were produced which, as you will recall, have only a few hundred elements.

High-level decisions are based on the analysis of a small number of small high-level representations. Once a decision is made, it must be carried out, and the process of carrying out a decision generally entails the conversion of a small high-level pattern, an **intention**, into a detailed low-level pattern for controlling individual muscles (during a movement) or individual storage locations (while recalling a particular word or event, for example). We therefore expect to see a very different organization for motor stores than we saw for sensory stores, and that is exactly what we saw.

When controlling a movement, a high-level intention, which is a small pattern (symbolized by a phrase such as "raise your arm") is used to access a large number of other patterns. Ultimately, individual muscles or groups of muscles are controlled. The configuration store illustrated in Figure 14.7 demonstrated the general principle of organization. The input and output pathways which convey preconfiguration patterns are small and comprise only a few hundred elements. The same is true for the pathways that convey motor patterns. The critical issue is that there are a large number of similar storage locations, each one controlling a small number of functionally related muscles. It follows for the motor store that if local damage destroys all storage locations that control a particular set of muscles, then the control function performed by that store on those muscles cannot be recovered.[5]

The fact that there is a divergence of information along the pathways of control implies that the same high-level control pattern must enable concurrent access to a large number of different low-level control patterns. I already showed how this was done: The configuration store uses one preconfiguration pattern to access a large number of components of the final configuration pattern. Thus the same preconfiguration pattern is replicated many times. When a preconfiguration pattern arrives along the input pathway, all storage locations containing a copy are activated, and simultaneous recall from all activated storage locations synthesizes a configuration pattern for the entire body. A general principle of organization for the motor system, then, is: *A small number of high-level representations enable access to a large number of low-level representations, and this general divergence of information along the pathways of control continues until the individual muscles are activated.*

CONTROLLING SIMPLE MOVEMENTS

Virtually all volitional movements can be decomposed into slow and ballistic components as described in the previous chapter. Slow or configurational movements are initiated by the relatively continuous action of the muscles of involvement, and they are generally regulated using visual or tactile feedback. Ballistic movements, in contrast, are initiated and terminated by sudden impulsive contractions of muscles and progress without sensory feedback. The following few sections describe the underlying mechanisms of slow and ballistic movements.

Configurational or Slow Movements

One way to initiate a movement is to recall a configuration pattern from memory and use it to replace the one in the configuration buffer. When a movement is controlled this way using only the configurational system, it is a **slow** or **configurational movement**. The speed of the movement is determined in part by how different the new configuration pattern is from the previous one, but it is also influenced by how quickly the configuration system can locate and recall configuration patterns from memory, how quickly the configuration buffer can be updated, and how quickly the motor system responds to changes in the configuration buffer.

---

[5]Since both right and left hemispheres of the brain can control both sides of the body to some degree, it is most likely that even if damaged, the brain would retain some control over each movement. Only with symmetrical bilateral damage of the motor areas would one expect irrecoverable paralysis of the target muscles.

A different way to control a slow movement, also using the configuration system, is to **adjust** the current configuration pattern rather than replace it with a new one from memory. An adjustment of the current configuration pattern causes a **relative displacement**, which is a movement relative to the current configuration, and hence the preconfiguration patterns for the movement is a set of **intended movements** of the body components of involvement. A relative displacement would be initiated, for example, when drawing a line between dots on a piece of paper or when raising the arm from a given position to a slightly higher one. In either case, the intended movement is used as a preconfiguration pattern to control the movement.

The motor system controls relative displacements by determining for each intended movement a **configuration adjustment pattern** for moving each desired body part. The particular configuration adjustment depends, of course, on the initial configuration of the body. For example, the required configuration adjustment for moving the hand as shown in Figure 14.9 depends on how the elbow is being held. Configuration adjustment patterns are therefore determined knowing both the intended movement and the starting configuration. When both an intended movement and starting configuration are presented to the motor system, a particular configuration adjustment pattern is determined, and if that pattern is used to adjust the pattern in the configuration buffer, the result will be the orchestration of the intended movement.

Movement stores are permanent memory stores for holding configuration adjustment patterns and their associated intended movement patterns. Movement stores are similar to configuration stores in three ways: They have a similar functional architecture; they process premotor patterns which have sensory origins; and they send their recalled patterns to the configuration buffer to be orchestrated. Movement stores differ from configuration stores in two ways: The premotor patterns have different sensory origins; and the configuration adjustments modify the pattern in the configuration store whereas configuration patterns replace them.

Configuration patterns and configuration adjustment patterns are conceptually different. Configuration patterns are motor patterns; hence they can be sent directly over the efferent pathways to control a configuration. Configuration adjustment patterns are not motor patterns; they are never transmitted over the efferent pathways. Configuration adjustment patterns are control patterns which regulate the activity of the configuration buffer.

The outcome of changing the current configuration pattern and adjusting it are similar: Both processes will initiate a movement. Moreover, if the current configuration and configuration adjustment are known, then the new configuration can be determined, and in the other direction, if the old and new configuration patterns are known, the configuration adjustment can be determined. Thus there are two major differences between configuration patterns and configuration adjustment patterns: (1) the sources of the sensory patterns, which

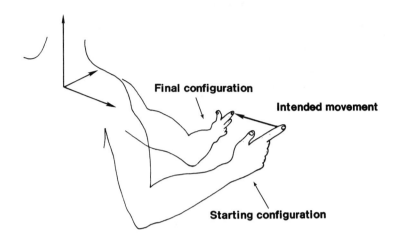

Final configuration

Intended movement

Starting configuration

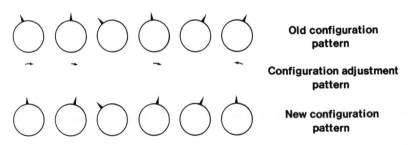

Old configuration
pattern

Configuration adjustment
pattern

New configuration
pattern

Figure 14.9. An arm movement and the configuration adjustment
required to change from the old configuration to the new one.

are used for acquiring them, and (2) how the configuration buffer processes
them.

Just like configuration patterns, configuration adjustment patterns have
sensory representations. This was illustrated earlier by the supraspinal control
loop which was used for holding a configuration in the presence of changing
external forces. The signals generated by the primary afferents were used to
adjust the pattern in the configuration buffer; hence they comprise a configuration adjustment pattern.

Preconfiguration patterns and intended movements generally have different
sensory origins. Preconfiguration patterns tend to be based on absolute sensory
measurements: the position, orientation, and size of an object. (Position is
measured with respect to the current orientation of the body.) Intended

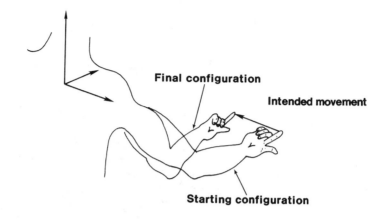

Final configuration

Intended movement

Starting configuration

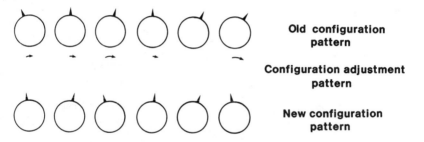

Old configuration
pattern

Configuration adjustment
pattern

New configuration
pattern

Figure 14.10. An arm movement going through the same spatial change as shown in Figure 14.9 only the arm is in different initial and final configurations. As a consequence, slightly different configuration adjustment patterns must be used.

movement patterns tend to be based on relative measurements: a displacement or a rotation.

These ideas are illustrated in Figures 14.9 and 14.10. Figure 14.9 showed the configuration adjustment needed for changing the configuration pattern for holding an arm in an initial and final configuration. Figure 14.10 illustrates the same arm and the same intended movement, only now the arm begins in a different initial configuration and ends in a different final configuration. As the figure shows, a different configuration adjustment is required. Figure 14.11 shows the relationships between configuration stores, movement stores, and the configuration buffer, and it illustrates that different types of spatial information are used for selecting patterns from within the configuration and motor stores.

Coordinate Systems and Coordinate Specification

Intended actions, such as grabbing a block or walking across a room, are initially represented with respect to the external world. The body profile system describes the current configuration of the body within the world, and the spatial system maintains the world model. Using these representations, the high-level control systems formulate the intended actions.

Intended actions are converted into intended movements prior to their orchestration. Suppose that the intended action is to grab a block which is within arm's reach. The visual and spatial systems together determine the intended movement of the hand to reach the block. The intended movement does not depend on the arm configuration; it only depends on the initial and final positions of the hand. The intended movement can therefore be represented as a vector in body-centered coordinates.

In order to move the hand to the block, a specific pattern of joint displacements must be initiated. However, there is generally not a unique pattern of joint displacements that will accomplish the intended hand movement. For example, the hand movement might be accomplished by a combination of the shoulder and elbow bends, or it might be accomplished by a combination of elbow and wrist bends. Moreover, the specific combination of bends will depend on the configuration of the body as a whole. The problem, then, is to convert the intended movement of the hand, given in body coordinates, to particular bends at each joint that will accomplish it.

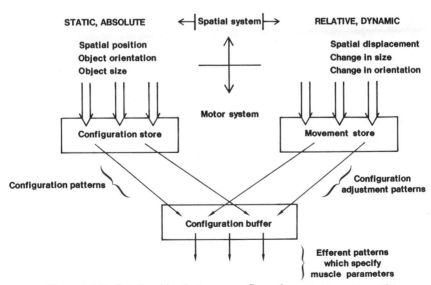

Figure 14.11. Relationships between configuration stores, movement stores and the configuration buffer.

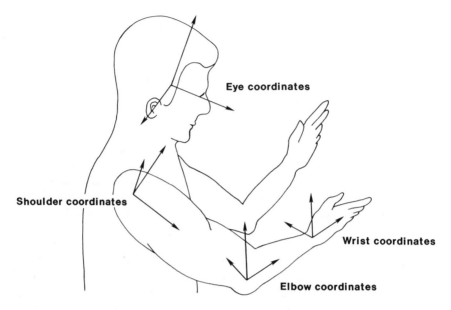

Eye coordinates

Shoulder coordinates

Wrist coordinates

Elbow coordinates

Figure 14.12. Various internal coordinate systems. Eye coordinates are body-centered. An intended movement, specified in eye-coordinates, also has representations in shoulder, elbow, and wrist coordinates. These representations indicate how the movement could be accomplished if it were to be performed with that joint alone.

There are many ways that intended movements specified in body-centered coordinates can be converted into particular intended joint displacements. One way, which will be described here, is to let the body profile system perform the transformations.

Consider the situation, illustrated in Figure 14.12, where each joint has its own coordinate system. The intended movement of the hand, specified in body-centered or eye coordinates also has a representation in each set of **joint coordinates**. When an intended movement is specified in joint coordinates, that specification indicates exactly what movement that joint alone must perform to accomplish the intended movement. For example, a movement specified in elbow coordinates is as if the upper arm and body are rigid in space and the eyes are located at the elbow.

Each representation in joint coordinates can easily be computed using the same strategy used by the profile buffer for updating surface patch vectors. The intended movement, specified in body-centered coordinates, is presented to a computational network which transforms it into shoulder coordinates. That transformation is passed along to a second computational network, which transforms it into elbow coordinates. The next network transforms that representation into wrist coordinates, and so forth. Although these transforma-

392

tions depend on the current configuration of the body, all relevant information (the angle of each joint and the position of the hand) is maintained by the profile buffer. Thus the transformations can be performed in real time and the intended movement, in joint coordinates of each joint, is available for determining specific displacements of each joint.

After the intended movement is transformed into joint coordinates for each joint, those representations are sent to their corresponding control groups in a motor store to locate motor patterns to orchestrate the movement. Thus the motor store determines for each joint whether it alone can perform the intended hand movement. The configuration of the body has already been taken into account. If, for a given intended movement, several different memory locations hold associated motor patterns, then orchestration of any one of them will accomplish the desired movement. In many cases, the intended movement can be accomplished by performing part of the movement with each limb. We do not know how the control system would divide the effort, however.

The situation is more complicated when none of the memory locations hold associated patterns but the movement can be accomplished by a combination of movements of several joints. For example, moving one's hand directly away from the body perpendicular to the chest can be accomplished only by an extension of the elbow together with a upper arm movement. One possible solution to this problem is to decompose the desired movement into parts, for example, its horizontal and vertical components, and then find movements of different limbs that will accomplish each of the component parts. We do not yet know how complex movements are orchestrated in general but some suggestions for particular types of movements will be made in the next chapter.

The High-Level Control of Simple Movements

The mental activity required for intentionally adjusting a configuration is far more complex than for holding one. Consider this example. Assume that a subject is attempting to hold his or her left arm in a horizontal position, and further suppose that it is not quite horizontal. The subject must first determine whether the arm needs to be raised or lowered and by how much. This knowledge is based on visual information (if the subject is looking at his or her own arm) or verbal information (if an observer says to raise or lower the arm). Suppose that the subject's arm needs to be raised by two inches and he or she knows that it needs to be raised. In either case, knowing that the arm needs to be raised by two inches means: (1) having a preconfiguration pattern which indicates an upward displacement; (2) having a parameter which specifies a movement magnitude of two inches; and (3) having attention focused on the arm. (The arm is a parameter to the movement.) Now suppose that the subject has already decided to raise the arm. The result of the decision is a high-level **intention** to adjust the configuration. The intention has three parameters: arm, upward, and two inches. In order to carry out the intention, only those local circuits in the configuration buffer which regulate the muscles which hold the arm up must have their values modified. Based only on the intention and its parameters, the configuration control system must select and adjust the correct circuitry in the configuration buffer by the correct amount.

The process of selecting arm circuits constitutes focusing the attention on the arm, and the process of increasing the existing values constitutes raising the arm. The intention is a high-level control pattern which controls the circuitry of the motor system. Carrying out the intention initiates at least the following processes: (1) Routing the upward movement preconfiguration pattern to the movement store which holds adjustment patterns for arm movements; the movement store will automatically analyze[6] the premotor pattern. (2) Routing the "two inches" parameter to the control system which regulates movement magnitudes. (3) Recalling the configuration adjustment patterns from the activated storage locations in the movement store. (4) Transmitting it to the configuration buffer. (5) Updating the pattern that is currently held in the configuration buffer; the result is an upward movement of the arm.

Notice that if while raising the arm the tension is increased by too much, the arm will overshoot the target position and the process will have to be repeated. Moreover, the change in tension depends on how far the arm must be moved and also how much weight is being held. If the motor pattern to the arm muscle specifies the desired change in muscle length, then the actual movements can be regulated effectively by the local circuits of the spinal cord which control the target muscle. This seems like one way the muscle circuits can be controlled.

The spatial system is instrumental in determining preconfiguration patterns for controlling movements. Once again, consider the process of raising an arm. By focusing attention on the arm, the spatial locations of the muscles of interest are made available by the spatial system. Those spatial coordinates can be used by the profile system to address the selected part of the arm. Once selected, the signals originating in the profile buffer can be routed to the configuration buffer just as if they had been generated by the primary afferents of the muscles themselves. The same circuitry that was described earlier for holding a configuration can therefore be used for adjusting a configuration.

Ballistic Movements

The ballistic system subserves the configuration system during most configurational adjustments. Consider the act of reaching for an object. The arm is first positioned by a ballistic movement, which places it in the vicinity of the object. Once the hand is close to the object, the final movement is performed slowly,

---

[6]Analysis of an input pattern by an associative storage system results in the activation of storage locations containing associated information. Refer to Chapters 3 and 4. Once a storage location is activated, its stored information is made available for recall.

with visual feedback. After the ballistic movement, the visual system analyzes the position of the hand relative to the object, informs the motor system of any disparity, and then the motor system adjusts the configuration (as previously described) to correct for any error. The initial ballistic movement gets the hand into the "ballpark" of the object while the final approach, a configurational adjustment, progresses with visual feedback.

The configuration patterns described earlier, and all of the machinery involved with their application, are concerned primarily with holding the body in a particular configuration, and even though a movement can be achieved by changing the pattern in the configuration buffer, the configuration system is concerned mainly with the **static** aspects of movements. In contrast, the ballistic system is concerned with the **dynamic** aspects of movements.

In theory, a movement could be initiated by activating the alpha motor neurons of the muscles of interest. However, as we have seen, this would cause a stretching of the intrafusal muscle fibers of the agonists and immediately activate the stretch reflex in opposition to the desired movement. In order to initiate a movement unopposed by the stretch reflex, the stretch reflex circuitry must be commanded not to oppose the desired movement. The stretch reflex must not be deactivated since it plays a crucial role in holding the current configuration. Instead, the equilibrium point of the stretch reflex must be adjusted to follow the trajectory of the intended movement. Any deviation from the intended movement would then be opposed (if the movement were progressing too quickly) or aided (if the movement were progressing too slowly) by the stretch reflex, but in the absence of a deviation, the movement would progress uninfluenced by the stretch reflex.

When either a new configuration pattern or a configuration adjustment pattern is used to initiate a movement, the goal is to bring the body into equilibrium at the adjusted position. If a second goal is to minimize the movement time, then it follows that the motor system should directly activate the alpha motor neurons and bring the mass of the muscle into activity. Since the change in the desired configuration is known (if a configuration adjustment is specified) or can be computed (if a new configuration is specified), the motor system can determine the required forces to accelerate the limb toward the desired new configuration and decelerate it as it approaches. These patterns are **thrust patterns**, time-varying patterns that regulate the dynamics of a movement. Clearly the application of a thrust pattern must be coordinated with a change in the configuration pattern so the stretch reflex will not impede the movement. Figure 14.13 illustrates some of the circuitry required for ballistic muscle control.

Trajectory Control

Complex movements can be controlled using sequences of configuration patterns to define the trajectory. Consider the process of grabbing an object. I

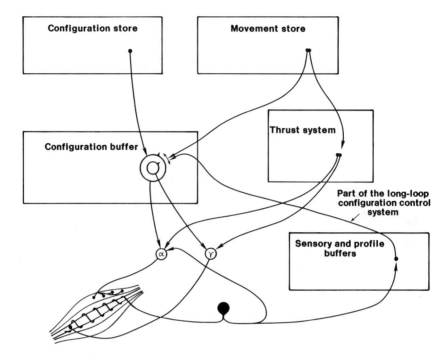

Figure 14.13. Some circuitry for thrust control. Any configuration adjustment must (a) coactivate alpha and beta motor neurons to initiate a thrust, and (b) modify the configuration pattern to hold the body in the new configuration. Changes to the configuration pattern must occur at the same rate that the muscles can respond to the current dynamic situation.

already explained how, by using various spatial representations, the appropriate configuration pattern can be located for holding the arm in the final position for grabbing the object. If, instead of focusing one's attention directly on the object to be grabbed, the focus shifts along a pathway toward the object, then a sequence of intended movements is made available to the motor system.[7] As a consequence, a sequence of configuration adjustment patterns can be located in configuration memory. If the configuration adjustment patterns in that sequence are recalled and applied, one after another, then the **trajectory** of the movement will be prescribed.

---

[7]This does not mean that the eyes must fixate at each point along the intended movement trajectory; only the internal focus of attention must shift. As a consequence of this process, obstructions along the intended trajectory will be detected, and a trajectory can planned which will avoid them.

396

The ballistic system takes a sequence of configuration adjustment patterns and computes an optimum thrust pattern for moving the body through each configuration specified by the sequence. Four parameters to the ballistic system are: (1) the initial configuration of the body, (2) the pattern of initial velocities of the body components at the onset of the movement, (3) the speed of the movement, and (4) the pattern of velocities of the body components at the end of the movement.

The intended speed of a movement is used to adjust the responsiveness of the muscle to movements and the thrusts required to animate the movements. Thus intended speed regulates several dynamic parameters. In addition, the intended speed regulates the rate of change of the premotor patterns for locating motor patterns for the movements. Hence intended speed is determined by a supervisory system. How the ballistic system computes the thrust pattern is an open question.

As a general rule, when adjusting a configuration, the ballistic system is subservient to the configuration system. When the configuration is to be adjusted, the intended movement is first determined. If the displacement is sufficiently small, there may be no ballistic component to the movement, but when the displacement is sufficiently large, the ballistic system automatically generates the required thrust pattern to orchestrate the movement. Thus, all movements have ballistic components.

There is conceptually no difference between configuration patterns and thrust patterns, as they both control muscle tensions. This does not mean, however, that they are equivalent: The efferent systems that orchestrate them have different static and dynamic behaviors and innervate different types of muscle fibers. The configuration system may never be able to initiate a ballistic movement whereas attempting to hold a configuration by the application of an unchanging thrust pattern may result in rapid muscle fatigue, tremor, or the like.

In order to illustrate these ideas, Figure 14.14 shows a mechanical arm with both configuration and thrust systems. The configuration is adjusted to hold the arm at its present position. The problem is to move the arm quickly to the new position illustrated in Figure 14.14b. The arm should not overshoot its target; hence it should arrive there with zero velocity.

The movement will be accomplished by applying the thrust pattern illustrated at the bottom of Figure 14.15 to the system while at the same time adjusting the configuration pattern to hold the arm in its new position. The illustrated thrust pattern initiates a ballistic movement. The flexors are momentarily innervated to their maximum tension while their antagonist extensors are relaxed. This impulsive force accelerates the arm. Just before the arm reaches its desired new position, the extensors are innervated and the flexors relaxed. This brings the movement to a halt at the desired new position, and the new configuration pattern holds it there. Notice that during the movement, the configuration pattern is continually being applied and it is continually changing. The thrust

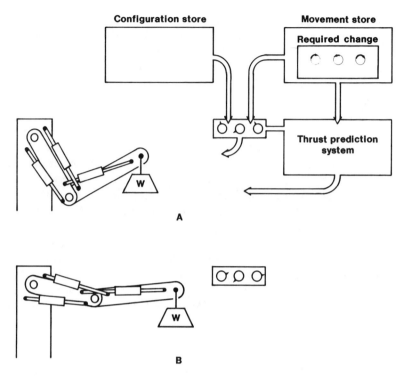

Figure 14.14. An arm control system. a. Initial configuration. b. Final configuration.

pattern, which propels the arm, was generated with prior knowledge of all forces required to move it through the intended trajectory. Had this not been the case, the additional forces resulting from the reflex circuitry would have caused the arm to overshoot or stop short of its target.

The difference between the ballistic system and the configuration system was illustrated by Kohout (1981), who described how a brain-damaged patient reacted when asked to perform certain tasks. When the patient was asked to reach as high as possible, he was able to reach just above his waist. When asked to touch a spot which was 10–12 centimeters above the highest position he just reached, he was able to touch the spot. However, he was unable to reach a point which was 10 centimeters above the spot. When asked to remove an object which was hanging from a hook as high as the point he could not reach, he was able to take the object down. When performing the first task, the patient appears to have initiated a configurational movement. He appears to have focused his attention on his arm and performed the movement under conscious control by adjusting the configuration pattern to move the arm. For the second task, he appears to have initiated both ballistic and slow movements. Touching the spot was apparently accomplished with a ballistic movement while attempting to reach above that spot was attempted with a configurational movement. Finally, he appears to have grabbed the object with a ballistic movement.

Hand-Eye Coordination

As a general rule, intended movements are automatically converted into movements. This means that the configuration adjustment required for the movement is available in the movement store. When the associations between intended movements and configuration adjustments are inappropriate, new associations must be learned. This section gives a brief indication of what takes place.

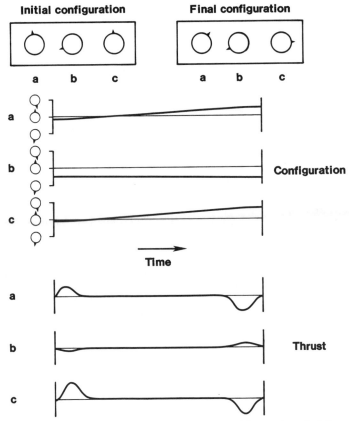

Figure 14.15. A changing configuration pattern (the upper set of three curves) and the corresponding thrust pattern (the lower set of three curves) to achieve the change. The thrust pattern needed to move an arm through a given trajectory depends on the weight of the arm and its load.

Learning to associate intended movements with configuration adjustment patterns is easy for most individuals, and you might like to try the following experiment. Draw a random figure on a piece of paper and then trace over it with the hand you use for writing. Although you will not be able to trace exactly over your initial figure, you will be able to trace over it with reasonable accuracy. Your eyes will follow along the intended path and extract the necessary intended movements to locate the required configuration adjustment patterns for the movements. You will use the resulting patterns to move your arm and hand. Now place a mirror in front of you and try to trace over your original drawing while watching your hand only in the mirror. The mirror systematically modifies the displacement vectors for the intended movements, and as a result, the visual system computes incorrect intended movement patterns. The motor system, using incorrect intended movements, accesses incorrect configuration adjustment patterns, and the arm obligingly moves in the wrong direction.

With practice, you can learn how to perform this task. While you are practicing, your motor system associates new configuration adjustment patterns with the relative displacement patterns determined by your visual system, and these new configuration adjustment patterns are made available when looking through a mirror and performing the given task. The mental process of paying attention to the motor act comprises routing the sensory and motor signals to the movement store, and initiating storage in unused storage locations of motor groups of the muscles of involvement. The configuration adjustment patterns come from the muscle spindles or other sensory apparatus of the arm and hence are immediately available to the motor system for storage, and the motor patterns are initiated by trial and error or other unknown control process and stored provided there is a successful outcome to the movement. More will be said about this in the next chapter. It is precisely the availability of both sensory and motor representations at the same time that learning of hand-eye coordination[8] is possible. (To convince yourself you have learned a new coordination skill, you might like to try the same task with a different random curve and compare your performance with your original attempt on your first random curve.)

SUMMARY

Both configuration and thrust are regulated by the sensory-motor system. Configuration is staged in the configuration buffer, which holds the patterns that dictate the instantaneous shape and rigidity of the body components.

---

[8]In Chapter 6 I described a patient who, after bilateral damage to the hippocampus and hippocampal gyrus, was unable to remember anything of his experiences since the damage occurred. That same patient was able to learn to perform a similar task to the one just described, and his improvement followed a normal learning curve. Even though the patient was unable to remember performing the task from day to day, his performance continually improved! (Milner, 1965.)

Changing or replacing the configuration pattern initiates a configurational movement, which is orchestrated by the gamma motor neurons and stretch reflex circuitry. Whenever a movement of sufficient magnitude is initiated, the ballistic system intervenes and initiates vigorous contractions which thrust the body components along the intended trajectory. This is a ballistic movement and involves coactivation of both alpha and gamma motor neurons. Thus both static and dynamic aspects of a movement are controlled.

Motor stores are functionally organized into control units which regulate the various parts of the body. This organization enables premotor patterns which have a small number of components to access motor patterns which have a large number of components. The result is that during the orchestration of a movement, there is a divergence of information from a small, high-level intention to a large, low-level motor pattern which controls individual muscles.

REFERENCES

Kohout, L. J. (1981). Control of movement and protection structures. *International Journal of Man-Machine Studies, 14*, 397-422.

Milner, B. (1965). Memory disturbance after bilateral hippocampal lesions. In P. M. Milner, & S. E. Glickman, (Eds.). *Cognitive processes and the brain.* New York: D. Van Nostrand.

Polit, A., & Bizzi, E. (1979). Characteristics of motor programs underlying arm movements in monkeys. *Journal of Neuropsychology, 42,*183-194.

Thompson, R. F. (1967). *Foundations of physiological psychology.* New York: Harper & Row.

SUGGESTED READINGS

Asanuma, H. (1972). Cerebral cortical control of movement. *The Physiologist, 16*, 143-166.

Bernstein, N. A. (1967). *The coordination and regulation of movements.* London: Pergamon Press.

Brand, M. (1984). *Intending and acting: Toward a naturalized action theory.* Cambridge, MA: Bradford Books.

Desmedt, J. E. (Ed.). (1978). *Progress in clinical neurophysiology, Vol. 4. Cerebral motor control in man: Long loop mechanisms.* New York: Karger.

Evarts, E. V., et al. (1979). Central Control of Movement. *Neurosciences Research Program Bulletin,* 9, No. 1.

Eyzaguirre, C., & Fidone, S. J. (1975). *Physiology of the nervous system. An introductory text (2d ed.).* Chicago, IL: Year Book Medical Publishers.

Gallistel, C. R. (1980). *The Organization of action: A new synthesis.* Hillsdale, NJ: Lawrence Erlbaum Associates.

Granit, R. (1970). *The basis of motor control.* New York: Academic Press.

Kelso, J. A. S. (Ed.). (1982). *Human motor behavior, An introduction.* Hillsdale, NJ: Lawrence Erlbaum Associates.

Prinz, W., & Sanders, A. F. (1984). *Cognition and motor processes.* New York: Springer-Verlag.

Schmidt, R. A. (1982). *Motor control and learning.* Champaign, IL: Human Kinetics.

15

THE HIGH-LEVEL CONTROL OF MOVEMENTS

INTRODUCTION

Many complex movements can be initiated and executed without paying attention to them, a fact which implies that detailed planning of movements is not always necessary. Instead, the sensory-motor system can execute complex movements by recalling and orchestrating stored sequences of premotor or motor patterns directly. This chapter describes the structure and organization of the storage systems which underlie the automatic control of movements.

In order to focus on particular aspects of skilled movements, the following activities will be considered: typing, handwriting, speech, and walking. Each activity demonstrates a different type of motor control and a different type of interaction with the environment. The principles that emerge convey a fairly comprehensive picture of the control structures involved.

PERCEPTIONS, DECISIONS, AND INTENTIONS

A great deal of mental activity consists of an unending repetition of the following four processes: (1) understanding what is to be done, (2) deciding how to respond and determining the expected outcome, (3) responding, and (4) comparing actual outcome with expected outcome. The following sections analyze understanding, decision making, and response production by describing the perceptual and control processes which take place when a person responds to a verbal command.

UNDERSTANDING

Consider the oral command "pick up the cup of coffee." The command must be understood both for content and for purpose. The auditory apparatus converts the sound patterns into primary auditory patterns which are analyzed by various

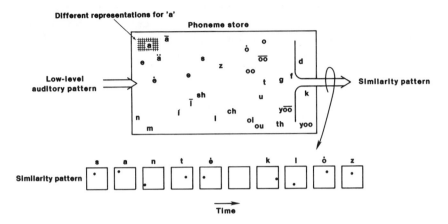

Figure 15.1. Top. The phoneme store showing a possible organization of phonemes. In the upper-left I have shown several memory locations to indicate that there may be many representations for the same sound. Bottom. The resulting similarity pattern for the word "Santa Claus." The intonation pattern, not encoded by the phoneme store, is analyzed by a different network which operates concurrently.

auditory stores. For content analysis, an auditory store which recognizes phonemes (or perhaps syllables) transforms the primary auditory pattern into an intermediate representation in which the presence of each phoneme is indicated by recognition signals from a set of memory locations and hence spatial positions in the store, as Figure 15.1 shows. The resulting similarity pattern is automatically sent to the naming store for further analysis.

The naming store analyzes the similarity pattern generated by the phoneme store and activates storage locations holding specific words and phrases such as "pick up," "cup," and "of coffee." Patterns in the activated storage locations are parameters to the mental procedures which are subsequently executed. While storage locations in the naming store are being activated, the similarity pattern being generated by the naming store is sent to the concept store for analysis.

The concept store analyzes the similarity pattern generated by the naming store and activates storage locations which hold various high-level mental procedures for responding to the utterance. The activated storage locations therefore encode possible meanings for the utterance. Recall and execution of a mental procedure from one of the activated storage locations initiates a response based on the assumed meaning.

Analysis of the contents of an utterance and analysis of its purpose occur concurrently. For determining purpose, intonation is analyzed. Intonation indicates whether the statement is rhetorical, a question, or a demand, and if a demand, how insistent the demanding person is on having the order obeyed.

403

(Will I be in danger if I don't do what he tells me?) The result of intonational analysis is the activation of storage locations which contain mental procedures for general high-level actions such as answering a question, obeying an order, or simply not responding at all. Hence the intonational content of an utterance plays a significant role in determining a response.

As a general rule, mental procedures are available which are not explicitly activated by perceptual analysis. For example, an individual may choose not to pick up the cup at all—he or she may simply be in an ornery mood. How an individual responds in a given situation is based on numerous factors, both obvious and hidden, and many responses do not depend on the current situation.

The storage networks of the brain are not as clearly defined as the above discussion suggests. Each storage network has physical limitations which organize stored information according to: (1) how long it lasts, (2) how quickly it varies over time, and (3) its spatial size. Phonemes, words, sentences, ideas, and themes all last for significantly different lengths of time; they all vary at vastly different rates, and as a consequence, no single storage system can process them all. To overcome this difficulty, a hierarchy of storage systems has evolved with each storage system in the hierarchy responsible for information which has different temporal and spatial characteristics. By integrating information over time, each storage system processes one type of pattern and generates a new representation whose physical properties are better suited for the next storage system in the hierarchy. I have assumed for clarity of explanation that phonemes, words, and sentences are the analyzed units of stored information, not because a storage system is restricted to that function. The perceptual stores may be viewed as a single, spatially distributed storage system with different regions having different spatial and temporal charac-teristics. As a consequence of each region's physical characteristics, information having matching characteristics is stored there, and it follows that regions tend to hold information of a particular syntactic type (phoneme, word, etc.)

The same is true for the control hierarchy. There is not a single decision and control system for all actions, but rather, a continuum of decision and control systems. Since we do not know their exact organization, I will assume the existence of particular types of networks having particular spatial and temporal properties. Such a description is only approximate and should be understood as such.

DECISION MAKING, INTENTIONS, AND PLANS

Deciding how to respond means choosing which mental procedure to activate. This may mean combining parts of different mental procedures and it may mean generating a new mental procedure.[1] For this discussion, I will assume that mental procedures are available for all acts under consideration. Moreover, I will assume that as a result of perceptual analysis, all storage locations whose response procedures are appropriate to the situation have been activated. Hence, **deciding** how to respond means choosing one of the activated storage locations, and **responding** means recalling and orchestrating the selected mental procedure.

The highest level of control must decide which procedure to activate. In order to make the decision, the individual must have some desires and some expectation as to the outcome of executing the selected procedure. The expectation may be a consequence of recalling an experience which followed a prior execution of the same mental procedure or it may be determined by predicting the outcome (such as predicting the future body image when given an adjustment to the current configuration). It may also be based on expected affect state as the following chapter suggests.

The **purposive system**, the highest level control system, decides which mental procedure to activate.[2] Once the decision is made, the individual has an **intention** for his or her actions. The intention includes the expected outcome of its performance. Recalling and executing the selected mental procedure constitutes **carrying out the intention**. (A person may intend to pick up the cup of coffee long before he or she actually picks it up!) The distinction between having an intention and carrying out an intention reflects both the structure of human storage systems and the distinction between static and dynamic patterns. An intention is a static representation. Once an intention is recalled, the resulting dynamic pattern of neural activity may be analyzed by other storage systems and hence cause other storage locations to be activated, or it may initiate and control various movements. Thus intentions are patterns which have associated expected outcomes and which control both mental and physical activity in an attempt to realize those outcomes. Carrying out an intention takes place when the static patterns are converted, during recall, into dynamic patterns which cause (effect) their own realization.

For the present, we simply do not know enough about how mental procedures are structured and encoded to know how their outcomes might be predicted. Thus we simply do not know how decisions are made, from the highest level, where the individual decides on a general course of action (to respond or not to respond) all the way down to the lowest levels, where the individual decides on

---

[1]This leads to a very natural question: What kinds of mental procedures combine and generate other mental procedures? At the present time, nobody knows. The highest levels of mental control are not yet understood, and there are currently no models for the processes which create and combine mental procedures.

[2]Various researchers have studied networks which (1) analyze patterns of signals and (2) select among them by competitive and cooperative processes. Consult, for example, Metzler (1977) or Amari and Arbib (1982).

a particular movement (which hand to use and what trajectory to follow). I will therefore assume that decisions are made wherever necessary and trace the course of events which follows each decision.

Plans

A mental procedure consists of the high-level specification of a sequence of actions (both mental and physical) which are to be carried out together with the expected outcomes of executing them. **Planning** is the specification of the details for each action in the sequence. For example, if the intention is to pick up a cup of coffee, high-level specifications include locating the cup of coffee to be picked up, moving toward it, reaching for it, grabbing it, holding it, and finally lifting it, while the expected outcome is holding the cup of coffee. At a lower level of control, the specifications for grabbing and lifting include the approach trajectory for the hand, the choice of grip, the forces to be applied, and the speed of the movement, and the expected outcomes are the visual and tactile consequences of each action. Specifications at this level for picking up a cup of coffee are based on the following sorts of considerations:

- Does the cup have a handle?
- If so, should the handle be used?
- If not, can the cup be grabbed directly? (If the cup is hot and does not have a handle, will grabbing it result in a burn?)
- Can the cup be grabbed in the usual way? (A cup made of styrofoam may collapse if grabbed as if it were a glass.)
- What surfaces will be grabbed, where are they located, and what are their orientations?
- How heavy is the cup, and hence how much force will be needed to pick it up?
- Are there any obstacles to be avoided?
- Once the cup is grabbed, might its contents spill if it is picked up quickly.

Experience plays a central role in planning a movement. For frequently performed actions, particularly skilled actions, there may be stored representations of previous similar intentions whose outcomes are known. As a consequence, prior plans can be used as specifications for current actions and prior outcomes become expected outcomes for the current plans. For intentions which are sufficiently complex, the verbal system plays a fundamental part in formulating the intended actions and expected outcomes. (See Vygotsky, 1978.) Depending on the activity, planning simple movements is often straightforward and will be discussed separately for each type of activity considered. Little is known at present as to how we plan complex actions, and this topic will not be discussed further.[3]

Once an action is planned, the sensory-motor system must orchestrate the plan. The plan itself is expressed as a premotor pattern for the intended action, and orchestrating the plan means: (1) converting the premotor pattern into a motor pattern for the action, and (2) transmitting the resulting motor pattern to the spinal circuits and muscles to animate the movement. The methods of orchestration will be a major focus in the remainder of this chapter.

Comparing Actual Outcomes with Expected Outcomes

The expected outcomes of an action at each level of control are automatically compared with the actual outcomes and the results made available to the system in charge of the action. The results may be used to terminate the current plan or simply to select among alternative actions within the definition of the plan. While typing, one high-level expected outcome is the production of a typed paper. If an incorrect letter is typed, the purposive system may initiate action to correct the mistake. At a lower level of control, the expected outcomes are the tactile sensation of squarely striking the key and the auditory sound of the key striking the platen. If these expected outcomes are not realized, typing may be interrupted and a low-level corrective procedure initiated. While walking, a certain feel of the pavement is expected. If an unexpected response is sensed, such as stepping off an unnoticed curb or stepping on a stone, the gait may be corrected to account for the changing pavement conditions. In this case the sensory outcome is used to select among alternate programs for walking and the individual may not even be aware of the change in gait. In either case, actual outcomes are compared with expected outcomes and the results are used to select among alternative future actions.

TIME AND THE CONTROL HIERARCHY

An action is rarely, if ever, fully planned before it is initiated. With reference to the previous example, a person may look for the cup of coffee before deciding whether or not to pick it up and he or she may start to reach for it before deciding how to pick it up. This section analyzes the relationship between time and the control of movement and shows that it is essentially the opposite of the relationship between time and perception. Speech understanding will serve as the example.

---

[3]Planning is an active area of investigation in artificial intelligence and I might suggest Nilsson (1980) or Rich (1983) as an introduction to that literature. For the cognitive science approach, consult Schank and Abelson (1977).

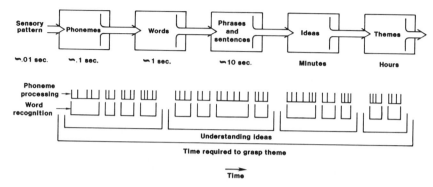

Figure 15.2. Each memory store in the sensory hierarchy recodes the incoming representation into a representation which varies more slowly in time. At the lowest levels we call understanding "recognition." We recognize phonemes and words provided we pay attention to them. At the highest levels we call understanding "generalization." Each store makes specific types of information available, is organized differently, and is controlled by a different level of control in the control hierarchy. The lower part of the figure indicates the relationship between time and recognition in the sensory hierarchy.

Each stage of speech understanding integrates information which lasts for a longer interval of time. Phonemes change most rapidly and last for the shortest length of time. Words generally last longer than phonemes, and sentences generally last longer than words. Through successive transformations, a sequence of rapidly varying, short, auditory patterns (the neural representations of the sounds) are transformed into a single, slowly varying, long-lasting sentence pattern. Note that each translation process depends on all stored patterns and hence on the individual's entire history of experiences! One high-level outcome is the activation of a set of storage locations in the concept store. Since the pattern of activated storage locations only changes when a sentence is recognized, it is the most slowly varying pattern so far in the sequence. Figure 15.2 illustrates the relationship between time and understanding.

An intention, such as "looking for the cup of coffee" or "picking it up," is a unit of mental activity which is constant over a long period of time—the time needed to carry it out. Carrying out an intention[4] means activating and recalling a mental procedure. This initiates a sequence of mental processes—attending the visual scene, locating the cup of coffee, deciding how to grab it, and then reaching for it and grabbing it. Each of these processes is shorter than the

---

[4]A person may intend to become rich and famous and spend years attempting to do so. My use of the term "intention" is restricted to short-term intentions. Schank and Abelson (1977) used the term "instrumental scripts" for similar types of activity.

controlling intention, and each varies more quickly than its controlling intention.

Each control pattern, beginning at the purposeful level, specifies the sequence of actions or mental processes which must be completed, and each action or mental process in the sequence takes less time to complete than its initiating control pattern. On the other hand, the control pattern that initiates an action or mental process at one level of control is generally smaller than the control pattern at the next lower level of control in the sequence. This divergence of information was discussed in the previous chapter. *The control patterns begin as small, slowly varying, long-lasting, high-level intentions and become rapidly varying, short, detailed, motor patterns as they are transformed by the storage systems along the pathways of control.* This, in essence, is the opposite of the sequence of perceptual processes which underlies understanding.

PROCEDURES AND SUBPROCEDURES

Each element of a mental procedure is a **subprocedure**. For example, "locate object X" is a subprocedure of the procedure "pick up object X." Each subprocedure is subservient to its initiating procedure. When the purposive system initiates a visual scan, the visual system, which is subservient to the purposive system, plans and carries out the scan. The purposive system may terminate the scan prematurely (for example, if it decides to do something else), in a normal way (if the sought-after object is found), or change the scan strategy (if the sought-after object is not immediately found). By executing a particular plan, the purposive system specifies the type of search and conditions for its normal termination.

Parameters to a procedure are available as a result of prior mental activity. When searching for a particular object in the visual field, the visual system uses information from storage locations which were activated earlier, and the recalled patterns are parameters for the search. When responding to "pick up the cup of coffee," storage locations activated by "cup," "coffee," and "cup of coffee" have visual representations which serve as test patterns for controlling the visual buffer, and they have control patterns which indicate where to look and how large an object to seek. These patterns are parameters to the search procedure,[5] and the expected outcome of a search is finding an object specified by a parameter. A search is satisfied when a high similarity signal is generated by the activated storage location which is holding the parameter to the search. The

---

[5]There are many different search procedures which differ in a variety of ways. A **directed search**, such as looking for a cup of coffee, uses parameters as I just described. An **undirected search**, where the gaze randomly selects objects to focus on, does not use parameters.

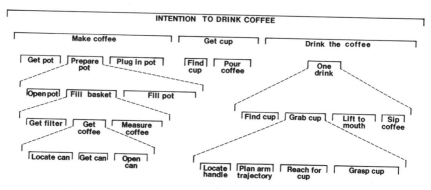

Figure 15.3. An intention to drink coffee may last for 30 minutes or more. The intention initiates a sequence of subintentions—getting the coffee, taking a sip from the cup, etc. Getting the coffee may entail finding the pot to make it in, preparing the pot, and then plugging it in. Preparing the pot reduces to a sequence of subprocesses, and so forth, until at the lowest levels, sequences of muscle contractions are initiated. Each subprocess is carried out by different mental and physical machinery and takes a different amount of time to perform. Subprocesses at different levels can be carried out concurrently.

purposive system, using information generated by the sensory and storage systems, decides when the sought-after object is located. The storage system compares the expected outcome with the actual outcome of the search, but the purposive system decides when the intended outcome has been realized.

Although visual scanning is a subprocedure of the initiating intention, the visual system, when carrying out the scan, initiates a number of its own subprocesses—transferring information between subsystems, controlling the focus of visual attention, directing the gaze, and so forth. Figure 15.3 illustrates the temporal relationships between a procedure and the subprocedures it initiates.

Well-learned procedures, which can be carried out automatically, are often executed concurrently. For example, when told to pick up a cup of coffee, and assuming the individual has decided to obey, he or she may look for the cup while at the same time move toward its expected location. If the cup is not seen, he or she must terminate the movement and decide on an alternate response. When looking for a lost letter amidst a pile of other papers, a variety of mental and physical processes must be carried out, including selecting a pile of papers to sift through, sifting through it while looking for the lost letter, and placing the inspected papers in a chosen location. Many of these actions occur simultaneously. In summary, a given procedure may have several subprocedures; some may execute in sequence while others may execute concurrently.

We currently do not know how decisions are made which initiate and terminate mental procedures. We do not know how intermediate results of a procedure are maintained, and therefore we do not know how, when a procedure is interrupted, it is able to restart (continue) where it left off. We do not know how a person knows when a desired object is located, and we therefore do not know how a search procedure is terminated. We do not know how the termination conditions are specified or interpreted or why a person gives up before finding a sought-after item. All of these high-level issues remain topics for future research.

THE DISTRIBUTION OF COMPUTATIONAL EFFORTS

The purposive system does not deal with detailed specifications of movement and it does not process low-level sensory representations. To do so would be computationally too demanding and inefficient.[6] When grabbing an object, the purposive system does not control individual arm muscles any more than it analyzes the position and surface orientations of the object being grabbed. Low-level systems do those things. The purposive system does not specify which storage locations to use when controlling a movement any more than it specifies which storage locations to use for storing current experiences. Once again, low-level systems do those things. In general, each perceptual and control system maintains autonomy over its own computational and storage systems and delivers only summary information (e.g. the result of a comparison) to the purposive system for processing.

The hierarchical organization of both the perceptual and control systems is a consequence of the computational requirements imposed on them. I have already explained how time enters into the hierarchy, and in the previous chapter I showed how, during the control of a movement, pattern size enters into the control hierarchy. The need to be able to store a large number of small perceptual patterns on the one hand, and to have small intentions regulate a large number of muscle fibers, on the other hand, has evolved into the hierarchical organization just described, where rapidly varying, highly detailed, large, perceptual patterns are transformed into slowly varying, small, highly encoded ideas during perception; and small, slowly varying, highly encoded intentions are transformed into large, rapidly varying, detailed motor patterns during performance.

The remainder of this chapter will focus on the control of movements. I will describe the organization of the motor stores and show how intentions are

---

[6]The purposive system can attend to low-level sensory and motor representations when they require high-level decisions. For example, an individual may focus attention on his or her pinkie and twitch it just a little bit. In general, however, the focus of attention is directed toward making high-level decisions; low-level decisions are automated by using prior stored patterns for their orchestration

converted into motor patterns which animate movements. I will no longer be concerned with the decision-making processes but will focus instead on the mechanisms of accessing stored motor patterns for controlling skilled movements. The analysis of current perceptual stimuli—tactile, kinesthetic, visual, and vestibular—plays a fundamental role in the control of movement, but the level of control, as you will see, is relatively low. The purposive system will have little to say about the details of individual movements.

MOTOR PROGRAMS FOR MOVEMENT CONTROL

A **motor program** is a time-varying pattern that animates and controls a movement trajectory. Motor patterns are very simple motor programs, and they have a functional role in motor control which corresponds to the role of phonemes during speech recognition.

Each motor program has a set of required **initial conditions** for its application, such as a specific body configuration, a specific intention, or a specific sensory signal. If an initial condition for a motor program is a configuration and the body has a different configuration than the required one, that particular motor program cannot be used since it cannot be activated. If it were used, the result of its application would be an unintended movement.

Each motor program has a set of **expected sensory outcomes** for its execution. If, during the execution of a motor program, the actual sensory outcome disagrees with the expected sensory outcome, a signal is generated which indicates the disagreement. The controlling system may then adjust the movement or terminate execution of the program.

Each motor program comprises both configurational and thrust subpatterns which regulate the static and dynamic components of the movement. The static component is the sequence of instantaneous configurations through which the body must pass, and its orchestration is effected by the gamma motor neurons as previously described. The static component is therefore a time-varying configuration pattern. The dynamic component is a time-varying thrust pattern which, assuming the configuration system cancels out static forces, specifies the additional tensions of the various muscles needed to propel the body through the desired trajectory. The configuration and thrust subpatterns are applied simultaneously during the orchestration of the movement.

A **premotor program**, the result of planning a movement, is a pattern that enables a complex motor program to be generated. When orchestrated, a premotor program is converted into a motor program for carrying out the intended action.

The only motor programs stored by the sensory-motor system are simple ones such as motor patterns; complex motor programs are created by uniting as many

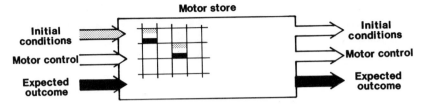

Motor store

Initial conditions

Motor control

Expected outcome

Initial conditions

Motor control

Expected outcome

Figure 15.4. Each motor store, including both configuration stores and movement stores, associates several modalities of information. For high-level motor stores, initial conditions are intentions. For low-level motor stores, initial conditions are sensory patterns (kinesthetic, vestibular, etc.). For high-level stores, expected outcomes are anticipated results. For low-level stores, expected outcomes are sensory patterns (tactile, kinesthetic, auditory, etc.).

simple motor programs as the situation requires.[7] In contrast, the sensory-motor system stores significantly more complex premotor programs whose resulting motor programs may last for many seconds (depending, of course, on the speed of orchestration). Each premotor program enables the generation of a corresponding motor program for a particular execution of the act.

A premotor program and its resulting motor program are often processed simultaneously. A premotor program specifies a complex sequence of movements which may take a long time to execute. The motor program which results when the first part of the premotor program is orchestrated can be executed while the remainder of the premotor pattern is being converted into a motor program. This is exactly analogous to the way subprocedures in a mental procedure execute concurrently with the mental procedure itself.

Premotor programs can be stored in premotor stores. Once a premotor program is stored, its orchestration consists of recalling and using it to generate a particular motor program for the action. One way a premotor program can be orchestrated is by using it to locate a sequence of motor patterns in motor memory. The motor patterns so located must have two properties: (1) each one must leave the body in the configuration required by the next one, and (2) the outcome of the sequence must be the intended action. Executing each motor pattern in sequence, then, results in the desired action. Hence the sequence of motor patterns obtained in this way is a motor program for the intended act.

Figure 15.4 illustrates the organization of a motor store. As the figure shows, each motor program has initial conditions and expected outcomes, and each

---

[7]For certain types of highly skilled movements, such as playing a Beethoven piano sonata from memory, the stored motor programs may be much longer than they would ordinarily be. Nonetheless, even for highly skilled movements, the sensory-motor system independently stores different parts of the complete program and applies them in sequence during the orchestration of the act.

storage location in the motor store holds all three types of patterns. When all initial conditions are realized, the storage location is activated and the associated stored motor program may be recalled and orchestrated. If, as a result of orchestrating the stored motor program, the expected result is realized, the storage location signals that fact. If the expected outcome for one motor pattern is also an initial condition for a second one, then the second one can be orchestrated provided the outcome of the first one is its expected outcome. It follows that with a suitable control system for motor memory, motor patterns can automatically be executed in sequence. Moreover, different sequences of motor programs can automatically be executed, depending on the outcomes of the actions they regulate.

Initial conditions and expected outcomes are concepts which apply to all levels of control. However, the representations differ at different levels of control and the length of time it takes to evaluate the expected outcomes differ. Nonetheless, the ideas are conceptually equivalent. Referring to the ongoing example, the statement "pick up the cup of coffee" is an initial condition for the activation of a procedure for picking up objects, and the expectation of holding the cup of coffee is the expected outcome of executing the procedure. If the expected outcome is not realized—for example, if the coffee spills—then failure of a match between the expected outcome and the actual outcome results in a signal which is used by the purposive system to execute a different mental procedure.

The following examples illustrate the principles that have been described so far in this chapter.

Typing

Typing was chosen as the first example of motor behavior because it has been studied in detail by other researchers (W.E. Cooper, 1983), it is a fairly simple process to understand, at least one mechanistic model of skilled typing has been proposed (Rumelhart & Norman, 1982), and many different perceptual and control processes are involved.

Typing, as with many skilled behaviors, requires the conversion of information from one high-level internal code, namely, the mental representation of a sequence of symbols, into a low-level motor code, a motor program which propels the fingers to strike the typewriter keys in the proper order. The processes which underlie the conversion will be the major focus of this section.

While typing, expert typists perform perceptual and motor processes at the same time and they process sequences of letters rather than single letters. They can type up to 200 words per minute, which, assuming on the average 5 letters per word, amounts to 1000 characters per minute or 17 characters per second or one character every 60 milliseconds. Since it takes much longer than 60 milliseconds to initiate and execute a motor command, it follows that skilled typists are generating the thrust pattern for one letter even before they strike the keys for the previous few letters. This illustrates the concurrency between the conversion of a premotor program into a motor program and the execution of the resulting motor program.

In order to give some insight into the mental processes which underlie skilled typing, I will first describe semiskilled typing. I will indicate the perceptual processes which take place while learning to type, and I will emphasize the interactions between perceptual and motor processes.

Semiskilled Typing

Not all typing is done by experts. I happen to be a semiskilled typist and on a good day I can type up to 60 words per minute. I use anywhere from 1 to 10 fingers, depending on circumstances, and I must frequently look at the keyboard or I will miss the keys. I often use different fingers to strike the same keys, and I only have to hunt for keys which I don't use very often (e.g., z, q, and j) or keys which have different positions on different computer terminal keyboards (e.g., ', ", +, :). In contrast, a beginning typist must locate each letter individually but quickly improves as his knowledge of the keyboard improves.

Learning Semiskilled Typing

In order to gain some insight into the perceptual and motor processes which underlie typing, imagine that you want to type a copy of the document presented in Figure 15.5 on the typewriter whose keyboard is also shown. I will assume that you already know the mechanics of the typewriter, that you have already placed a piece of paper in it, and that you have decided to begin typing. The following sequence of mental activities is typical:

1. You look at the text for the first symbol to be typed and attend to it. Both a permanent record of the symbol will be made in experiential memory and a temporary record will be made in spatial memory. If the text symbols are familiar, you may remember a sequence of them.[8] (Consider the text and keyboard shown in Figure 15.6.)
2. Next you scan the keyboard for the symbol or symbols just noted. The way that you scan the keyboard depends on how you encoded the

---

[8]If, for example, the text is in English, you may read and remember one or more words and use your verbal knowledge to extract from memory the proper sequence of letters to be typed. If you are familiar with the symbols—for example, they are letters of the alphabet, you may verbalize them and remember their names rather than their images. The central issue is that you will create an appropriate internal representation so that you can find the proper keys on the keyboard. Once the keys are located, the sensory-motor system takes charge of the typing process.

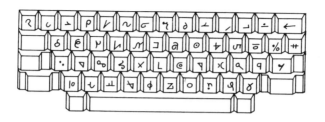

ſⴐ◖ ∴⊃Ϲ ∴ ⊥Ⳁⵘ⊥ⵊⴰⴈⴖ-Φⴈ∴ⴑⵗ ⴈⵗ Ƶ⊙ⵅⳐſ◖ ∴Ƶⵗ ⵜ∴⊃◖
ⴹⳐⴈⴈ ⵜⴈ◖ſⵗⵇƵⵀ ⴹⵗſⳐ ⵕⴰ◖Ƶ ⵜⴈⴖ ⴖⵕ◖ⴈ⊥ⴈ◖ ◖ⵅ∴⊃◖
ⴹ⊙ſⳐⴈⴖ ∴Ƶⵗ ſⳐ⊙ſⳐⴈⴖ ⵕⴈ◖ⴈ◖ ∴Ƶⵗ ⵕ∴ſⴈ◖ ∴Ƶⵗ ◖∴Ϲ∴⊃◖
∴Ƶⵗ ⴈƵⴈ Φⴹ ⴈƵⴈ Φ∴⊥ⴈ ⵕƵ ſⳐⴈ ⊥ⵅⴈⴈⴈⴈ Ϲ∴⊃◖

Figure 15.5. A typewriter keyboard and document to be typed.

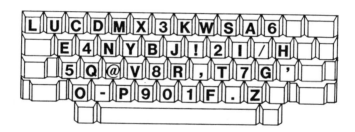

**51@ 2BQ 577 Q!PR 5 @N72P5BN 05751PN
BR5B BRN Q/IYB IV 21V212BJ 829NQ
N-/NPB5 B2I1Q 4N R59N P51 7N5@ @I41 BRN /5BR
4RNYN BR5B @N927 @2QPI!Y58NFN1B 729NQ**

Figure 15.6. A keyboard and document having familiar symbols.

symbols: visual code, verbal code, or whatever. Both scanning the text for the symbol to be typed and locating it on the keyboard are visual subprocesses and will not be further discussed here.

Once you have found the key, you must press it. The spatial location of the key is determined by your visual and spatial systems and made available to your sensory-motor system. Thus the requirements on your sensory-motor system are

416

3. to select a particular finger to use[9] and

4. to generate a motor program which, when executed, will move the selected finger at the correct speed to the spatial location of the key to be depressed. (The existence of the key is now irrelevant. The sensory-motor system can only move the finger to a specified location; if that location is correct, the correct symbol will be typed; if not, a typing error will result.)

    Depending on the location of the selected key relative to the current positions of your hands, you must

5. decide on which motor procedure to initiate. If the key is close to your finger, you might

6a. initiate a simple ballistic movement to strike it. If your finger is a significant distance from the key, you might

6b. initiate a ballistic movement to get your finger close to the selected key (the expected sensory outcome), then perhaps

6c. adjust your configuration using visual feedback, and finally

6d. initiate a ballistic movement to strike the key.

7. After the key is struck you must relax your fingers and withdraw your hands from the keyboard so that you can search for the next key.

Once you have generated a motor program to press the key (step 6a or 6d) and perhaps even before you initiate the movement, you will begin to look for the second key to press. If you remember the second symbol from before, you may only need to scan the keyboard for it; otherwise you will need to rescan the text. In either case, your focus of attention must shift from the first symbol to the second.[10]

Typing each subsequent symbol would proceed in much the same way except for the fact that your knowledge of the symbols and keyboard improves while you process each subsequent symbol. While scanning the keyboard to find the first symbol, you begin to create a spatial representation of the keyboard in your spatial memory. At the same time, you begin to create a permanent represen-

---

[9]The choice of finger may have been made in advance. For example, you may already have decided to use your index finger or, if you are already an expert typist, you may use the proper finger for the keyboard you are familiar with.

[10]The visual system needs to know the symbol just typed in order to locate the next symbol to type. If the symbol just typed also appears nearby in the text, the visual system may locate the wrong text occurrence. This may result in a typing error. Double letters are particularly problematic. In order to compensate for the difficulty, double letters are encoded by a special "double indicator" preceded or followed by the code for the letter to be doubled. When double letters are typed, the double indicator is interpreted by the sensory-motor system as a command to execute the corresponding motor program twice. Occasionally the doubling operation is applied to the wrong motor program and the result is a doubling error: "giibs" may be typed instead of "gibbs" and "scrren" may be typed instead of "screen".

tation in your experiential memory and perhaps in other permanent stores as well. The permanent representations not only contains pictorial (iconic) representations of the symbols, but they also contain the spatial locations of the corresponding keys on the keyboard. The spatial locations are specified relative to the keyboard—they are object-centered. By the time you are ready to type the second symbol, you can use stored information to improve your performance.[11]

Stored information can reduce the time it takes to locate each subsequent key on the keyboard. If, while looking for the first key, you saw the second key to be typed, you will use your knowledge of its spatial location to direct your gaze to the correct (or a nearby) position on the keyboard. If you did not see it, you will use that fact to direct your gaze where you have not yet looked. In either case the search will be sped up.

Stored information can also be used to improve motor performance. If you know the approximate location of the next key to be pressed, you may begin to move your hands in its general direction even before you locate it.

Finally, both relative displacements (intended movements) and the motor programs used to accomplish them will be stored along with the tactile and auditory responses of striking the key. The relative displacements will become initial conditions for the motor program, and the associations between the relative displacements and motor patterns will be used to automate them. The tactile and auditory responses will also be associated with the motor patterns to be used as expected outcomes for later executions of the motor procedure. Hence the sensory outcomes will be used to signal a successful performance of the act.

After sufficient practice, the visual system is able to scan the text and, using its detailed internal representation of the keyboard, deliver to the sensory-motor system the sequence of relative displacements of the keys to be pressed. The generation of relative displacements for the word "cherish" is illustrated in Figure 15.7. At this point, a detailed representation of the keyboard is no longer being constructed; instead, the existing representation is being used to translate **automatically** between symbol and key location. The internal representation of the symbol is presented to the storage system, and associated information, the location of the key relative to the keyboard, is immediately recalled. Differences between subsequent key locations are determined, and the result is the sequence of intended relative displacements for the keys to be pressed. Since new memory traces are no longer being made (e.g., learning is no longer taking place), the associated information can be recalled immediately. This represents a change from a learning mode, where the store is used as an associative store, to one of

---

[11]This is only partly true. Consolidation of permanent information takes time, and access to permanent traces is denied until consolidation is complete.

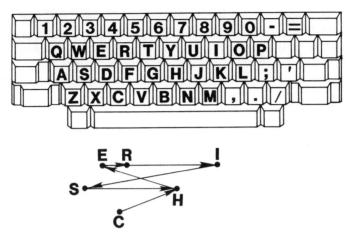

Figure 15.7. A standard QWERTY keyboard and the displacement pattern for the word "cherish."

skilled performance, where the store is used as an association store.[12] (Typing is not yet skilled; what is skilled is getting the location of the key when given its symbol.)

After sufficient practice, the sensory-motor system is able to accept the sequence of relative displacements and use it as a premotor program to generate an appropriate motor program for typing the letters. The sequence of relative displacements is the premotor program for the text to be typed, and its orchestration results in the text being typed. The translation between premotor program and motor program is performed by the motor store in the same way that the translation between key symbol and key location is performed by a premotor store. The motor store is used as an association store, and the performance is skilled.

There is a fundamental difference between translating from symbol sequence to displacement sequence and translating from displacement sequence to motor program. The difference is that the first process has no constraints while the second process is constrained by the fact that the final configuration of each motor pattern must be the initial configuration for the next motor pattern. The sequence of motor patterns must be **united**. It is not known how this is done.

---

[12]The use of two associative stores as one association store was described in Chapter 3. When using this type of association store, if an input is not recognized or is recognized by two different storage locations, a control error occurs and the access control network must decide what to do next. When using a simple association store, nonrecognition and multiple recognitions do not occur. The store delivers some output, and if it is wrong, a typing error occurs which must subsequently be corrected.

Learning[13] semiskilled typing encompasses learning several diverse subtasks. (1) The visual system must learn to scan the text for the letters to be typed, and (2) translate their visual representations into the verbal representation used by the visual and motor systems.[14] The verbal representation may be a visual code, a verbal code, or some other internal format. (3) The visual system must build the keyboard representation which enables symbols to be translated directly into spatial locations, and it (4) must learn to use the keyboard representation. (5) Finally, it must learn to take the resulting sequence of spatial locations and translate it into a sequence of relative displacements. The sequence of relative displacements is the premotor program for typing. (6) The sensory-motor system must learn to convert the premotor program into a motor program. That is, it must store associations between premotor and current configurations and motor patterns for the intended movements. If a single finger is used for typing, the relative displacements are converted into arm movements which move the finger into position to strike the next key, and the key-striking movement is initiated in conjunction with the arm movement so the finger will strike the key at the proper time. The key-strike program contains the tactile representation of a normal key strike, which is the expected outcome of the action. When more than one finger is used, the sensory-motor system, knowing both which finger was last used and the relative displacement of the next key, must determine which finger to use next and the arm movement to position it to strike the next key. The finger motion for striking the next key is coordinated with the arm movement. See Figure 15.8. When both hands are used, the pattern of relative displacements is broken into two subpatterns, one for each hand, and their orchestration is coordinated so that the sequence of key strikes is the correct one. Exactly how this is done remains an open question.

For many frequently typed words (or letter sequences), the verbal representation of the word is the premotor pattern for typing it. When that premotor pattern is used to control a movement, the entire word is typed without any intervening decision: The process is automatic.

Tactile information is used both for specifying initial conditions and for specifying expected outcomes. In the first place, the feel of the keyboard is used to determine the type of key-striking movement to be initiated: A much stronger striking movement is initiated for typing on a typewriter that has hard-to-press keys than on a typewriter that has easy-to-press keys. In the second place, for each key-striking movement there is an expected tactile response. If the actual

---

[13]Learning in the sense used here is like learning to hold a configuration. By some process which we don't yet understand, particular control patterns are generated for controlling the networks under consideration. The control patterns become associated with the intention of performing the indicated act, and later, when performing the intended act, the control patterns can be recalled and applied automatically. More will be said about learning in Chapter 17.

[14]In some cases this may entail reading the words of the text and using knowledge of their spelling for obtaining the verbal representations of the letters from memory.

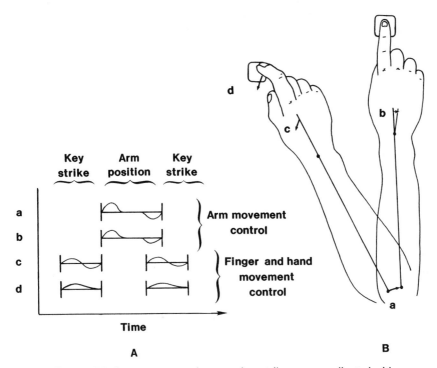

Figure 15.8. Arm movements between key strikes are coordinated with key-striking movements. Arm movements comprise a) movements of the elbow and bending of the elbow to position the wrist, and b) horizontal flexion of the wrist to position the finger. Key-striking movements include c) vertical flexion of the wrist and d) a striking thrust of the fingers. A key-striking movement may begin before the hand reaches its final position.

outcome agrees with the expected outcome, the key has been properly struck and subsequent actions proceed uninterrupted. However, when the actual response disagrees with the expected outcome, for example, if two keys are struck simultaneously, due to an error in the arm or finger movement, the ongoing actions may be interrupted and a corrective procedure initiated.

The role of tactile feedback changes as performance improves. For the novice typist, when tactile feedback indicates a successful key-strike, the motor program for the following key stroke may be activated. Thus the tactile pattern is a precondition for typing the next symbol. As performance improves, the motor programs for several letters may be initiated before tactile feedback from the first program can be evaluated. As a consequence, several letters may be typed after an error occurs but before the mistake is detected. It follows that the successful outcome for typing one symbol cannot be used as an initial condition for typing the next symbol, and the responsibility of timing subsequent key strokes is delegated to a higher level of control.

Learning to Touch-Type

When learning to touch-type, the process is quite different. First, the hands are placed in a specific configuration with the left index finger on the letter "f" and the right index finger on the letter "j" (assuming a standard American QWERTY keyboard). This is the **home position** and is the starting configuration for each movement sequence. Each finger is assigned to a specific set of letters, and only the assigned finger will press its letters.

When learning to touch-type, each key to be pressed is located in the same way that I described for semiskilled typing. Tactile information is used the same way for skilled and semiskilled typing and will not be further mentioned. However, that is where the similarity ends. Now, the learner focuses his or her attention on the particular finger that must be used and on the trajectory of the movement. The movement is therefore performed under conscious control. After pressing the key, the hands are purposefully returned to the home position. This establishes the exact trajectory for the intended movement, and because the focus of attention is on the movement, a stored representation of the motor program and its tactile response can be made. The premotor pattern associated with a motor pattern is the verbal or visual representation of the symbol being typed. When the hands are in the home position, orchestrating the stored motor pattern will cause the proper finger to strike the intended key and the hands to return to the home position. Once the stored engrams are available, focusing the visual attention on a given symbol gives immediate access to a motor pattern for typing it, and typing is accomplished by recalling the stored motor pattern and sending it directly to the motor apparatus for orchestration. This is possible because the initial condition for the motor pattern, hands in the home position, is automatically satisfied. This differs from semiskilled typing, where focusing the attention on the symbol gives access to the spatial location of the key for that symbol. The spatial location is a premotor pattern, not a motor pattern, so a further translation into a motor pattern is still required.

The fact that a visual presentation of a symbol can give immediate access to the motor pattern does not mean that the motor pattern will be recalled and orchestrated. The motor control system controls orchestration. Moreover, the fact that the symbol is visually attended does not mean that the motor pattern will be activated. Before that can happen, high-level control circuits must route the visual representation to the verbal networks for an initial translation into a verbal code, and the control networks must route the verbal code to the motor store for analysis. It follows that learning to type entails:

1. Storing mental procedures for scanning the page and attending the symbols,
2. Setting up control patterns for routing the visual representations of the attended symbols to the verbal stores for analysis,
3. Setting up control patterns for routing the resulting verbal representations to the motor stores for analysis,
4. And commanding the sensory-motor system to recall and orchestrate the motor pattern, which is activated by the verbal representation. All this is in addition to
5. Holding the hands in the home position.

These five control processes become part of the mental procedure associated with the "typing intention."

INTENTIONS AS INITIAL CONDITIONS

There may be many different motor patterns associated with the same external symbol. For example, the name of the symbol can be spoken, it can be typed, it can be printed, and it can be written in cursive, and each of these processes requires a motor program for its animation. When typing, it has been assumed that the representation of a symbol activates only the motor pattern for typing that particular symbol. Since several different motor programs for hand movements may be associated with each symbol, additional initial conditions must be associated with them which will prevent them from becoming activated except while typing.[15] A likely possibility, illustrated in Figure 15.9, is that the "typing intention" is associated with each motor pattern or program for typing as an initial condition. The only time a motor pattern or program for typing can be activated, then, is while the "typing intention" is active: while typing. Motor patterns or programs for typing would be unavailable at other times.

The coordination between hand movements and eye movements is crucial during skilled typing. I have already indicated that several letters are processed concurrently, with each letter in a different stage of processing. Just as soon as the visual system scans a letter, the sensory-motor system begins to generate a motor pattern for typing it. Long before the letter is typed, however, the visual system scans for the next letter and the sensory-motor system starts to generate its motor pattern as well. There may be as many as seven or eight letters in various stages of processing at the same time, as Figure 15.10 shows. (This is

---

[15]The need to distinguish between the motor programs for writing and typing stems from the fact that hands are used for both processes. Since different muscles are used to control vocalization, speech and writing (or typing) can occur simultaneously.

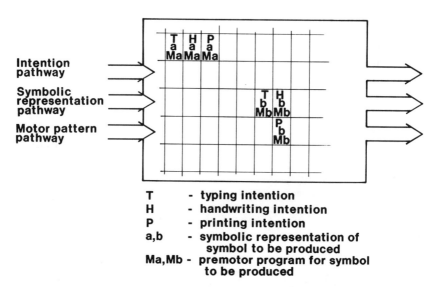

T — typing intention
H — handwriting intention
P — printing intention
a,b — symbolic representation of symbol to be produced
Ma,Mb — premotor program for symbol to be produced

Figure 15.9. Part of the motor store which associates premotor patterns (programs) with symbols to be produced and the intentions for producing them. The premotor patterns are spatial patterns which orchestrate the movements. The recalled premotor patterns are temporarily stored (buffered) prior to their orchestration.

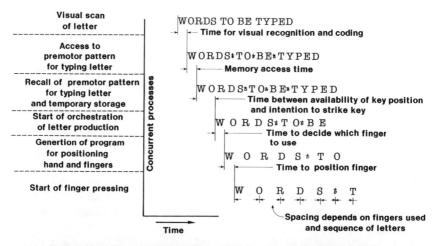

Figure 15.10. Some of the stages of processing required for typing. Note that by the time the finger-pressing starts for the letter "W" (bottom line), orchestration has already begun for the letter "O" (two lines up) and the visual system is already scanning the letter "R" (top line).

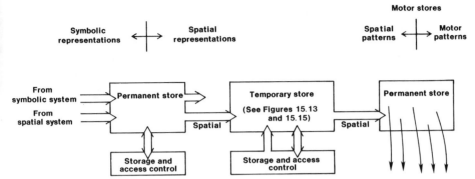

Figure 15.11. Relationships between the permanent store for premotor patterns, the temporary store for premotor patterns, and the permanent store for motor patterns. Note that representations are symbolic prior to the generation of premotor patterns, and representations are spatial prior to the generation of motor patterns.

called pipelining in computer parlance.) Part of skilled typing, then, is the ability to coordinate the processes of scanning and visual attention with the processes of generating motor programs and orchestrating them.

A temporary storage system is needed for holding sequences of premotor patterns prior to their orchestration so that they can be orchestrated at different speeds and so that the orchestration can be interrupted and resumed at a later time. The placement of the temporary store for premotor patterns is illustrated in Figure 15.11. An association store is used for translating the verbal code for each letter into its premotor pattern.[16] The resulting sequence of premotor patterns is stored temporarily in a storage system. While typing, the patterns in the temporary premotor store are sequentially recalled and transmitted to the motor store for orchestration. The speed of recall from the temporary storage system is variable, and recall can begin with any location in the store. Thus the speed of the final movement is determined by the speed of recall from the temporary store. Moreover, if orchestration of the stored sequence is interrupted by another high-level process, orchestration can be resumed where it left off.

Figure 15.12 illustrates how motor patterns might be held temporarily prior to their application. (Whether or not they are is an open question at present.) Since each motor pattern controls specific muscles, the temporary storage system must be organized like other motor stores. That is, it must be spatially distributed, with specific locations holding the motor patterns for specific

---

[16]The temporary premotor store was not mentioned while discussing semiskilled typing because each intended displacement was immediately orchestrated and hence the store was not needed for that discussion. Once sequences of letters are typed, the temporary store is needed, but those issues were omitted for clarity of the earlier presentation.

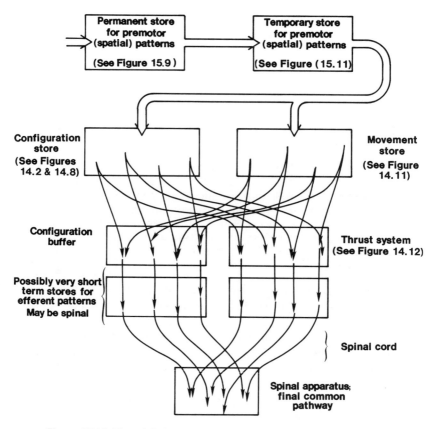

Figure 15.12. The global architecture of the motor system. Note that none of the storage control systems are illustrated.

muscle groups. Because motor patterns vary rapidly over time, one would expect such a store to act like a buffer rather than a temporary storage system, and its use would be for smoothing actions over very short time intervals—milliseconds—rather than longer intervals, such as seconds. A motor buffer would function during movement in much the same way that a sensory buffer does during perception, and the temporary store for premotor patterns would function during movement like spatial memory or the body profile system does during perceptual analysis.

Handwriting

I have chosen to discuss handwriting as the second example of skilled behavior for two reasons. First, the perceptual processes are similar for typing and handwriting so we may assume the high-level encodings are the verbal

426

representations of the letters to be written; we need not consider low-level perceptual processing any further. Second, both processes are generally animated with hand movements; thus the same sensory-motor systems are involved and we can focus on the similarities and differences between the two processes.

In order to focus on the similarities and differences, assume the following: (1) An individual who is skilled in both processes is going to write and type the same sentence; (2) He or she has the sentence in mind; therefore, perceptual processes need not be considered;[17] (3) The perceptual apparatus is not involved except as a feedback mechanism during the movements, and (4) The same premotor representation is used for both processes—namely, a verbal code for the letters of the sentence. The only differences, therefore, are in the ways the verbal code is converted into a motor program to control the hands. Assume (5) that while typing, a "typing intention" is active so that only motor programs for typing are available, and (6) while handwriting, a "handwriting intention" is active so that only motor programs for handwriting are available. (7) While typing, the hands are in the home position, and (8) while writing, the writing hand is holding a pencil in a normal position for writing, with the pencil point at the proper place to start. These configurations are held by the "typing intention" and "handwriting intention," respectively. Finally, assume (9) the only purpose for writing is to produce the written form of the sentence, not to convey the mood, intent, or personality characteristics of the writer.

When handwriting, the verbal representation of each letter is first converted into a pattern of relative displacements,[18] a premotor pattern for the letter being produced. The premotor pattern is stored in the temporary storage system for premotor patterns as illustrated in Figure 15.13. During orchestration, the premotor pattern is recalled from the temporary store and transmitted to the motor stores for conversion into a motor pattern. The pattern of relative displacements is converted by the motor stores into a sequence of muscle contractions which move the arm, hand, and fingers. Figure 15.14 illustrates the computational architecture, and Figure 15.15 illustrates the premotor pattern for the letter "b."

The patterns of relative displacements for each letter are learned when the individual first starts to write. Since the same pattern is used whenever the individual writes the letter, the appearance of the letter is the same regardless of how it is orchestrated—normal handwriting, writing with arm movements, writing with a pencil held between the teeth, or whatever.

---

[17]For example, I will not consider the verbal process of translating from a word to its spelling.

[18] Relative displacements are also used when an individual copies a figure that he or she sees in his or her visual field. A sequence of points is selected along the symbol as the focus of visual attention scans it, and the relative displacements are extracted and used as a premotor pattern for copying the symbol. This premotor pattern, a sequence of relative displacements, is analogous to the premotor patterns for letters and the same motor patterns can therefore be used for orchestrating it that are used for handwriting.

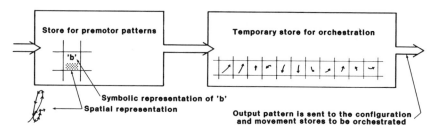

Figure 15.13. The premotor store which translates the symbolic representations of letters to be handwritten into premotor patterns is shown at the left. The symbolic representation for the letter "b" is translated by this store into a time-varying spatial pattern, shown to the left below the store. This pattern, when recalled, is stored in a sequence of storage locations in the temporary store shown at the right. The sequence can be recalled at any speed for orchestration.

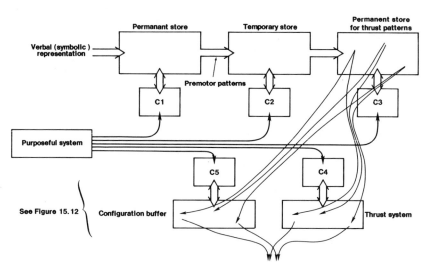

Figure 15.14. The architecture of the motor system.

The appearance of a given letter depends on the letter to its immediate left. For example, the appearance of the letter "b" in the sequence "ab" differs from its appearance in the sequence "ob." This suggests three possibilities: (1) There are two different representations for each letter, depending on whether the previous letter ends in a high stroke (b, o, v, and w) or a low stroke (all remaining letters); (2) There is a separate representation for the beginning of each letter and a separate representation for its body (refer to Figure 15.16); and (3) There is one representation for each letter and the premotor patterns are modified to unite two adjoining letters. Probably all three possibilities are realized, with the choice depending on many factors including speed of writing and the particular letter combination. The possibility that the beginning segments have separate representations from their bodies seems to have some support by considering the appearance of letters at the beginnings of words. Some samples of my own writing, illustrated in Figure 15.17, indicate that the transition segment often does not appear at all. When writing very quickly, letters are automatically united, a fact that suggests different stored representations may be used, depending on the previous letter. Finally, when writing very slowly and deliberately, the quality of the union between letters is notably improved, a fact that suggests that an independent process may be used for smoothing out the strokes.

Assume, now, that a premotor program for each word is constructed in the temporary premotor store and only needs to be orchestrated. A fundamental question is, how is the sequence of relative displacements, which specifies a letter or word, converted into a pattern of muscle contractions which moves the

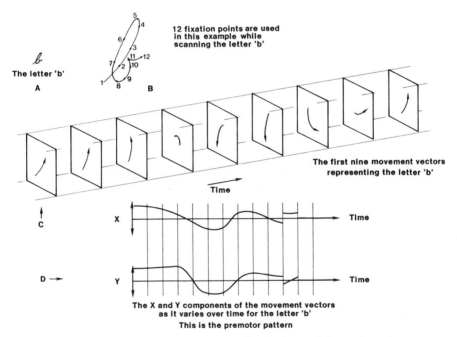

Figure 15.15. The premotor pattern for the letter "b" consists of a sequence of intended spatial displacements. The corresponding motor pattern consists of a time-varying pattern of movements, resolved along the axes of an appropriate coordinate system. a. The letter. b. A sequence of fixation points used to create the sequence of intended movements for the letter. c. The resulting time-varying sequence, shown symbolically. d. The same time-varying pattern decomposed into its horizontal (X) and vertical (Y) components.

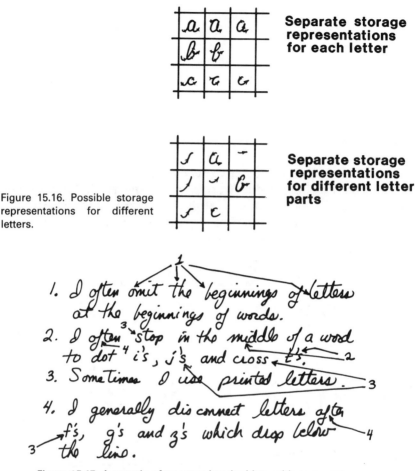

Figure 15.16. Possible storage representations for different letters.

Separate storage representations for each letter

Separate storage representations for different letter parts

Figure 15.17. A sample of my own handwriting, with comments.

pencil through the intended trajectory to produce the letter or word? The answer depends on several factors and differs from time to time even for the same individual. The following four parameters must be considered: (1) the intensity of the letters to be written and hence the pressure on the pencil point, (2) their size, (3) the speed of writing, and (4) the slant of the letters.

When writing, a very natural way to hold and control the pencil is illustrated in Figure 15.18. The pencil is held by clamping it between thumb and the index and middle fingers. If the pressure exerted by the thumb is sufficiently strong, it is also opposed by the ring and little fingers. This configuration is held throughout so the movements particular to writing are adjustments to the configuration. We may assume the configuration is held by the "handwriting intention" and needs no further consideration.

430

The intensity of the written letters depends on a constant downward pressure exerted by slightly twisting the wrist as shown in Figure 15.19, which increases the pressure on the pencil delivered by the thumb and index fingers. This constant pressure is also configurational and therefore needs no further consideration.

The movements that create the letters are the combined movements of the fingers, wrist, and arm, with the effort shifting from fingers to arm as the size of the letters increases. For small letters, the movement consists mainly of flexing and extending the index and middle fingers and thumb and rotating the wrist about the two axes shown in Figure 15.20. Arbitrary letters can be written by using the X and Y components of the spatial representations (shown in Figure 15.15d for the letter "b") as premotor patterns for controlling the wrist and finger movements. The X component of the spatial representation is used to control the thumb and finger movements (Figure 15.20b) while the Y component is used to control the wrist (Figure 15.20a).

When learning to write, associations are made between intended displace-

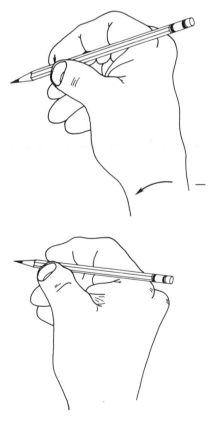

Figure 15.18. Holding a pencil for writing.

Figure 15.19. Intentity is increased by increasing the pressure of the pencil point against the paper. This is done by increasing the torsion on the hand and exerting more force on the pencil.

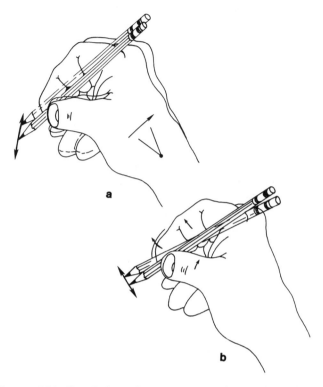

Figure 15.20. Two independent movements for cursive writing. a. Movement of the wrist causes an arc-like movement of the pencil point on the paper while, b. flexing and unflexing the thumb and fingers which hold the pencil causes an almost perpendicular linear motion of the pencil point.

ments of the pencil point, motor patterns which effect the movements, and the tactile responses of the pencil and paper. The intended displacements are measured relative to the current position of the pencil point.

While writing, the intended size specifies the ratio between the intended displacement and the actual movement that is produced. Because the directions of all movements are controlled by the intended displacement patterns and the magnitudes of all movements are regulated by the intended size parameter, the result of orchestration is the production of the same letter at a size specified by the intended size parameter. The tactile response probably enters into the regulation of displacements, but how is an open question. How intended size regulates the muscle contractions is also an open question.

The physical characteristics of the hand limit its ability to determine the size of the handwriting. At one extreme, the letters become so small as to be unintelligible. At the other extreme, the movement is so great that the thumb and fingers can no longer hold the pencil. The largest letter that can be efficiently produced by finger movements alone is about an inch tall and wide.

When the intended size is beyond an inch, the type of movement changes from one animated primarily by finger movements to one animated primarily by arm movements. For very large letters, writing is done entirely with arm movements. In general, writing combines both types of movements and the proportion of the movement allocated to the arm and fingers is regulated by the size intention. Refer to Figure 15.21. When the intended size of the letters is small, the motor store that converts intended displacements into motor patterns for arm movements is given a small ratio, perhaps zero, while the motor store that converts intended displacements into finger movements is given a large ratio, one that will produce letters of the desired size. As the intended size increases, the ratios are modified, and for very large letters, the ratio for finger

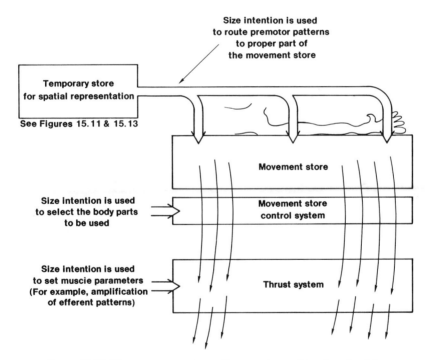

Figure 15.21. The same premotor pattern can be sent to all parts of the movement store. The premotor pathway determines the spatial direction of the movement when orchestrated by the selected body part. The size intention determines which body part will be used by (a) transmitting the premotor pattern along the correct pathway, and (b) by informing the movement control system of the selected store (not shown here). The size intention is also used by the thrust system when it determines movement parameters for the intended movement.

movements is small while the ratio for arm movements is chosen to produce letters of the desired size.

In the previous chapter I indicated how relative displacements are translated into arm movements for positioning the hand. These movements were learned as a child and are not specialized for writing. Nonetheless, the sequence of intended displacements, which is used as a premotor pattern for controlling finger movements during writing, can be used as a premotor pattern for controlling arm movements without additional learning.

The premotor program that controls the fingers, hand, and arm while writing can also be used to control the movement of any other body part. If the pencil is held between the teeth, for example, and the motor program orchestrated through the muscles of the neck and trunk, the same letter will be produced. The central point is that *premotor programs for writing are sequences of intended spatial displacements.* They are translated into actual movements by the motor stores which control the affected body part. As a consequence, the appearance of the writing is similar for a given individual, regardless of how she or he animates the writing.

The speed of writing is controlled by the speed with which premotor patterns are recalled from the temporary premotor store. When orchestrated at a very slow speed, the movements may be configurational. When orchestrated at a fast speed, the movements are ballistic. The dynamics of the movement are regulated by the thrust system, which analyzes the intended displacements and produces the appropriate motor patterns for the intended movements.

The slant of the letters is determined by the premotor patterns that are sent to the motor store for orchestration. If each intended displacement vector is systematically rotated about a vertical axis, the letters produced by the modified premotor patterns will have a different slant. Thus a systematic transformation of the premotor program determines the slant of the writing. These transformations may be done by the spatial system prior to their orchestration, or they may be performed directly by the motor system as the premotor patterns are orchestrated. How the premotor patterns are transformed remains a mystery.

Phonation

Phonation is the production of speech sounds and, like handwriting, entails the translation of a verbal representation of the intended utterance into muscle contractions that produce the desired sounds. This section suggests how the sensory-motor system controls the speech apparatus during phonation. (See, for example, MacNeilage, 1983.)

The vocal machinery comprises the abdomen, larynx, pharynx, neck, oral cavity, and lips. Refer to Figure 15.22. The muscles in the anterior wall of the abdomen control the rate of air expulsion and hence determine loudness. The

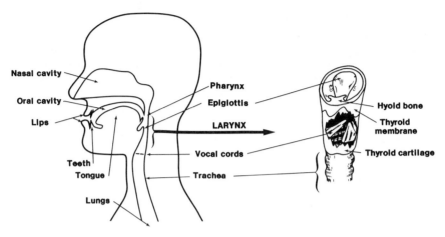

Figure 15.22. The vocal apparatus.

larynx contains the vocal cords which regulate pitch and also the onset of voicing in sounds such as "u" in "under." The pharynx regulates air passage into the mouth and nose and controls nasal sounds. The oral cavity, including tongue and mouth, regulates timbre, which is critical for producing vowel sounds. Finally, the lips stop and modify air flow during sounds such as "b," "p" and "v." In all, more than 100 muscles are controlled during phonation.

The rate of syllable production during speech varies from a few hundred syllables per minute to perhaps 500 when reciting well-known clichés. This means that one syllable is produced every 12 to 29 milliseconds. These speeds are comparable to those of typing, and it follows that the motor patterns for articulating a given syllable must be produced even before previous syllables are spoken.

The control pathways for the motor patterns that regulate the vocal apparatus originate at different places on the motor cortex and convey patterns with a variety of speeds, hence delays. Because of these differences, timing of signals along the pathways is critical. This section will describe the networks that produce the motor programs for speech and control the synchronization between articulatory events.

In order to focus on the similarities between speech and handwriting, assume the following: (1) An individual already has in mind a sentence to be uttered. (2) The perceptual apparatus is not involved except as a feedback mechanism during speech. (3) The premotor patterns for speech are the verbal representations of the words to be spoken. Hence the speech system only needs to convert them into the appropriate motor patterns to produce the desired sounds. (4) Finally, the only purpose of the speech is to produce the sounds of the words, not to convey mood or purpose of utterance.

435

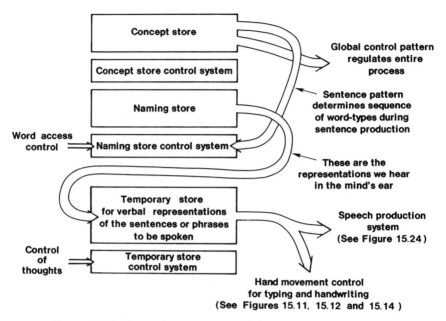

Figure 15.23. The major systems used for converting the internal representation of a concept into its verbal representation. Outputs from this system go to the hand movement control system and the speech production system.

Figure 15.23 shows some of the stages in the translation of an idea into a spoken representation of the idea. The first few stages are mentioned here for completeness only. At the highest level of control, an intention to convey an idea initiates a mental procedure that creates the internal or verbal representation of the sentence to be uttered. The idea is expressed as a sentence pattern or sequence of sentence patterns. Each sentence pattern initiates recall of a particular sequence of words from the naming store. The recalled words are ones which were activated by prior mental activity and are parameters to the sentence pattern. (See Baron, 1974a, 1974b for computer simulations of this process.) (In this context, each sentence pattern is a high-level procedure for expressing in words the idea it represents.) The sequence of recalled words from the naming store comprises the verbal representation of the sentence to be spoken. The verbal representations are stored in a temporary storage system as shown in Figure 15.23.

The next stage in the production of speech is the conversion of the verbal representation of the sentence into a **prevocalization pattern**, a premotor pattern for the sounds to be voiced. Although the representation of the prevocalization pattern may vary from individual to individual, it is likely that for most of us it is an auditory representation of the sounds to be spoken.[19] The translation from verbal representation to prevocalization pattern is accomplished by an associative store in the same way that the verbal representations of letters are translated during handwriting into the sequences of intended displacements that specify them. The prevocalization patterns are not motor patterns; they are an intermediate representation and are stored temporarily prior to their application to produce the sounds of speech.

The motor stores that control the vocal apparatus will be called **vocalization stores**. They are functionally divided according to the particular organ being controlled. This is exactly analogous to the division of the motor stores that control handwriting into independent control sections that regulate the fingers, wrists, and arms. Each vocalization store associates the patterns for particular movements with the premotor patterns that require those movements.

When speaking, the prevocalization patterns are transmitted to all vocalization stores simultaneously. Each vocalization store analyzes the incoming prevocalization pattern and generates the appropriate motor pattern for regulating the organ that it controls.[20] It follows that the timing of articulatory events is not an issue: The motor pattern associated with each prevocalization pattern already incorporates any delays due to speed of conduction along the motor pathway and time required by the apparatus to produce the desired movement. Figure 15.24 illustrates the major systems used for speech production. Neither the configuration system nor the sensory systems whose inputs are used to regulate speech are illustrated.

There are at least three parameters that regulate the outputs of the vocalization stores: intended loudness, intended pitch, and intended enunciation. These parameters correspond loosely to intended size, intended intensity, and intended slant of letters during handwriting. The speech parameters regulate the ratio between movements specified by the prevocalization patterns and the actual movements produced during phonation.

Intended loudness regulates the volume of the speech. The prevocalization pattern that controls the diaphragm and abdominal muscles determines how quickly air is expelled during phonation. Each stressed syllable is caused by an

---

[19]**Echolalia** is a clinical syndrome in which a brain-damaged patient mimics—echoes—the speech of another person without conscious attention. This suggests that auditory codes can be translated directly into articulatory codes and hence that auditory codes are premotor patterns for articulatory codes. In addition, the fact that delayed auditory feedback, listening to one's own speech with a delay of a few milliseconds, severely interferes with speech production also suggests that auditory signals are the modality of initial conditions and expected outcomes for articulation.

[20]The regulated parameter is not known for certain, but many linguists believe it to be the target positions of the various articulators—hence their configuration. When a target position is unattainable—such as when a subject holds a small block of wood, a bite block, between his teeth— adjustments made to the intended configurations enable the subject to continue speaking without a significant performance deficit.

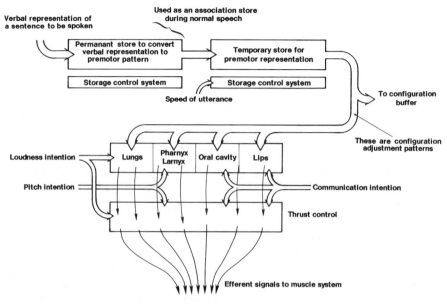

Figure 15.24. The major storage systems used during speech production. Compare this figure with Figure 15.2. Not shown are the configuration system and the sensory signals which regulate breathing.

increase in tension of the muscles in the anterior wall of the abdomen, which in turn expels air more rapidly. It follows that intended loudness increases the ratio between contractions specified by the prevocalization patterns and the actual contractions of the corresponding muscles. Thus intended loudness serves the same role as the volume control does on an audio amplifier.

Increased rate of air expulsion is accompanied by a change in the entire pattern of breathing. Inhaling becomes more frequent and therefore the number of interruptions in vocalization increases. Speech is interrupted when the lungs are low on air; speech is resumed after sufficient air is inhaled. An interruption in speech is accomplished by halting recall of the prevocalization pattern from the temporary memory store which holds it prior to its application. When recall of the prevocalization process is halted, all speech stops. The special adaptations of the respiratory system for speech are discussed at length by Lenneberg (1967, pp. 76–89) and will not be reproduced here.

Intended pitch regulates the tension of the vocal cords. As vocal cord tension increases, so too does the frequency of their vibrations and hence the pitch of the speech sounds. By regulating both pitch and loudness, the speech envelope is determined. The speech envelope conveys information such as whether the statement is a question. How motivational and emotional information is used to determine the speech envelope is a topic for future research.

To a limited extent, intended enunciation controls the style of speech. When

438

speaking, we each have our own style of enunciation and emphasis which is determined by the prevocalization patterns in much the same way that writing style is determined by premotor patterns. The relaxed style that each of us uses can be modified by exaggerating movements of the lips and oral cavity or by emphasizing various syllables. Movements of the lips and oral cavity are determined by how the muscles respond to the prevocalization patterns. If the responsiveness of the muscles is increased, so that each intended movement is amplified, and if at the same time vocalization is slowed down, the result is clearly articulated speech. Such a style might be initiated when lecturing to a large audience or while speaking to a deaf person who only reads lips. In the latter case, loudness might be decreased and only the lip movements and facial expression exaggerated. Syllables are emphasized by increasing their loudness, hence increasing the responsiveness of the abdominal muscles. In either case, the control circuitry which effects the emphasis is independent of the circuitry which generates the speech sounds and can be regulated by independent systems.

In summary, the principles that apply to typing and handwriting also apply to phonation. There are differences in the number and variety of systems involved, but not in the nature of translation from verbal code into muscle pattern to accomplish the desired output.

Locomotion

Typing, handwriting, and speech are all similar processes, and the patterns of expected outcomes are used primarily to detect performance errors and initiate corrective actions. In the absence of performance errors, the processes continue to be directed from centrally generated motor programs.

Locomotion, the focus of this section, illustrates a distinct change in the method of control. During locomotion, sensory signals play a fundamental role in the control of movements. Sensory signals are used both as initial conditions and expected outcomes, and their sources are much more varied and specialized. Vestibular signals are crucial in maintaining posture and balance. So are visual signals, particularly visual flow, which indicates movements of the body relative to the world. Kinesthetic signals as well as tactile signals also play important roles in locomotion and balance.

Although sensory signals are important for locomotion, nonetheless the principles and organizations of the motor stores are remarkably similar to those already described. This section, then, focuses on the architecture and control structures of the systems that control locomotion.

The Normal Walking Gait. The normal walking gait has been studied in considerable detail (Inman, Ralston, & Todd, 1981; McMahon, 1984a,b; Saunders, Inman, & Eberhart, 1953) and can be characterized as a **compass gait**

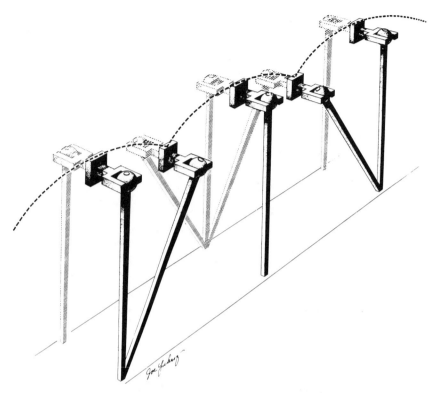

Figure 15.25. The hypothetical compass gait. The center of gravity moves along a sequence of arcs. (Reproduced, with permission, from J. B. deC. M. Saunders, V. T. Inman, & H. D. Eberhart, The major determinants in normal and pathological gait. *Journal of Bone and Joint Surgery*, 35-A, 1953, 543-558.)

with five refinements as described below. The compass gait, if it could be performed, would comprise walking with knees held rigid and pelvis remaining horizontal with its center in the plane of movement. Refer to Figure 15.25. The figure shows that the movement of the center of the pelvis follows a sequence of arcs whose radii equal the lengths of the legs. Since the mass of the body is supported by the pelvis, the center of mass of the body rises and falls by a considerable amount, which means the potential energy of the system rises and falls by a considerable amount. Moreover, since the center of mass is not above the stance leg, a torque would be exerted about the stance point, which would move the center of mass to the right or left of the plane of movement, depending on which leg is the support leg. Since we have assumed that the pelvis remains in the plane of movement, the compass gait is impossible and serves only as a theoretical starting point for understanding the normal walking gait.

While walking normally, the pelvis neither remains horizontal nor does it remain in the plane of the movement. Figures 15.26, 15.27, and 15.28 show that the pelvis rotates about a vertical axis and also about the horizontal axis in the plane of movement. These two refinements to the compass gait are called **pelvic rotation** and **pelvic tilt**. Both pelvic rotation and pelvic tilt flatten the arcs of the compass gait and reduce the changes in potential energy of the system. The arcs of the compass gait are further flattened by two additional refinements to the compass gait: **knee flexion** and **ankle flexion** of the stance leg as shown in Figure 15.29. Finally, as I described earlier, the pelvis cannot remain in the plane of movement because of the torques exerted about the

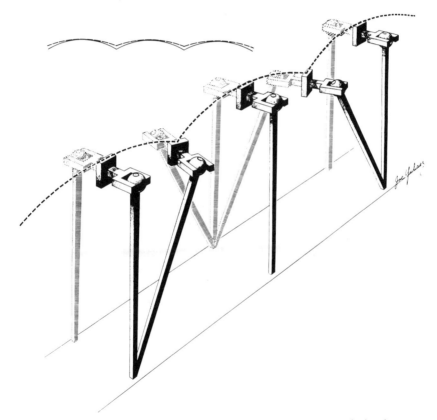

Figure 15.26. Pelvic rotation. The pelvis turns about a vertical axis, lengthening the steps and flattening the arcs by increasing the effective length of the legs. The solid line represents the dashed curve shown in Figure 15.25. (Reproduced, with permission, from V. T. Inman, H. J. Ralston, & F. Todd, *Human Walking*. Copyright © 1981 by Williams & Wilkins. Adapted from J. B. deC. M. Saunders, V. T. Inman, & H. D. Eberhart, The major determinants in normal and pathological gait. *Journal of Bone and Joint Surgery*, 35-A, 1953, 543-558.)

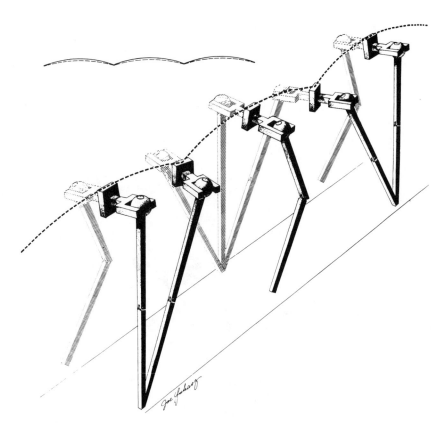

Figure 15.27. Adding pelvic tilt to pelvic rotation flattens the arcs further. Just before toe-off, the pelvis is lowered abruptly on the swing leg side, then raised slowly until heel strike. Knee flexion of the swing leg is necessary so the foot will clear the ground. The solid line represents the dashed curve shown in Figure 15.26. (Reproduced, with permission, from V. T. Inman, H. J. Ralston, & F. Todd, *Human Walking*. Copyright © 1981 by Williams & Wilkins. Adapted from J. B. deC. M. Saunders, V. T. Inman, & H. D. Eberhart, The major determinants in normal and pathological gait. *Journal of Bone and Joint Surgery*, 35-A, 1953, 543-558.)

stance points. The pelvis, in fact, moves laterally from side to side as shown in Figure 15.30. **Lateral movement** of the pelvis is the fifth refinement to the compass gait.

In addition to the component movements of the legs and pelvis, the arms generally swing forward and backward to counteract the movements of the opposite legs. Also, the ankle of the stance leg is extended and the knee is straightened as the center of mass of the body passes over the stance point.

442

These extensions propel the body forward and overcome frictional and viscous energy losses of the system.

Controlling the Walking Gait.   The motor stores that hold the programs for walking are functionally divided according to body part. For example, one motor store holds the patterns that control the ankle, another the pattern that controls the knee, another the thigh, and so forth. The premotor patterns comprise (1) the intention of walking, (2) the direction and type of step (forward, left, or right; leg raised to avoid an obstacle, etc.), and (3) sensory patterns which serve as initial conditions. The sensory patterns will be described shortly. Although the walking intention and type of step may be common premotor patterns for all motor stores, the sensory patterns differ for each motor store.

Walking is a periodic activity: Aside from small deviations, the trajectory of each limb repeats during each cycle of movement. (One cycle is the time

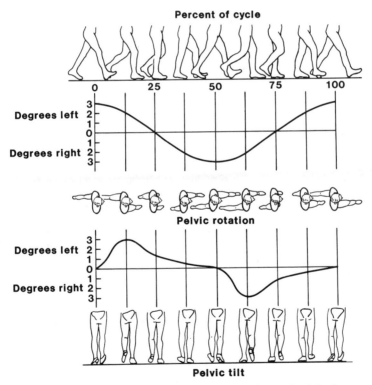

Figure 15.28. An illustration showing pelvic rotation and pelvic tilt as a function of percent of walking cycle. (Adapted from Thomas A. McMahon, *Muscles, Reflexes, and Locomotion*, Figures 8.5 and 8.6. Copyright © 1984 by Princeton University Press. Used with permission.)

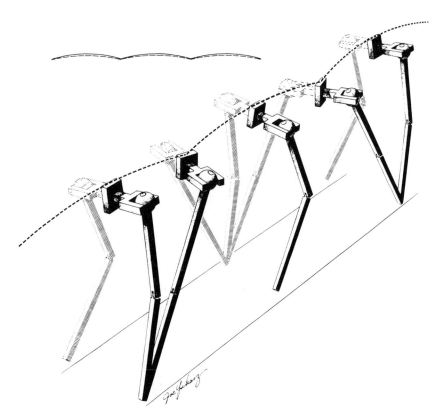

Figure 15.29. Knee flexion combines with pelvic rotation to achieve minimum vertical displacement of the center of gravity. The solid line represents the dashed curve shown in Figure 15.27. (Reproduced, with permission, from V. T. Inman, H. J. Ralston, & F. Todd, *Human Walking*. Copyright © 1981 by Williams & Wilkins. Adapted from J. B. deC. M. Saunders, V. T. Inman, & H. D. Eberhart, The major determinants in normal and pathological gait. *Journal of Bone and Joint Surgery*, 35-A, 1953, 543-558.)

between occurrences of the same event, such as the right heel striking the ground.) If the motor pattern for each body part is stored for one cycle, then walking could be controlled by periodically orchestrating each of the motor patterns, beginning when the cycle begins for the particular body part. (See Grillner & Wallen, 1985.) This is not how walking is orchestrated, as you will see. Note that if the motor pattern for flexing the right ankle begins when the right heel strikes the ground, and the motor pattern for flexing the left ankle begins when the left heel strikes the ground, then the cycles are out of phase and the motor patterns must be orchestrated at different times.

The motor patterns that control walking, however, are not necessarily stored for an entire cycle of movement. Each leg goes through a swing phase, where it is lifted from the ground and swung forward until it is again planted on the ground, and a stance phase, where it supports the weight of the body. The motor patterns that control each phase may be stored in different storage locations and orchestrated in sequence. Moreover, the number of stored patterns comprising one cycle may differ for each body part. The important issue is that by uniting

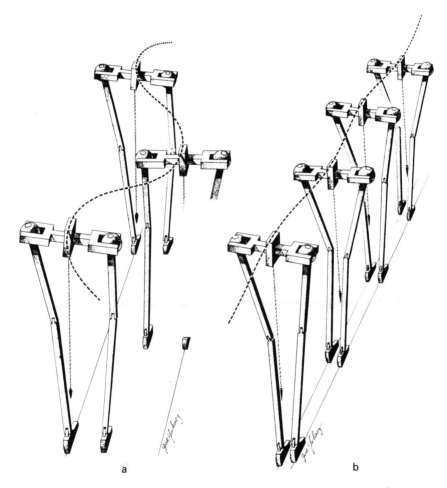

a   b

Figure 15.30. a. If the limbs were parallel there would be excessive lateral displacement of the center of gravity. b. Through the influence of a tibiofemeral angle and of adduction of the hip joint, excessive lateral displacement is corrected. (Reproduced, with permission, from J. B. deC. M. Saunders, V. T. Inman, & H. D. Eberhart, The major determinants in normal and pathological gait. *Journal of Bone and Joint Surgery*, 35-A, 1953, 543-558.)

each body part's motor patterns for each phase of one complete cycle, a motor program can be generated which controls the entire body while walking.

Motor patterns for different body parts are coordinated by storing as initial conditions the sensory signals that are generated at the beginning of the cycle for that body part. For example, the motor pattern for flexing the right ankle might be initiated by the tactile signal generated by the right heel contacting the ground. If the heel is struck too soon or it does not contact the ground at all, either a different motor pattern would be executed (if one is available for the current sensory signals) or a signal would be generated to inform the purposive system that no appropriate motor program is available. In that case, the purposive system must intervene, and this is the only time that it must intervene to coordinate low-level motor events.

The expected sensory outcomes for the motor programs depend on the body part and are stored with the motor patterns for that body part. For example, shortly after the heel of the right foot contacts the ground, the ball of the right foot contacts the ground. The tactile response is therefore an expected sensory outcome for the event, and the expected time of contact within the cycle is specified by the stored sensory pattern. If, because of a change in the pavement surface, the ball of the foot does not contact the ground at the expected time, the outcome is unexpected and the generated program would be interrupted. Figure 15.31 illustrates part of the configuration pattern for one cycle of walking, assuming that joint angle is the controlled parameter.

Walking is not orchestrated by periodically executing fixed motor patterns for each cycle of movement. A large collection of motor patterns are available, which differ, depending on the intended step type, sensory conditions, and intended speed of orchestration. Since the motor stores for the different body parts are independent, different motor patterns can be recalled and orchestrated for one body part without changing the ones orchestrated for other body parts. If, for example, there is an obstacle that the right foot must step over, the motor pattern for properly lifting the right leg will be utilized without necessarily changing the motor patterns used by other body parts.

The control of locomotion is a distributed process shared by all involved motor stores. When the high-level intention of walking is active, those storage locations of each motor store which controls walking are active. The high-level system analyzes the situation and, using spatial information, generates a high-level plan of movement. The high-level plan comprises the sequence of intended body movements in space. The plan is further refined by subprocedures into a sequence of intended steps for moving the body in the intended way. At any given time, the low-level plan might only guide the body for a few steps, and while that part of the plan is orchestrated, the high-level system will plan the next few intended movements. Thus the high-level system intervenes on occasion, and in general only momentarily, except under unusual circumstances.

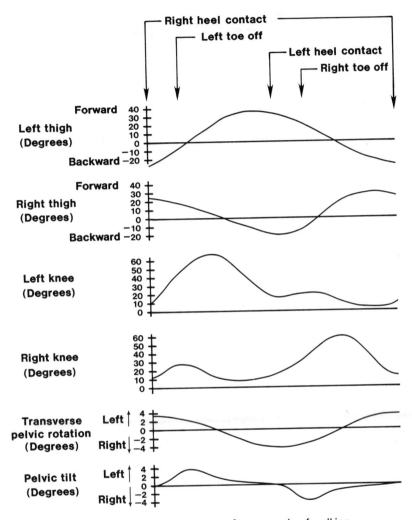

Figure 15.31. The configuration pattern for one cycle of walking.

Sensory signals together with high-level intentions are sufficient to control all low-level aspects of locomotion. Each motor store controls a particular body part and analyzes the intention, step type, and sensory signals. Analysis isolates the motor patterns required for controlling the particular body part. The sensory signals serve as initial conditions for selecting one storage location for recall. The motor pattern from the selected storage locations is recalled and orchestrated when the initial conditions are satisfied, and hence the next part of the walking cycle for the given body part is performed automatically. Since all body parts are independently controlled in the same way and coordinated by a

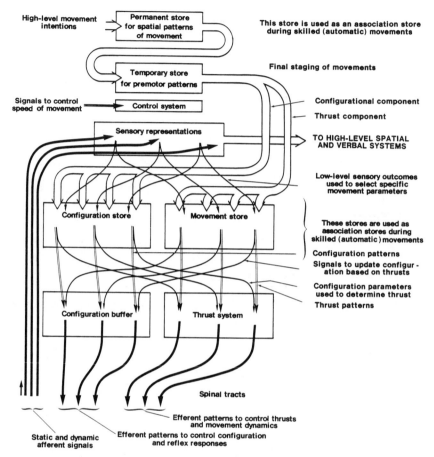

High-level movement intentions

Permanent store for spatial patterns of movement

This store is used as an association store during skilled (automatic) movements

Final staging of movements

Temporary store for premotor patterns

Signals to control speed of movement

Control system

Configurational component

Thrust component

Sensory representations

TO HIGH-LEVEL SPATIAL AND VERBAL SYSTEMS

Low-level sensory outcomes used to select specific movement parameters

Configuration store

Movement store

These stores are used as association stores during skilled (automatic) movements

Configuration patterns

Signals to update configur-ation based on thrusts

Configuration parameters used to determine thrust

Thrust patterns

Configuration buffer

Thrust system

Spinal tracts

Efferent patterns to control thrusts and movement dynamics

Static and dynamic afferent signals

Efferent patterns to control configuration and reflex responses

Figure 15.32. Some of the networks and their interconnections required for controlling locomotion. Compare with Figures 15.12, 15.14, 15.23, and 15.24.

combination of intentions and sensory signals, walking is automatic and the purposive system is free to do other things.

Figure 15.32 illustrates the storage systems required for skilled (automatic) movements. As the figure shows, the high-level intentions are converted into premotor patterns which are temporarily stored in a temporary premotor store prior to their orchestration. The premotor patterns held by the temporary store comprise the current low-level plan of movement. This includes step type, such as a high step for stepping over an object. When orchestrated, the components of the plan are transmitted to the motor stores (configuration store and movement store) where they activate storage locations holding motor patterns for carrying out the plan. Sensory signals select among the active memory locations and initiate recall of the proper motor patterns at the proper time for orchestration. The configuration component selects the proper configuration patterns while the thrust component selects the proper thrust patterns. The configuration buffer and thrust system generate the final efferent patterns which are sent over the spinal pathways to control the gait.

Sensory Signals for Locomotion.   The principal sources of sensory information for locomotion are vestibular, visual, tactile, and kinesthetic.

Because the head moves with the body, vestibular signals indicate both linear and angular acceleration of the body as well as its orientation relative to the force of gravity. A small pattern of vestibular values stored during an ideal walking cycle, therefore, can serve as a pattern of expected vestibular signals for future cycles of walking. Deviations of the actual vestibular signals from the expected ones initiate corrections to the gait, which are either reflexive, if the deviations are small, or controlled by the high-level system, if the deviations are large.

Linear and angular velocities and linear and angular accelerations can also be determined by the visual system using the visual flow pattern. Moreover, the visual system can determine the uniform linear motion of the body relative to its environment,[21] a value which cannot be derived by the vestibular system.

Hence, visually determined information is crucial for locomotion.[22]

Tactile information, particularly contact with the ground and forces on the sole of the foot, are used to control various parts of the gait as described earlier. Moreover, the tactile pattern for an ideal cycle serves as an expected outcome during following cycles of walking. Deviations of the actual tactile responses from the expected ones initiate adjustments to the gait or select among alternative motor programs for orchestration.

---

[21]The motion of an individual relative to her or his environment is sometimes called egomotion, and the determination of egomotion and relative depth from visual flow patterns is a topic of current research in computer vision. See Prazdny, 1980; Hildreth and Ullman, 1982; Horn and Schunck, 1981.

[22]Uniform movement can also be derived by the kinesthetic system. When walking, the speed of movement is determined by the speed of the gait. When the visual and kinesthetic systems determine different values for the movement, for example, when walking up an escalator which isn't moving or when walking along a moving sidewalk such as found in many airports, the result is the illusion of floating in space. When the visual and vestibular systems derive different values for angular rotation or linear acceleration, the result is the sensation of dizziness. As a child, did you ever spin around on the same spot and then stop, only to find that the world seems to continue spinning? The vestibular system adapts to the rotational movement and when the rotation stops, the vestibular system generates a signal which is interpreted as a rotation in the opposite direction. The vestibular signals control spatial memory, and when the vestibular signals cause a shift of the image in spatial memory, the current image, which is not moving, shifts out of registration with the incoming visual image. As a result, a visual flow pattern is generated which is interpreted as a rotation of the body within the world.

Finally, kinesthetic patterns specify the expected instantaneous configuration of the body while walking and regulate the stretch reflex. Deviations from the intended configuration are countered by changes in the muscle tensions that propel the body toward the intended configuration and stabilize the gait. This is the dynamic counterpart of holding a configuration, which was described in the previous chapter.

Motor Patterns for Locomotion. Motor patterns for locomotion comprise several subpatterns which control the body. These are the efferent patterns, which actually control the muscles and their receptors. The configuration subpattern specifies the intended instantaneous configuration of the body and comprises all instantaneous configuration subpatterns for the involved body parts.[23] The thrust subpattern specifies the expected forces required to hold or propel the body through the intended movement and comprises all thrust subpatterns for the involved body parts. Finally, the pattern of responsiveness values specifies how reactive the stretch reflex will be to deviations from the intended configuration.[24]

In the absence of external obstacles, orchestration of the motor patterns for walking will completely control the gait and overcome slight deviations in movement due to muscle fatigue, minor changes in the pavement surface, minor resistance due to wind, and so forth. When there are significant obstacles present, such as walking up or down a hill or across a sloping surface, stepping over a pothole, or climbing stairs, the high-level system must intervene.

At the highest level, the choice of a motor program depends on the movement intention—walking at a normal gait, walking quickly, running, and so forth. As soon as the initiating intention changes, the motor programs accessed by the initial conditions (the sensory signals specified by the motor programs) change and a new set of motor programs is orchestrated. The purposive system may not need to do any more than change the initiating intention. On the other hand, if there are no available motor programs which satisfy the intention and current sensory conditions, the purposive system must become directly involved. How and when the purposive system interacts during locomotion is an open question.

---

[23]Some parts of the body, particularly the head, may be controlled primarily by reflex actions which are not specified within the motor patterns. The relationships between controlled movements and reflex movements are not yet known.

[24]I am sure that you have all experienced what happens when you climb up or down stairs and, not paying attention, you inadvertently step one step beyond the top or one step below the bottom of the staircase. The incredible jolt initiated by your reflex system occurs either because the expected muscle tensions were not needed or they were needed and not present. This phenomenon is a good indication of how sensory signals and reflex actions interact during the automatic performance of a simple motor act.

SUMMARY

The automatic control of movement is possible once the motor stores have stored sets of constituent motor patterns for the underlying units of motion. Each motor pattern not only specifies the trajectory of the movement, but also the thrust pattern required to propel the body through the trajectory. The motor patterns also specify initial conditions for their execution and expected sensory outcomes. Premotor patterns, stored with the motor patterns, are often high-level intentions, such as handwriting or walking.

When an intention is active, those memory locations holding the constituent motor patterns for the actions become available. When, in addition, the correct sensory patterns are elicited, the proper constituent motor patterns are recalled from the motor stores and orchestrated. Because different body parts are controlled by independent motor stores, the sensory signals needed for controlling them can be different. Movements are controlled automatically when the sensory signals are able to select the proper constituent motor patterns to orchestrate the intended movements. When this happens, the entire movement can be orchestrated without conscious control.

Sensory signals not only serve as initial conditions to initiate movements, but they are compared against stored sensory patterns which specify the expected outcomes of the movement. When the actual and expected sensory patterns disagree, a signal is generated which notifies the purposive system that it must intervene in the control of the movement. In the absence of a signal of disagreement, the movement can progress automatically. Because the sensory signals can select among alternative motor patterns, movements can be controlled automatically even while the goals of the movement are changing. When walking down the street, the intention to turn right selects motor patterns which, without any further conscious control, cause a right turn to be made. Thus, except under unusual conditions, the purposive system is not directly involved.

Parameters to motor programs enable the same motor programs to be used under a variety of different situations. Parameters modify the responsiveness of the muscles to motor patterns. This often entails modifying the responsiveness of the muscles to signals along the reflex pathways. For example, the weight of an object is a parameter to the procedure for lifting objects and the size of a letter is a parameter to the procedure for writing the letter. These parameters are held in a temporary storage system during the orchestration of movements and they determine how the muscles respond to the same motor pattern. Parameters may be modified if the actual movements are performed incorrectly, and once modified, the new values are held during the orchestration of the action. If, for example, an object is heavier than expected, all appropriate muscle tensions can be increased. Once the new parameter is established, that is, once the intended muscle tensions are increased, the intended actions can be carried out without further attention.

Mental procedures control movements at the highest level and consist of the control patterns which establish the pathways for the sensory signals to follow, the pathways for the control patterns to follow, and so forth. Mental procedures also specify conditions under which the purposive system must interrupt them. When scanning the visual field for a particular object, locating the object terminates the scan. Finally, mental procedures establish the intentions which are analyzed by the motor stores for selecting among alternative sets of motor patterns. It is not known how mental procedures are selected for execution, how they are terminated, and how they are resumed if temporarily interrupted. These, and many related decision and control processes, are topics for future research.

REFERENCES

Amari, S., & Arbib, M.A. (1982). *Lecture Notes in Biomathematics, Vol. 45*, S. Levin (Ed.), *Competition and cooperation in neural nets.* New York: Springer-Verlag.

Baron, R. J. (1974a). A theory for the neural basis of language. P. 1: A neural network model. *International Journal of Man-Machine Studies, 6*, 13-48.

———(1974b). A theory for the neural basis of language. P. 2: Simulation studies of the model. *International Journal of Man-Machine Studies, 6*, 155-204.

Cooper, W. E. (Ed.). (1983). *Cognitive aspects of skilled typewriting.* New York: Springer-Verlag.

Grillner, S., & Wallen, P. (1985). Central pattern generators for locomotion, with special reference to verterbrates. *Annual Review of Neuroscience, 8*, 233-261.

Hildreth, E. C., & Ullman, S. (1982). The measurement of visual motion. A.I. Memo No. 699, Artificial Intelligence Laboratory, Massachusetts Institute of Technology, Cambridge, MA.

Horn, B. K. P., & Schunck, B. G. (1981). Determining optical flow. *Artificial Intelligence, 17*, 185-203.

Inman, V. T., Ralston, H. J., & Todd, F. (1981). *Human walking.* Baltimore: Williams & Wilkins.

Lenneberg, E. H. (1967). *Biological foundations of language.* New York: John Wiley & Sons.

MacNeilage, P. F. (Ed.). (1983). *The production of speech.* New York: Springer-Verlag.

McMahon, T. A. (1984a). Mechanisms of Locomotion. *Robotics Research, 3*, 4-28.

———(1984b). *Muscles, reflexes, and locomotion.* Princeton, NJ: Princeton University Press.

Metzler, J. (Ed.) (1977). *Systems neuroscience.* New York: Academic Press.

Nilsson, N. J. (1980). *Principles of artificial intelligence.* Palo Alto, CA: Tioga.

Prazdny, K. (1980). Egomotion and relative depth map from visual flow. *Biological Cybernetics, 36*, 87-102.

Rich, E. (1983). *Artificial Intelligence.* New York: McGraw-Hill.

Rumelhart, D. E., & Norman, D. A. (1982). Simulating a skilled typist: A study of skilled cognitive-motor performance. *Cognitive Science, 6*, 1-36.

Saunders, J. B. deC. M., Inman, V. T., & Eberhart, H. D. (1953). The major determinants in normal and pathological gait. *Journal of Bone and Joint Surgery, 35A*, 543-558.

Schank, R. C., & Abelson, R. P. (1977). *Scripts, plans, goals and understanding. An inquiry into human knowledge structures.* Hillsdale, NJ: Lawrence Erlbaum Associates.

Vygotsky, L. S. (1978). *Mind in society. The development of higher psychological processes.* Cambridge, MA: Harvard University Press.

16

SENSATIONS, AFFECTS, AND BEHAVIOR

INTRODUCTION

The previous chapters have described several computational and storage networks of the brain and the representations they use. No attempt was made to relate them to the mind: That is one goal of this chapter. Another goal is to describe how the mental state of a person is regulated by memory and environment and how mental state influences one's behavior.

In order to describe the relationships between mind and brain I will correlate physiological processes with associated mental sensations. For example, in Chapter 7, I indicated that according to Land's theory of color vision, the physiological correlate of the sensation of color is the pattern of activity in triples of cells which encode normalized integrated reflectance values obtained by the red, blue, and green color receptors of the eye. Whether or not normalized integrated reflectance values are actually encoded by the eye (or higher visual networks) is still an open question, but even if they are, it is impossible to prove that such a pattern causes a particular color sensation. Still, most of us recognize that specific patterns of retinal activity result in specific color sensations, and based on what we presently know about the retina and about colors, the correspondence suggested by Land is the best we have for the time being.

SENSATIONS, FEELINGS, AND EMOTIONS

A **sensation** is a sensory impression derived as an immediate reaction to stimulation of a sensory organ; hence the sensations of sound, sight, touch, temperature, pain, and so on.[1] An **emotion** is a mental state such as love,

---

[1]Low-level damage to the visual or auditory systems may render a patient incapable of understanding sights and sounds. Speech sounds appear like "the rustling of leaves" and objects may

fear, anger, jealousy, and hate. A **feeling** is an awareness of a sensation or emotional state; hence consciousness. An **affect** is any mental state that biases a behavior. Sensations and emotions are affects, as are hunger, thirst, and sexual arousal. Finally, **consciousness** is an awareness of one's own sensations and feelings resulting from storage of information in a storage system. Consciousness will be the first topic of this chapter.

Consciousness

In Chapter 6, I suggested that the physiological correlate of consciousness is the storage of information in a memory store. I also suggested that the physiological correlate of focusing the attention is selecting a stimulus event or modality for permanent storage. Let me elaborate on these two points.

Storage systems fall into four major classes: sensory buffers, temporary stores for static patterns, temporary stores for dynamic patterns,[2] and permanent stores. Sensory buffers are temporary storage systems with adaptive memory traces. They hold sensory impressions for a few moments, and as computational networks they make explicit a variety of attributes of the physical world. Among the sensory buffers already described are the visual, auditory, and kinesthetic buffers. Temporary memory stores hold static patterns for an extended period of time, often many minutes, but when the focus of attention shifts, all information is lost. Two examples are the stores of current experiences described in Chapter 6, and the stores described in Chapter 15 which hold premotor patterns prior to their orchestration.

Spatial memory is a temporary storage system which holds dynamic patterns—mental images. Mental images, if you recall, are independent of their location in spatial memory and float throughout the storage system as the focus of visual attention shifts. The configuration buffer is also a temporary memory store which holds a dynamic pattern: the current configuration pattern for the body. In contrast to mental images, however, configuration patterns never move. Each pattern component regulates the muscle tension in the particular muscle controlled by that buffer location. Object buffers are also examples of temporary memory stores, and like the profile buffer, their representations do not move around. Permanent memory stores with nondegrading memory traces comprise the fourth class of storage system. Included in this category are thestores of experience, naming stores, concept stores, stores for mental procedures, premotor stores, and motor stores, to name just a few.

---

appear as unrecognizable patterns of light and dark. Still, the sensations of sight and sound remain. What lacks are the sensations of familiarity, understanding, and recognition which result when the low-level encodings are analyzed and stored by the permanent storage systems.

[2]Static patterns are spatially distributed patterns of synaptic parameters within a storage system, whereas dynamic patterns are depolarization patterns. Both static and dynamic patterns represent information which changes over time. Refer to Chapter 2.

Since consciousness is the sensation associated with information storage in a memory store, it follows that the existence of different types of memory stores means that there may be a variety of different levels of consciousness. Indeed that seems to be the case. Associated with each sensory modality is a sensory buffer, and also associated with each sensory modality is a set of physical sensations for the sensory impressions of that modality. Awareness of those sensory impressions is the sensation that results when the sensory encodings are stored in a sensory buffer. Awareness of color is just one example among many in the visual system; awareness of movement, of increasing or decreasing brightness, of the existence of surfaces, and of the existence of objects are other examples in the visual system. I already showed that these perceived attributes correspond to features which are made explicit and stored temporarily in the visual buffer.

In addition to the sensation of sight, we can focus our attention on a particular object, color, shape, surface or movement. Once we do, that attribute enters the main stream of our consciousness. It is then that the storage representations of the selected attribute are sent to the permanent stores of visual experience for storage and analysis. We become conscious of them precisely because their representations are stored in one or more storage systems. Focusing the attention selects a stimulus for permanent storage and consciousness is the sensation that results when storage takes place.

Note that the sensation of sight is the physiological correlate of temporary storage, not permanent storage. The physiological correlate of permanent storage is the awareness of the selected object, color, or whatever. To understand the distinction, consider the numerals "A" and "B" shown in Figure 16.1. By paying attention to the "A," its representation momentarily enters the focus of visual attention, hence the main stream of consciousness, and the figure is recognized as an "A." At that moment, the "B" is no longer in the focus of attention. Still, we do not lose sight of its presence, only of its "B-ness." Its representation is still being stored in the visual buffer so it remains in sight.[3] This is the mechanism which underlies many well known visual illusions which deal with visual ambiguity. Refer to Figure 16.2. When we imagine things and see them in the mind's eye, their representations are sent from spatial memory to permanent memory for storage. They enter our stream of consciousness because they are permanently stored. Since they are not stored in the visual buffer[4] we do not see them. Since they are stored in permanent memory they

---

[3]For patients with simultaneous agnosia, a clinical syndrome described in Chapter 6, there is a loss of awareness of all objects in the visual field except the one currently occupying the focus of attention. This suggests that the underlying cause is damage to the visual buffer but not to the pathways that send visual information to experiential memory for permanent storage.

[4]Some individuals appear to see the images recalled from permanent memory. The famous Russian psychologist Luria (1968) described such an individual in great detail. Perhaps for him and others like him, the recalled visual representations are sent to the visual buffer where, when they are stored, they are once again seen.

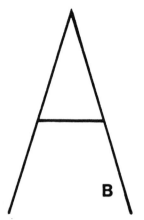

Figure 16.1. Two letters, A and B. When paying attention to the letter A, the letter B no longer occupies the focus of attention, and vice versa. Still, the letter not being attended remains visible.

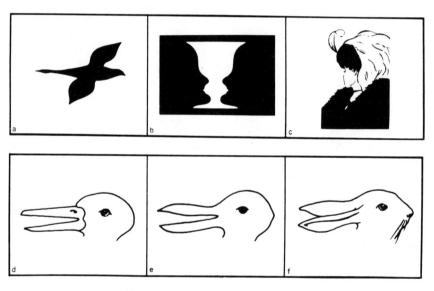

Figure 16.2. Ambiguous figures. Notice how your own attention shifts when the interpretation changes from one meaning to the other. (Reproduced, with permission, from John P. Frisby, *Seeing. Illusion, Brain and Mind.* Copyright © 1980 by Oxford University Press.)

occupy the focus of attention and we are aware of them. It is precisely because of that awareness that we see them in the mind's eye.

A similar argument can be made for the arena of sounds. We are aware of sounds because their low-level representations are stored in our auditory buffers. The auditory buffers make explicit a variety of high-level auditory representa-

456

tions. What we focus our auditory attention on—those sounds that we choose to select for permanent storage—those are the particular sounds which enter the main stream of our auditory consciousness.

During times of learning, for example, when learning a skill such as playing the piano, one's attention is focused on a combination of sensory and motor events. One must focus on a particular note on the musical score and then on the finger needed to strike the corresponding key on the keyboard. It is then that permanent memory traces are made which will later enable the visual representation of the notes to access the motor programs for striking the keys. As a consequence, while learning, we are conscious of our actions. Later, when performance is controlled by the memory traces, new memory traces are not made and we are unaware of what we are doing. The movements are automatic; they are not under conscious control. The actions are unconscious precisely because they do not result in the creation of new memory traces.[5,6]

Familiarity

Each associative storage system is a computational network which compares its current input pattern with all stored patterns. The result is a similarity pattern. The components of the similarity pattern, the similarity values from the individual storage locations, indicate how similar the input pattern is to the pattern stored in that location, and the physiological correlate of familiarity is rapid activity in the similarity cells of an associative storage system. High similarity values indicate that the current input pattern was previously stored; hence it is familiar.

The physiological correlate of *déjà vu* is rapid activity in the pathway which delivers similarity activity from the stores of experience when the current event is in reality unfamiliar. The similarity signals may be generated by a pathological condition or they may be generated because part of the event is familiar but not familiar enough to enable access to prior related experiences. In either case, the sensation of familiarity occurs even though the current experiences never happened before.

---

[5]One may pay attention to one's intention, for example, dealing cards, without paying attention to the resulting movements. One may also pay attention to the movements themselves. Paying attention to an intention or movement selects it for permanent storage and hence the intention or action is made conscious.

[6]Even though the actions are unconscious, the access parameters to the memory traces may be modified during performance. Hence one's performance can improve. Said another way, one can learn even though one is unconscious of the actions which are taking place.

AFFECT CENTERS

Physical sensations derived from external stimulation of the body—sight, hearing, touch, and so on—have obvious origins, and the patterns which represent them are slowly yielding to analysis in the laboratory. In time, we will understand them completely.

Certain physical sensations, such as hunger and thirst, also have physiological origins. Deep within the older parts of the brain—the limbic system—are highly organized networks of neurons called **centers** whose activity correlates with hunger and thirst. Laboratory animals with lesions to one part of the hunger center eat incessantly and soon become obese while animals with lesions to a different part stop eating altogether and would die if not force-fed. Although there is considerable controversy as to how the lesions modify the affect (e.g., by changing the hunger drive or by altering the taste sensation and therefore the pleasure response), nonetheless the existence is well accepted of specialized networks whose computations either control or modulate a particular behavior or affect.

Specialized centers have been found for a variety of affects, including hunger, thirst, sexual arousal, aggression, fear, and pleasure, and the fact that the brain is organized into affect centers is not entirely unexpected. Many behaviors or tendencies are innate—preprogrammed—so that when a situation arises that triggers one of them, the individual behaves (makes decisions, alters his or her posture or facial expression, etc.) in a stereotyped way. Preprogrammed patterns of behavior include fighting, laughing, crying, fear, loving, and lust. In order to elicit the appropriate pattern of behavior, one would expect a variety of specialized systems for evaluating the state of the body and the state of the environment, and as a consequence, one would expect to find centers whose activity elicits or inhibits a particular pattern of behaviors. That is exactly what has been found.

Sensory receptors are monitors of the environment. The retina monitors incident light. The cochlea monitors movements of the fluid in the inner ear, hence it indirectly monitors rapid changes in air pressure—sounds. The olfactory bulb monitors the chemistry of the air, and various receptors of the skin monitor temperature, physical distortions (tickle, prick, pressure, etc.), and damage (chemical, thermal, and mechanical).

Affect centers are neural networks which monitor the chemistry of the body as well as activity of the brain. Just as the sensory receptors monitor the environment and generate sensory patterns which enter our awareness (sight, hearing, touch, etc.), the affect centers generate affect patterns which enter our awareness (pleasure, anger, rage, familiarity, and so on). Figure 16.3 illustrates the fact that a pattern of activity is continuously generated by all the various affect centers. Moreover, the components of that pattern describe the various affects. When the hunger center is active because of a physical need for

458

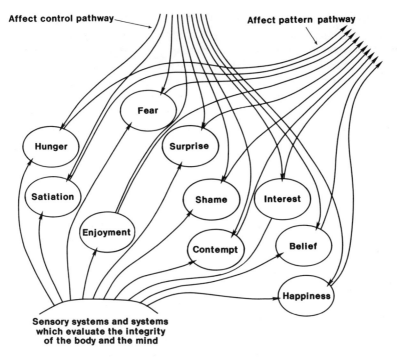

Affect control pathway

Affect pattern pathway

Fear

Hunger

Surprise

Satiation

Shame

Interest

Enjoyment

Contempt

Belief

Happiness

Sensory systems and systems
which evaluate the integrity
of the body and the mind

Figure 16.3. Components of the affect system.

nourishment, the components of the pattern originating in the hunger center become active. After eating, when the need for nourishment diminishes, the activity in those pattern components decreases.

Although there is probably not a single localized pathway that conveys affect information, nonetheless for the sake of convenience, I will call the set of cells conveying affect information the **affect pathway** and the pattern conveyed by it the **affect pattern**.

The affect pattern is part of the information stored in the permanent stores of experience, and the physiological correlate of each affect is a particular affect pattern or subpattern. When hungry, those components of the affect pattern signaling the need for food are active and the corresponding sensation is hunger. When frightened, those components of the affect pattern signaling danger become active and the corresponding sensation is fear. The same is true for other emotions and affects.

Bear in mind the fact that there may be no center for a particular emotion even though it may be felt. The correspondence is true for color: There is no receptor for the color red even though we perceive red. Redness is mediated by a characteristic pattern[7] in a set of cells, not by the activity of a single cell. Some affect states, such as hunger, have associated affect centers. Others do not. Each emotional state is mediated by a characteristic pattern of activity generated by all affect centers, not by the activity of a single center or cell. Where there are affect centers for certain affects, the correspondence between affect and its underlying physiological basis is clear. Where there is no affect center, such as for jealousy, which is a combination of envy, fear, and rage, the underlying physiological basis for the affect may not be evident. Yet we know there must be an underlying representation; it is just that we do not yet know what it is.

CONTROL OF THE AFFECT STATES

Figure 16.3 shows the **affect control pathway**, a pathway which conveys information—affect patterns—to the various affect centers. The cells comprising the affect control pathway are in one-to-one correspondence with those of the affect pathway. As a consequence, if the affect pattern which occurred at an earlier time is transmitted over the affect control pathway, the various affect centers are informed of the state they were in when that affect pattern occurred. Whether or not the incoming affect pattern alters the affect state is up to the various control systems that regulate the affect centers.

Because the affect state is stored with each experience, when we remember an event we can determine how we felt at the time. Moreover, since the stores of experience are associative, current affect information can be used to locate past events. ("The last time I was this hungry was when we were canoeing down the Mississippi"; "I haven't felt this good since I got an 'A' in anatomy"; "It made me furious to do business with him"; "I didn't believe her when she told me she didn't love me any more.") I'm sure that each of you knows how it feels to hear the songs that were popular when you were dating your high school sweetheart. Listening to them elicits strong similarity signals from the memory locations holding the memories of those experiences; the similarity signals synthesize the old affect patterns and cause them to be brought to mind.

PRIMARY AFFECTS

There are a number of affects which are considered by many to be primary, although there is not complete agreement as to what they are. Table 13.1 indicates the current beliefs of three prominent theorists (Mandler, 1984, p. 36).

---

[7]A given color is characterized by the set of ratios between the normalized integrated reflectance values. Thus many different patterns are seen as the same color depending on the absolute level of illumination. Raising or lowering the light level does not change the color.

TABLE 16.1
Fundamental or Primary Emotions Listed by
Three Leading Theorists

Tomkins	Izard	Plutchik
Fear	Fear	Fear
Anger	Anger	Anger
Enjoyment	Joy	Joy
Disgust	Disgust	Disgust
Interest	Interest	Anticipation
Surprise	Surprise	Surprise
Contempt	Contempt	
Shame	Shame	
	Sadness	Sadness
Distress		
	Guilt	
		Acceptance

Although not included in any of the above lists, happiness and self-esteem are also fundamental affects. Happiness is a state of mind that cannot be equated with any of the positive affects listed above, including joy. Many physical sensations are enjoyed: the smell of a rose, a chocolate bar, sexual pleasure, a Beethoven sonata. None of these things bring happiness although they may bring pleasure. Happiness is a state of mind which is brought about by several factors including control of oneself, control of one's life, a sense of direction, and a sense of sharing. Actions which may reduce one's happiness are avoided even though they may give immediate pleasure. One does not steal a candy bar even though it may taste good at the time. In the first place being caught is embarrassing. In the second place being imprisoned diminishes control over one's life and hence threatens happiness. Happiness, therefore, biases decisions which determine a person's long-range plans. This is in contrast to the primitive affects which tend to bias a person's immediate actions.

Beliefs and Certainty

A **belief** is the mental acceptance of something even though there may be no proof of its certainty, and the **belief system** is the affect system which evaluates assertions and assigns acceptance values to them. Belief states range from positive (belief or acceptance) to uncertainty and skepticism, whereas disbelief in a state or condition is the same as belief in the opposite state or condition. This section introduces the belief system and suggests its role in behavior.

The fact that our beliefs play a role in everyday behavior is illustrated by this simple example. When we recognize a friend, we act in a certain way because we believe the person is that friend. Our belief is based on the assumption that the

461

individual is not an impostor; hence we generally decide to whom we are talking based on the most casual glance. If there is any doubt, we look very carefully at facial details, body features, clothing, and gait in an attempt to determine whom we are talking to. Sooner or later, for some unknown reason, we either believe the person is our friend or we don't. If we do, we behave in one way. If there is even the slightest uncertainty, however, we behave in an entirely different way. Imagine how you would act in a society where you don't know whom to trust and whom not to trust. Your behavior would change drastically!

A change in mental state occurs when we suddenly accept something which we did not previously believe or understand. This is particularly true when there is a well established system of proofs for assertions. Consider this assertion:

> A steel band is stretched tightly around the earth at the equator so that it touches the ground everywhere. It is then cut and lengthened by 10 inches, which is 20 millionths of one percent of its original length. The modified steel band will rise by an average of more than 1.5 inches off the ground!

It is hard to believe that lengthening the band by only 10 inches would increase its average height by more than 1.5 inches but that fact is easy to prove.[8] If you understand and believe the proof, you will accept the validity of the statement; until then you will either accept the statement on blind faith, accept it because you already understand the principles, you will not accept it, or you will believe it to be improbable. When you do accept it there will be a sudden but perceptible change in your mental state indicating the transition from uncertainty to certainty; from skepticism to acceptance. That difference in mental state plays a fundamental role in behavior.

The belief system modifies virtually every type of behavior. Lack of confidence in oneself degrades one's personality; confidence leads to assertiveness. When looking at home for a lost article which you believe you misplaced at the office, it is often overlooked even when in plain sight. It is well known that children live up to your expectations of them. The positive attitude you convey to the child when you believe he or she can get the job done is often sufficient to impart the confidence necessary for success.

The belief system requires the symbolic analysis of (thought about) each

---

[8]The circumference of a circle is related to its radius by $C = 2 \times PI \times R$, where C is the circumference, R is the radius, and $2 \times PI$ is approximately 6.283. A change in radius corresponds to a change in height. Dividing by $2 \times PI$ we derive the relationship $C/6.283 = R$. If we add 10 to C we get $(C+10)/6.283 = R$ or $C/6.283 + 10/6.283 = R$. Since C/6.283 is the old radius, adding 10 to the circumference increases the radius by 10/6.283 or approximately 1.59 inches. Thus the steel band must rise by that amount. For those of you who still don't believe the statement, there is another way to look at it. Rather than cutting the band in one place and inserting 10 inches, cut it in quarters and insert 2.5 inches at each cut. As Figure 16.4 shows, this must lift the band off the surface of the earth by at least 1.25 inches everywhere. The fact that the actual height is over 1.5 inches should now be believable.

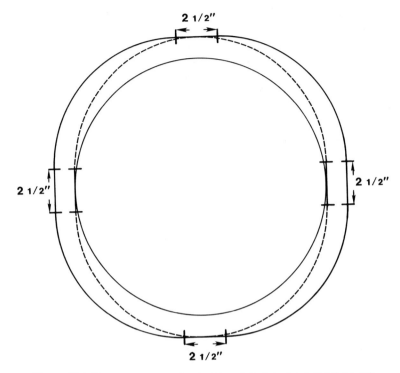

Figure 16.4. The appearance of a steel band stretched around the earth after adding ten inches to its length. Dashed lines show its appearance after adding two and one half inches at each side where it crosses the equator.

assertion. This differs from the systems regulating the more primitive affects, such as happiness, fear, pleasure, hunger, and thirst, which neither require symbolic evaluation nor yield to it. Regulation of the primitive affects is innate. In contrast, when we believe something, it is because we processed a considerable amount of symbolic information in forming that belief.

The belief system plays a regulatory role in most day-to-day activities. When we are hungry we seek food. The way we go about it often involves a considerable amount of symbolic processing, planning, and numerous assumptions. For example, we might decide to eat hamburgers and plan to go to the store to shop for food. We assume that we can get to the store, that we have the money to purchase the food, that the store will have the food, and so forth, all as part of the long-range goal of satisfying both the hunger drive and the pleasure drive. None of the intervening activities satisfy either drive; hence it is the symbolic thought that leads us to the belief that a more satisfactory state will result if the plan is carried out. The credibility assigned by the belief system to each step in the plan is crucial to choosing the plan as the course of action.

Our knowledge of the belief system is in its infancy. We know little about how it works, and one should expect the belief system to be the topic of considerable investigation in the coming years.

Self-esteem is belief in oneself. Self-esteem, like happiness, influences a person's long-range plans. I am writing this book because I believe the theories are correct and because I believe other people will find them interesting. Moreover, I believe this work will establish a good reputation for me. All of these things increase my self-esteem and hence my happiness. Having people read and share my ideas, of course, are also important to my happiness and self-esteem as well.

Affects and Neurochemistry

Many affects either trigger or are triggered by specific chemical systems. For example, when threatened with physical harm, hence frightened, adrenalin is released into the bloodstream. Either the increased heart rate caused by the adrenalin is sensed and the individual feels aroused, the adrenalin is sensed, or one of the altered physiological states is sensed. In any case, the physiological correlate of arousal is increased sensory activity directly or indirectly caused by adrenalin in the bloodstream. Since adrenalin lasts only for a few minutes, the state of arousal lasts only for a few minutes.

The length of time during which an affect biases a behavior depends on the particular affect and the chemical systems involved. A novel stimulus provokes interest, a state which may last from a few minutes to several hours depending on the stimulus and the individual. The depression that results from the loss of a loved one may last for years. Although the biochemistry of depression is only beginning to be understood, the fact that depression lasts for a much longer time than interest suggests the two affects are subserved by different chemical systems. In addition, the fact that interest is a positive affect and depression a negative one suggests that different affect centers are responsible for evaluating the conditions that lead to them.

There is a considerable amount of research on mind-altering drugs, including antidepressants, antischizophrenics, and antianxiety drugs, to name a few. As we better understand the chemical bases for the various affects and the structure of the systems that process them we should gain considerable insight into the control of affects and how they in turn control behavior.

Affects and Memory

While affect patterns are part of each stored experience, different components of the affect pattern are stored in different memory stores.

Sensory patterns are stored in the lowest level storage systems along with affect patterns for affects which change quickly. Low-level sensory patterns are high-resolution representations which vary quickly in time and space. Phonemes are one example. Phonemes are stored in the phoneme store, which is used to recode the auditory representation during the first stage of speech analysis. Letters are a second example. They are the corresponding low-level visual representations stored by a permanent visual store and used to recode written text during the first stage of reading. Phonemes and letters are rarely if ever associated with any affects, but certain low-level visual and auditory patterns are: Visual representations of spiders and snakes elicit fear as do certain sounds, such as the rattle of a rattlesnake. These representations are innate—they are genetically stored prior to birth. Whether they are stored in the same storage systems as sensory data or in special storage systems is not known.

The system for recognizing facial expressions is also innate. Facial expressions are part of a nonverbal communication system for conveying emotions: anger, happiness, fear, love. Many facial expressions are universal. People of all cultures express happiness and pleasure with a smile and recognize the smile as an expression of pleasure. Although certain types of brain damage alter both the production and recognition of facial expressions, we presently do not know whether the underlying system is specialized or general, where it is located, or how it works.

Affect patterns for affects which regulate our daily lives are stored with the records of our experience. These affects include enjoyment (pleasure), interest, surprise, shame, fear, anger, and so on.

When a particular event is associated with a strong affect, the recurrence of that event automatically elicits the affect. As an example, if either a very good or a very bad experience takes place at a particular restaurant, sight of the restaurant or even just thinking about it (such as when friends are discussing it) brings the associated positive or negative affect to mind. That affect biases any decisions relating to the restaurant—such as whether or not to go there for dinner. It is by this mechanism that prior experiences influence behavior. Since, as a general rule, negative affects occur faster and are stronger than positive affects, a single bad experience is often sufficient to deter repeating it. One particularly unpleasant experience at a restaurant generally keeps a person from going there again.

As I pointed out time and again, storage representations of an event are comprised of sequences of patterns which represent the focus of attention from moment to moment during the event. Although an experience is never repeated, the components of the storage representation recur. They are the individual patterns selected for the focus of attention which are formed with the explicit purpose of enabling the storage system to recognize similar components at a later time. Because the individual patterns in the sequence are canonical, they are immediately recognized by the storage systems. When the eyes glance at a familiar place or object, the visual encodings are immediately recognized

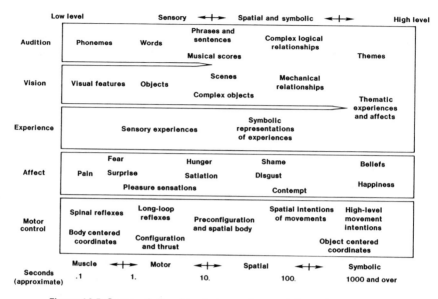

	Low level		Sensory ←—+—►		Spatial and symbolic ←—+—►		High level

Figure 16.5. Some relationships between time and the various processing systems.

and the associated affects brought to mind. Since the affects are brought to mind without intervening control, those parts of the storage system which hold them must operate as an association store rather than an associative store. It is by this mechanism that prior affects become available and are used to bias decisions which determine future actions.

As experiences unfold, places in the storage system where similar patterns were stored evaluate the similarity and generate strong similarity signals. Strong similarity signals enable access to memories of prior events. Just as the similarity signals from the sensory buffers are combined and selected to form storage representations, the similarity signals from the experience stores are combined and selected to form high-level representations of the experiences. This hierarchy is illustrated in Figure 16.5. The high-level representations produced in this way no longer encode specific events. Instead they encode the affect state of the individual and the places in his or her memory where events having similar affects occurred. Moreover, just as the patterns in each stage of the storage hierarchy vary more slowly than the patterns in the previous stage, these high-level patterns vary more slowly than the ones which represent the experiences. It is at this level that slowly varying affects such as happiness and self-esteem are stored, and hence the store which holds them will be called the **affect store.**

466

Affects and Behavior

The affect system plays a fundamental role in behavior. When hungry we seek food to eat. When tired we seek a place for sleep. When sexually aroused we seek a partner for lovemaking. Our actions are determined to a large extent by our affect state. This section describes how the affect system restricts our choices of action, predicts the changes that will occur to the affect state when an action is performed, and shows how the expected changes to the affect state bias the decision.

The affect system biases our choices for action long before a decision is made among them. Since the affect pattern is an input pattern to the stores of experience, it influences which storage locations will be activated by current experiences. When hungry, those memories whose affect states indicate hunger are more likely to be activated than those which indicate satiation. Since actions are governed by mental procedures (plans for action), a mental procedure which is not activated is never even considered. It follows that the affect system influences behavior by preventing some actions from being considered in the first place.[9]

The affect system also biases the way we carry out programs of behavior. Although we might choose to do the same thing when happy or when sad, our posture, movements, facial expression, body gestures, vocal expressions, and so forth, are all influenced by the affect system. This is because affect patterns are stored with low-level patterns such as configuration patterns and motor patterns and bias which of them will be used as well.

Stored affect patterns form the basis for predicting future affect states. When a particular event results in severe pain, the encodings of the initiating stimulus, together with the resulting affect pattern (which indicates pain and distress), are stored as part of the memories of the event. When a similar event occurs later, strong similarity signals are generated by the storage location holding the memories of the former event. The affect pattern is automatically synthesized and sent along the affect control pathway to the fear center, which evaluates the signals and, recognizing the potential for pain and distress, immediately activates the fear response.

Affect patterns also bias decisions. Suppose that several different actions are under consideration and a decision must be made among them. Suppose also that there is an expected outcome for each action. The expected outcome is the actual outcome for prior executions of the same action and hence the affect

---

[9]A chess player rarely analyzes every legal move before choosing the best one he thought about. Instead, only potentially good moves are analyzed; poor moves never come to mind. The set of potential moves forms a decision tree, and failing to consider various possibilities at the beginning is called **forward pruning** of the decision tree. Clearly a person does not consider all things he or she might do when deciding to act. Instead he or she considers only a small subset of the possibilities. The affect system, in essence, does forward pruning on the decision tree.

states which resulted before are stored with those memories. Prior resulting affect states become the expected affect states for the current action. Hence changes for each affect can be determined by comparing initial and final affect patterns for the past experiences.

One way to model the decision process is to assign a weight to each affect state and establish an ideal affect value for each affect. That action would be chosen for which the expected affect state is closest to the ideal. For example, suppose an action reduces hunger. Further suppose that the values assigned to the various degrees of hunger are given in Table 16.2. A negative number implies an undesirable state, one that should be reduced (made less negative). I will choose 0 as the ideal value for each negative affect. Eating reduces hunger so that if hunger is the only affect considered, the individual would seek food to eat.

In general, decisions are based on numerous affects.[10] Table 16.2, motivated by Schank (1975), indicates several affects and an arbitrary set of affect values for them. When making a decision, the weight given to a particular affect, the amount of influence it has on the decision, depends both on the affect and on the state of that affect. A choice is made based on a combination of affects, affect changes, and the weights given to each of them. The weight given to hunger in a decision which involves eating is much greater when hungry than when satisfied, and the weight given to fear generally exceeds the weight given hunger.

The tendency to choose an action is governed by each affect that changes and whether the expected change brings the value of the affect closer to or further away from its ideal. The neural machinery which makes decisions combines values from all changing affects and determines whether the affect pattern moves closer to or further away from its ideal. That action is chosen whose expected affect state is closest to the ideal.

As a specific example, consider only the affects given in Table 16.2. The values are arbitrary, as are the affect patterns, changes to them, and weights given in the following example. Particular values were chosen to illustrate the ideas. The ideal state is (no appetite, satisfied, unconcerned, calm, OK, quiet, neutral, cool) = (0,0,0,0,0,0,0,0). Suppose that a college student has an exam the next day and is hungry and anxious. Hence his affect state is (−3,0,−2,0,0,0,0,0). He is considering three actions: (1) studying for the exam, 2) eating a pizza, and (3) visiting his girlfriend. Studying for the exam will increase hunger by 1 unit, decrease fear of failure by 2 units, and increase happiness by 1 unit. Eating a pizza will decrease hunger by 4 units, increase fear by 1 unit, and increase happiness by 1 unit; and visiting his girlfriend will increase hunger by 1 unit, increase fear by 1 unit, and increase happiness by 4 units. For this individual, hunger has a weight of 2, satiation a weight of 2, fear

---

[10]Decision making is unconscious. Although we may be aware of some of the factors which enter into a decision, the instant of choice—the moment of truth—is hidden from consciousness.

TABLE 16.2
Arbitrary Numerical Values for Various Affects

Affect	Affect state	Affect value
HUNGER	starving	− 8
	ravenous	− 6
	"can eat a horse"	− 5
	hungry	− 3
	no appetite	0
SATIATION	satiated	− 9
	stuffed	− 6
	full	− 3
	satisfied	0
FEAR	terrified	− 9
	scared	− 5
	anxious	− 2
	unconcerned	0
ANGER	furious	− 9
	enraged	− 8
	angry	− 5
	irked	− 3
	upset	− 2
	calm	0
DEPRESSION	catatonic	− 9
	depressed	− 5
	upset	− 3
	sad	− 2
	OK	0
JOY	quiet	0
	pleased	2
	happy	5
	ecstatic	10
DISGUST	nauseated	− 8
	revolted	− 7
	disgusted	− 6
	bothered	− 2
	neutral	0
SURPRISE	cool	0
	surprised	5
	amazed	7
	astounded	9

a weight of 1, and happiness a weight of 1 so he would choose to eat a pizza based on the following considerations. If he studies for the exam his state will become $(-4,0,0,0,0,1,0,0)$, which is $(-3,0,-2,0,0,0,0,0) + (-1,0,2,0,0,1,0,0)$. If he eats the pizza his state will become $(0,-1,-3,0,0,1,0,0)$, which is $(-3,0,-2,0,0,0,0,0) + (3,-1,-1,0,0,1,0,0)$; and if he visits his girlfriend his state will become $(-4,0,-3,0,0,4,0,0)$ which is $(-3,0,-2,0,0,0,0,0) + (-1,0,-1,0,0,4,0,0)$. Note that in the second example, decreasing hunger by 4 units actually adds 3 to hunger and subtracts 1 from satiation. If we assume a linear combination of affects, we can derive an **overall satisfaction** for each state under consideration. The original state has an overall satisfaction of $2 \times (-3) + 1 \times (-2) = -8$. If the student studies, his expected overall satisfaction will become $2 \times (-4) + 1 \times 1 = -7$. If he eats pizza, his expected overall satisfaction will become $2 \times (-1) + 1 \times (-3) + 1 \times 1 = -4$, and if he visits his girl, his expected overall satisfaction will become $2 \times (-4) + 1 \times (-3) + 1 \times 4 = -7$. Since the expected overall satisfaction after eating pizza is least negative, the student would eat pizza. Continuing with the same example, if the student gives[11] hunger, satiation, and fear a weight of 1 and joy a weight of 2, he will visit his girlfriend, and if he gives hunger, satiation, and joy a weight of 1 and fear a weight of 2, he will study for the exam. Thus the particular choice an individual makes is determined by his or her own priorities even though they may not be available for his conscious inspection.

The weight given to an affect may change from time to time. For example, the weight given to one affect may depend on the value of another affect. A person may prefer one kind of music when happy and a different kind or no music at all when sad. Drugs can modify the weights given to the various affects as can the affect state itself. A person just frightened will not seek food, but if he or she is sufficiently hungry and the threat has persisted long enough, he or she may eat.

In summary, the affect system influences behavior in two different ways: restricting the choices of what to consider, and biasing the decision process itself.

TIME AND THE AFFECT HIERARCHY

Long-term and short-term affects govern behavior in different ways. Happiness and self-esteem do not strongly influence moment-to-moment decisions although, as I already indicated they limit what we consider doing by preventing

---

[11]The choice of weights is not a conscious decision. The system which evaluates affects and makes decisions implements the decisions in neural circuitry. The coupling weights, which are the weights given to each affect, are determined throughout the individual's history based in an unknown way on his entire history of actions and thoughts.

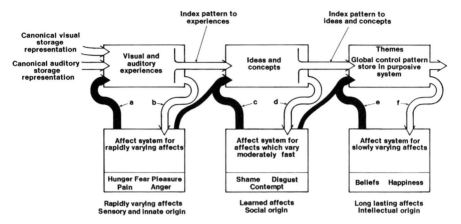

Figure 16.6. Some relations between sensory and symbolic representations and the affect system. Example patterns: a. pain; b. fear of something which caused pain; c. repulsion from seeing someone killed; d. shame resulting from the realization of being seen naked; e. happiness derived from getting a new job; and f. the pattern which increases one's self-esteem from getting a new job.

some possibilities from ever being considered. In contrast, although hunger, thirst, fear, and pleasure strongly influence moment-to-moment decisions, they do not have much influence on long-term decisions, such as the choice of a career or mate.

Both the stores of experience and the stores which control our behavior are organized into hierarchies. Low-level stores hold rapidly varying patterns which don't last very long while high-level stores hold slowly varying patterns which last a long time. The stored affect patterns have similar temporal properties. In the control hierarchy, the highest-level stores hold patterns which vary slowly and last a long time while the lowest-level stores hold patterns which vary quickly and don't last very long. It is for this reason that slowly varying affects have the greatest influence on high-level decisions while rapidly varying affects have the greatest influence on low-level (moment-to-moment) decisions.

Figure 16.6 shows three memory stores in the storage hierarchy and how they store both sensory patterns and affect patterns. Each store has different storage parameters; still, the stored patterns all represent experiences. Since the storage control system for an experiential store chooses contiguous storage locations for sequential events, stored memories become organized according to their time of occurrence. In particular, time progresses systematically from one storage location to the next along the pathways which encode time of experience.

Because each storage location in the low-level experiential store holds memories which last for several seconds, the storage system can predict future

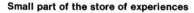

Small part of the store of experiences

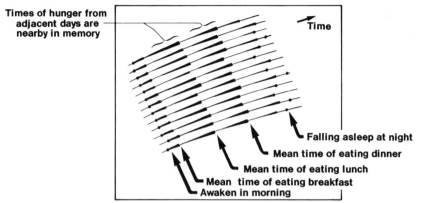

Times of hunger from adjacent days are nearby in memory

Time

Falling asleep at night
Mean time of eating dinner
Mean time of eating lunch
Mean time of eating breakfast
Awaken in morning

Figure 16.7. If time is organized along parallel paths in memory, and corresponding times from adjacent days line up, then affects related to daily cycles will be systematically organized. As a consequence, simple circuitry can be used to predict affects and control them. (The parallel lines representing days should be right next to one another. Thus the illustrated paths might represent the same day of each week or the same date of each month.)

events and future affect states. For short-term predictions, if an event is recognized by one storage location and the affect pattern is synthesized from the same storage location, the synthesized affect pattern is a prediction of the affect state which will occur in the next few seconds. If recall is initiated from that storage location, the recalled event is the expected consequence of the current event. Hence the organization of experiences into packets enables the prediction of imminent events and their outcomes.

The fact that each storage location holds patterns which last as many as 15 or 20 seconds can be concluded from the studies of Penfield and his colleagues showing the effects of electrical stimulation to the exposed cortex. Refer to Chapter 6. If recognition by one storage location enables recall of information from several of the following storage locations, then the recalled information predicts both the affect state and the coming events for the next several minutes. The farther along the pathway of events that recall is initiated, the longer-range the prediction.

The question remains, how can predictions be made for longer spans of time? Figure 16.7 shows one possibility. If the sequences of storage locations which encode time are systematically arranged so that corresponding times from different days are close to one another, then consecutive storage locations either hold events which occurred nearby in time or events which occurred at similar times on consecutive days. If recognition of one event enables recall of events which are stored in nearby storage locations, a mechanism is provided for controlling cyclical and habitual behavior.

Habits and Cycles

Suppose that memories are automatically recalled from storage locations which are near the ones storing current experiences. Suppose also that the recalled affect patterns are used to control the affect state. Since nearby storage locations hold memories of events which occurred at approximately the same time on previous days, the current affect state will tend to repeat the affect state from the previous day. Since our current actions are controlled by motor programs which are activated during the normal course of activity and there is an increased likelihood that yesterday's motor programs will be reactivated because of the affect state, there is a tendency to repeat those actions which we performed at the same time on the previous day. This is precisely what is meant by a habit. We tend to eat at the same time each day, do the crossword puzzle at the same time each day, expect the kids home from school at the same time each day, and so on, and although many of these events are governed by the clock, the storage system still predicts each event that will occur. When an expected event does not occur or when an expected activity is not carried out, a state of anxiety results. Anxiety is a negative affect, so the natural tendency is to act to reduce the anxious state. Hence there is an automatic bias toward repeating the previous activity. This reduces the anxiety and strengthens the habit.

ARCHITECTURE OF THE STORES OF EXPERIENCE

When we see or hear something familiar which previously caused a sudden change in our affect state, the affect system is immediately and automatically alerted to the event. For example, if we saw a dog which we thought was friendly

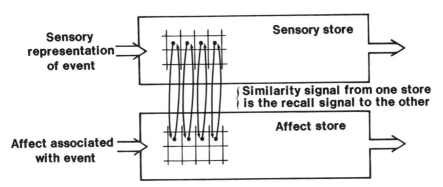

Figure 16.8. One possible architecture which allows sensory patterns to automatically synthesize affect patterns, and vice versa. Also refer to Figure 3.17.

but when we approached it suddenly attacked, we are immediately frightened when we see the dog again. Sight of the dog causes fear without intervening control. That is why I previously indicated that the portion of experiential memory which holds affect patterns acts like an association store rather than an associative store.

One way to build an association store is illustrated in Figure 16.8. As the figure shows, the store is functionally divided into two parts. One part, the sensory substore, holds the sensory storage representations produced by the low-level sensory networks. The second part, the affect substore, holds the corresponding affect patterns. Command inputs always initiate storage in both parts of the store. As the figure also shows, the similarity signal from a storage location in the sensory substore acts as a recall signal to the corresponding storage location in the affect substore, and the similarity signal from a storage location in the affect substore modifies the recall parameters in the sensory substore. As a consequence, a familiar sensory stimulus automatically invokes the affect pattern which occurred during the event, and events having the current affect state are easier to remember than events having different affect states.

Because of the functional architecture illustrated in Figure 16.8, the sensory and affect stores can be physically isolated from each other. The only requirement is that the control neurons that regulate each substore be function-ally tied together as the previous figure showed. As long as the storage substores are functionally tied together, the sensory substore can be located in one part of the brain and its corresponding affect substore in the other. Since opposite points of each cerebral hemisphere are functionally connected by neurons whose axons comprise part of the corpus callosum, the sensory and affect substores can even be located on opposite sides of the brain. If this turns out to be the case, then damage to the corpus callosum would prevent the patient from remember-ing what his affect state was during prior events.[12] It would also make it difficult or impossible for him to learn to avoid stimuli which changed his affect state. (Consult Tucker, 1981, for evidence of emotional lateralization in the human brain.)

SUMMARY

Various mental sensations can be equated with physiological activity. Con-sciousness corresponds to the storage of information in a memory store. Certain physical sensations, such as colors, sound, touch, and pain, correspond to

---

[12]If the subject thought about his or her mood, he or she might know that he or she was happy at the time. Still, the sensation of happiness would not be stimulated when thinking about the event. This is somewhat like patients with brain damage to the right hemisphere who are able to describe a smiling face as happy because the teeth are visible and the mouth curves upward, not because they recognize that the facial expression conveys happiness.

storage of low-level patterns in sensory buffers; feelings such as "squareness" and "4-ness," and the gestalt recognition of a friend, correspond to storage of information in high-level stores and recognition of those patterns by the stores. Familiarity and *déjà vu* correspond to rapid activity in the cells which convey similarity information from various storage systems, and focusing the attention corresponds to the selection of information for permanent storage in the stores of experience.

Within the brain are centers which evaluate the states of the body, environment, and mind and encode those states by specific patterns of activity called affect patterns. Affect patterns not only control decisions but they are the physiological correlates to a variety of mental states, such as fear, pleasure, happiness, hunger, thirst, and so forth.

Affect patterns describing the current state are stored with the current representations of the experience and can be used later to locate the experience in memory. They are also synthesized when a later experience is similar to the current experience. Because of the structural organization of the experiential storage system, prior affect states alter the current one, enable the formation of high-level reflexes, and tend to promote the formation of habits and cyclical behaviors.

The substores which hold affect and sensory patterns may be physically separated, and when the pathways connecting them are severed, predictable syndromes in behavior result. The structure and functioning of the affect centers is currently not known but will be the topic of vigorous research in the coming years.

REFERENCES

Luria, A. R. (1968). *The mind of a mnemonist.* New York: Basic Books.

Mandler, G. (1984). *Mind and body. Psychology of emotion and stress.* New York: W. W. Norton.

Schank, R. C. (1975). *Conceptual information processing.* Amsterdam: North-Holland.

Tucker, D. M. (1981). Lateral brain function, emotion, and conceptualization. *Psychological Bulletin, 89,* 19-46.

SUGGESTED READINGS

Andreasen, N. C. (1984). *The broken brain.* New York: Harper and Row.

Eccles, J. C. (1966). *Brain and conscious experience.* New York: Springer-Verlag.

Hilgard, E. R. (1977). *Divided consciousness: Multiple controls in human thought and action.* New York: John Wiley & Sons.

Smith, A. (1984). *The mind.* New York: Viking Press.

17

THE THREE
COMPUTATIONAL SYSTEMS
AND LEARNING

INTRODUCTION

In previous chapters I described the brain's various sensory and motor systems. In this chapter I will group them together into three coordinating systems, according to the types of computations they perform. The three systems are the **spatial system**, the **symbolic system**, and the **purposive system**. I will indicate how the systems interact and relate them to the brain's architecture. I will describe innate capabilities of the brain, and finally, I will suggest how, because of these innate capabilities, a child is able to learn.

COMPUTATIONAL SYSTEMS OF THE BRAIN

The three computational systems are illustrated in Figures 17.1 and 17.2. Figure 17.1 indicates the purposive system and shows most of the spatial system. The heavy arrows indicate that the purposive system maintains control over all networks within the spatial system. The visual system, shown in the upper-right of Figure 17.2, is part of the spatial system. It is shown in Figure 17.2 because of the structural parallel it has with the auditory system. The visual system includes the eyes, masking and disparity networks, the visual buffer, spatial memory, and the stores of visual experience. Figure 17.2 shows most of the symbolic system, parts of the purposive system (again), and some avenues of communication between them. The affect system is part of the purposive system; the vestibular system and body sense experience system are part of the spatial system. The control networks have been omitted from these figures for clarity.

The three computational systems are characterized by the kinds of computations they perform. The following three sections describe them, suggest some ways they interact with one another, and indicate the kinds of computations they perform. These sections are not presenting models for them

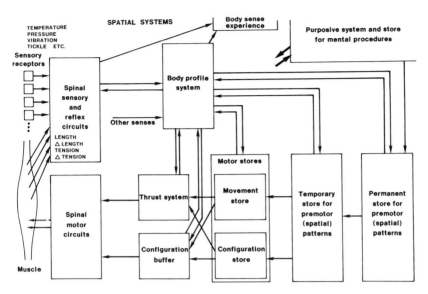

Figure 17.1. Many components of the spatial system. The visual system and spatial memory are shown in Figure 17.2. The control networks are not shown.

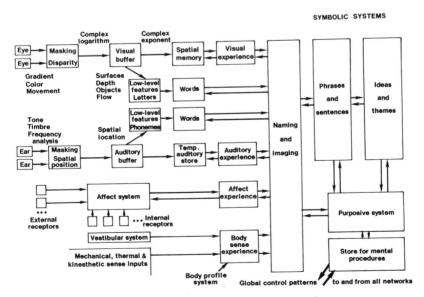

Figure 17.2. The symbolic and purposive systems and the visual components of the spatial system. The control networks are not shown.

but rather are suggesting general principles of organization which may, in the future, lead to a sufficiently detailed understanding so that computational models can be presented.

The Spatial System

The **spatial system** includes much of the visual system, the vestibular system, the tactile system, the body posture system, object buffers, and those parts of the sensory-motor system not concerned with vocalization. It creates, maintains, and processes the **world model**, the **postural model**, and object representations in **object buffers**.

The spatial system manipulates analog spatial information. It represents both physical objects and the world and it simulates physical interactions between them. The underlying computations are those of coordinate transformations, spatial transformations, perspective transformations, simulation of physical interactions, and so forth.

Visual inputs are the primary source of external spatial information. In the absence of visual inputs, tactile and kinesthetic inputs become primary. Inputs from the auditory system are secondary and indicate the spatial coordinates of sound sources. Finally, the various storage systems supply the spatial system with representations of objects and places which were previously experienced. All of these inputs enable the spatial system to create and maintain the world and postural models.

It is the spatial system, not the visual system, that relates the body to the world. In order to understand the difference, close your eyes and get yourself a glass of water. Even with your eyes closed you know where you are and where objects are around you. By reaching out and touching things, you can update your knowledge of your location, and assuming you don't trip and fall down, you can get the water without difficulty.

The spatial system plans many movements, and it is used by the symbolic system for planning other movements. When movements are accomplished without prior verbal thought, they are planned and executed by the spatial system. This happens, for example, when a person walks down the street but has his mind on something else, perhaps his girlfriend. During the orchestration of movements, the spatial system predicts their outcome. It determines which body parts will collide with themselves or with nearby objects, and if such a collision would result, the spatial system informs the purposive system of that fact. The purposive system will then formulate an alternative plan or the spatial system will formulate alternative movements for the same task.

The spatial system maintains the mental map used by the symbolic system while planning the route for a trip. Memories of experiences are coded with the spatial coordinates of where they occurred, and those spatial coordinates can be used to access the memories. This process was described earlier. When planning a route between two places, the symbolic system first accesses memories of them. The recalled memories are sent to spatial memory where they are stored as icons representing the places themselves. Using the spatial coordinates from their storage representation, the spatial system inserts the icons so as to preserve the spatial relationship between the places. The resulting mental image, a **mental map**, is used to plan a route between the two places.

While traversing (scanning) the mental map, the spatial coordinates of intermediate places are computed and used to access additional experiences. These experiences are recalled and icons for them inserted in spatial memory maintaining their correct spatial relationships to existing icons. This mental process elaborates and refines the existing mental map. We do not know which system controls this process but clearly the symbolic and spatial systems cooperate throughout.

As new icons for places and objects are recalled and inserted in the mental map, specific facts about them (such as road hazards, construction zones, traffic signals, and stop signs) are also recalled from the experiences. The affect patterns (such as the frustration of frequent stops along a stretch of highway or the pleasure derived from a friend who lives there) are also recalled.

While the spatial system creates the mental map and traverses alternative routes, the purposive system analyzes the affect states which are recalled. Based on its evaluations, the purposive system decides which route to follow. Once the decision is made, the symbolic and spatial systems once again scan the route and convert it into one of two types of plans, depending on which system is in control: a spatial plan consisting of a sequence of directions, distances, and expected landmarks; or a symbolic plan consisting of a sequence of verbal descriptions (such as "Go two blocks to the stop sign, then turn right and go two traffic signals. . . . "). The symbolic plan, if created, is created as the symbolic system analyzes the sequences of iconic representations extracted by the spatial system as it mentally scans the selected route. Thus a symbolic plan is the verbal description of a spatial plan. Whichever plan is generated becomes the intention and is used by the system in charge of the action for controlling it.

There are many things we do not know about the spatial system. We do not know how it integrates information from different sensory modalities to create the world model. We do not know how it represents objects. We do not know how it manipulates the body profile nor how it creates mental images from the body profile. We do not know what coordinate systems it uses, and we do not know how it manipulates them.

On the other hand we are beginning to understand the underlying principles of spatial modeling. We know how to manipulate analog spatial representations and we know something of the computations to simulate physical processes. We know how to represent position, surface orientation, and movement vectors in a variety of coordinate systems, and we know how to translate representations between coordinate systems. We are beginning to understand how to represent objects and bodies and how to model the world, and we are learning how to relate them to each other. And we are learning how neural networks which resemble and model the brain's networks can implement them. Perhaps most important, we are learning about the organization of the subsystems of the spatial system, how they interact with each other, and what parts of the brain are responsible for those functions.

The Symbolic System

The symbolic system processes symbolic information. It processes tokens and makes their sensory representations available. It analyzes sensory and control patterns and makes tokens for them available. The tokens include the internal representations of the words of natural language, of concepts and ideas, of mathematical and logical symbols, or of the symbols of a musical score.

One of the principal responsibilities of the symbolic system is processing natural language, including both the analysis and production of speech and writing. In this regard, the symbolic system converts speech and writing into internal representations of concepts and ideas (e.g., sentence patterns) and it generates verbal descriptions from them.

Symbolic tokens are the constituents of symbolic thought just as icons are the constituents of spatial thought. Symbolic tokens are the components of the dialogues we have with ourselves when we think, the components manipulated by our minds when we plan actions and predict their outcomes, the patterns which the naming stores convert into icons when we imagine what we are thinking about, the patterns which the vocalization system converts into motor programs when we speak, and the patterns which the spatial system converts into motor programs when we write. In this capacity, symbolic tokens are premotor patterns for speech and writing.

Just as the spatial system receives and processes information from a variety of sensory sources, so too does the symbolic system. The auditory encodings of phonemes, words, and sometimes phrases are inputs to the symbolic system. So are the visual encodings of letters and words. Not only do the visual and verbal systems make inputs into the symbolic system, so does the affect system. We can verbalize that we are hungry, thirsty, angry, or jealous. We can describe the sensations we feel when we touch something hot, fuzzy, or sharp. We can describe pain, and we can name where and how hard our body is touched when an object contacts us. Since the symbolic system gains access to the symbolic tokens representing these physical and mental qualities, their sensory representations must be inputs to the symbolic system.

The naming stores interface the symbolic system with the spatial system and hence are part of both systems. The naming stores associate symbolic tokens with sensory representations and convert between them either by imaging or by naming. I have already described both process in detail. In general, verbal tokens enable access to a variety of sensory representations of each object, and when one is recalled and stored in another storage system, we see, hear, or feel (in the mind only) the same sensations we did when the object was originally experienced. (The sensations are not ones of sight, sound, and touch, but of seeing, hearing, and feeling in the mind's eyes, ears, and body.) Moreover, once we have thought about objects of a certain category such as chairs, the token ("chair" in this case) may become associated with a characterization[1] rather than a specific instance. The naming stores hold these characterizations and bring them to mind when we think about the class of objects.

The symbolic system utilizes the spatial system in a variety of computational processes: planning a route before a trip, deciding among alternatives, understanding complex grammatical constructions, understanding complex mechanical relationships, understanding physical cause-and-effect relationships, and so forth.

When trying to understand how a mechanical linkage works, for example, images of the mechanism are manipulated by spatial memory and the resulting icons inspected by the mind's eye[2] to determine the physical relationships. We **understand** the mechanism when we can mentally simulate it in spatial memory without violating any known physical laws. (Consider how peddling your bicycle makes it go forward or how the lockset on a door holds the door closed.)

The following demonstration should help you think about interactions between your own spatial and symbolic systems. I will try to explain to you how the escapement mechanism of a pendulum clock works. You should try to determine the exact moment when you feel you understand it. Refer to Figure 17.3.

Consider the situation illustrated in A. The escapement wheel is driven to rotate clockwise by the weights and pulleys of a clock (not shown). Although it can rotate a little, tooth number 4 is about to contact the left pallet on the ratchet arm. Notice that the ratchet arm is connected to a swinging pendulum. The situation at the moment of contact is illustrated in B. As the escapement wheel continues to rotate, gear tooth 4 pushes up on the left pallet. This moves the ratchet arm and left pallet upward. The movement imparts energy to the ratchet arm which in turn pushes the pendulum and keeps it swinging. Inset C

---

[1]A chair can be characterized as a plane surface about 16 inches square held parallel to the ground at a height of about 16 inches by four legs, together with a second surface which is held perpendicular to the first surface by extensions of two of the legs. This characterization is generated from the surface orientation representation and need not be a verbal characterization.

[2]The mind's eye is not a homunculus. Quite the contrary. The mind's eye corresponds to the pathway that delivers information from spatial memory to the memory stores of the high-level visual system for storage and analysis. The same stores analyze mental images that analyze current representations of the visual field. When I refer to the mind's eye I mean only that the representations originate in spatial memory rather than in the low-level visual system. Thus the analyzed patterns are imagined rather than in sight.

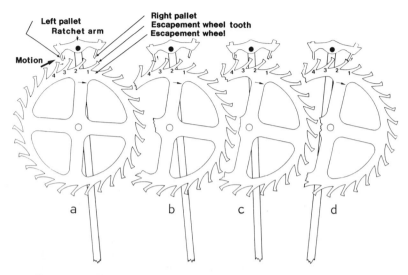

Figure 17.3. The escapement mechanism of a pendulum clock.

in the figure shows the situation just as the tooth 4 is about to slip past the left pallet. As the left pallet moves up and out of the way of tooth 4, the right pallet moves down to block tooth 2 on the escapement wheel. The moment of contact of tooth 2 on the right pallet is shown in D. Now tooth 2 pushes up on the right pallet, imparting energy to the ratchet arm, until it can slip by the right pallet. This pushes the pendulum in the opposite direction. As you can see from D, tooth 4 is now past the left pallet so that when tooth 2 slips by the right pallet, the left pallet blocks the movement of tooth 5. The process repeats. The rocking movement of the ratchet arm is determined by the speed of the attached pendulum, which determines the speed of the escapement wheel and hence clock, and the energy imparted by the escapement wheel teeth pushing up on the pallets overcomes frictional losses within the clock mechanism.

In this example, several physical laws must be understood. Gears, ratchets, and pallets are rigid; hence their icons are not allowed to change in size or shape during an imagined movement. Two physical parts cannot pass through one another. Thus before the escapement wheel can move, the pallet blocking it must move out of its way. Gears rotate on axles so the teeth of the escape wheel are constrained to a circular path in spatial memory. Finally, under the influence of gravity, the pendulum swings back and forth. These physical laws, maintained either in symbolic form by the symbolic system or in some analog form by the spatial system, are converted into control patterns, which constrain how the spatial system manipulates the icons it is processing. Although we do not yet know how physical laws are represented, current researchers are investigating a variety of possibilities.

482

Now think about how you related the written description of the escapement mechanism to the iconic representations shown in Figure 17.3 and how you manipulated your spatial representations while you looked at it. The words "clockwise," "slip past," "upward," "contact," "blocked," "rocking," and "pushes" were converted into control processes for spatial memory. Each of them named specific allowable physical interactions and hence operations in spatial memory. The words "escapement wheel," "ratchet arm," "pallet," and "tooth 5" were used as search parameters when you scanned and rescanned the figure. The fact that you could identify the named components of the clock implies that you could segment the figure into objects and focus your attention on them. It is precisely when you focused your attention on one of them that a representation was created for it in an object buffer and an icon was created for it in spatial memory. If, when you looked at B you understood how the movement of tooth 4 would push up on the left pallet, thereby moving the right pallet down to block tooth 2 of the escapement wheel, then you understood specific physical properties and interactions and were able to simulate them in your mind—specifically, in your spatial memory. It was then that you understood the mechanism.

There is a continual interplay between the symbolic system and the spatial system while planning an action, and the naming stores translate the tokens used by one system into the tokens used by the other. When the symbolic system plans a sequence of actions such as those involved in rearranging the furniture in a room, two different types of plans are manipulated. One plan consists of a sequence of verbal tokens, such as "move the sofa against that wall (pointing to show the location), then move that chair (again pointing) over there . . . " The second plan is the sequence of spatial representations of the pieces of furniture and how they are moved by the body. When generating the verbal plan, the spatial system is used extensively for manipulating the icons representing the room and furniture. When the mental images are inspected by the mind's eye, the icons are converted into a symbolic description of the intended movements—the verbal plan. The naming stores perform this translation. Carrying out the plan requires conversion of the tokens back into their spatial representations so that the sensory and motor systems can generate appropriate motor programs for moving the pieces of furniture. The naming stores perform this conversion also.

We are a long way from understanding how the symbolic system actually processes the tokens of thought. Although we have some insights into how simple sentences might be processed and understood by neural networks, we have few insights into how complex grammatical constructions can be processed. Although we know how to translate between symbolic token and icon or sensory representation, we do not yet know any of the details of either underlying representation. We have little understanding of how we represent and manipulate logical relationships, mathematical equations, or beliefs, to name just a few. Thus we have a long way to go to understand the symbolic system.

The Purposive System

The purposive system controls all information-processing systems, including itself, and it makes all decisions. It determines when information should be stored and when it should be recalled. It determines which systems should store information and therefore determines what occupies the focus of attention. It determines when to initiate an action and what action to initiate. It regulates each information-processing network by specifying what computation to perform, and it regulates information transmission along the various pathways.[3]

The purposive system is the decision making system of the brain. It chooses actions and behaviors that will satisfy the needs of the animal, both physical and emotional, and therefore its computations predict cause and determine effect.

The affect system is a major component of the purposive system. Affects bias all decisions. To the mind, nothing is neutral. Associated with the representations of each object and place are affect patterns which relate them to human needs and desires. When deciding among alternatives, the associated affect patterns are synthesized and used to bias the decisions that are made. This happens at all levels of control, including the lowest level, where anger, frustration, and pleasure are expressed, to the highest levels, where the belief system determines acceptance values and biases the outcomes of all high-level decisions.

Mental procedures are the sequences of mental processes which underlie our thoughts and actions and global control patterns are the patterns which specify the corresponding mental procedures. Thus one component of a global control pattern might command a particular storage system to initiate storage while another component might initiate a transfer of information along a particular pathway. Using computer terminology, mental procedures are the mind's algorithms while global control patterns are the brain's code.

The store for mental procedures holds global control patterns and associates them with affect patterns. The associated affect patterns are those patterns which were active before and after the mental procedure's previous uses. For a given mental procedure, the affect pattern which was active before its use is a precondition for its use. The affect pattern which was active after its use is a

---

[3]Have you ever been reading only to discover that your mind had wandered off and was thinking about something entirely different? During the process, your visual system unconsciously (automatically) scanned the words of the text while your motor system unconsciously (automatically) mumbled them. What happened was that information was no longer routed from the visual system to the high-level symbolic system for analysis; those pathways were blocked. Instead, information was routed from that part of the symbolic system which manipulates internal representations—thoughts—to that part of the symbolic system which analyzes them.

prediction of the affect state that will result if it is used to control a mental procedure. In essence, the associated patterns **index** the global control store according to physical and emotional needs and their satisfaction. When we are hungry we seek food in one of a relatively small number of ways (e.g., buying food, stealing food, bargaining for food, etc.); when anxious, we seek emotional relief in one of a small number of ways (e.g., withdrawal from the source of anxiety, coping with the situation by problem solving, repressing the source of anxiety, etc.). The hunger and anxiety affect patterns enable access to the mental procedures for these behaviors.

Looking at the situation from the opposite point of view, global control patterns are associated with those affect states which can be modified by their application. The associated global control patterns can therefore be used to satisfy the needs signaled by that affect state, for example, to reduce hunger or reduce anxiety.

The computations performed by the purposive system are quite different from those of the spatial or symbolic systems. The purposive system does not manipulate symbolic tokens nor does it manipulate sensory or iconic representations. The patterns it manipulates are of two types: control patterns, and affect patterns. The operations it performs on control patterns include starting them (e.g., transmitting them over the appropriate control pathways), stopping them, interrupting them, putting several of them together, modifying them, and so forth. We have no knowledge of how or where these operations are performed. The operations it performs on affect patterns are comparing them, evaluating them with respect to current and future needs, and choosing among alternatives based on them. We are just beginning to understand the structure of the purposive system. (See, for example, Faught, 1977.)

THE COMPUTATIONAL TOPOLOGY OF THE BRAIN

Although we do not yet know the correspondences between the anatomical networks of the brain and the computational networks illustrated in Figures 17.1 and 17.2, numerous sources, primarily from the clinical literature, suggest the following general principles.

The cerebral cortex is the principal storage organ of the brain. It comprises the sensory and motor buffers, all temporary and permanent memory stores, and various processing networks, such as spatial memory, object buffers, and the postural buffer. Structures deep within the brain control the cortical storage and processing networks as well as information transmission along the various pathways. They also analyze the current states of the body and mind and generate affect patterns describing those states. As a consequence, the structures closest to the surface of the brain comprise the storage and analysis systems while those structures which lie deep within the brain regulate all computational activities.

The sensory projection areas of the cortex (primary visual cortex, auditory cortex, and sensory areas of the sensory-motor cortex) comprise the sensory buffers for the corresponding sensory modalities. They therefore process temporary dynamic information patterns. The sensory projection areas may also comprise other computational networks as well. For example, several pieces of evidence presented earlier suggest that spatial memory resides in the primary visual cortex; however, this possibility is far from certain. Still, if spatial memory does not share the primary visual cortex with the visual buffer, it most likely resides nearby since there is no evidence that cortical areas distant from the visual cortex process low-level visual patterns.

The motor areas of the cerebral cortex also process temporary dynamic patterns. The significant differences between the temporary patterns processed by the sensory buffers and those processed by the motor buffers (e.g., configuration store) have been explored in detail in previous chapters and will not be repeated here.

Areas of the cerebral cortex not devoted to processing low-level sensory or motor patterns (e.g., sensory or motor buffers) either comprise temporary memory stores, permanent memory stores, or both.

There is a well-known asymmetry between the right and left halves of the human brain. (See, for example, Springer & Deutsch, 1985.) For most individuals, the right half dominates for spatial processing (including most mathematics), music (except possibly the perception of music by a musically experienced person), gestalt recognition (immediate recognition of faces, for example), and emotions, while the left half dominates for processing logical and analytical relationships, symbolic thought, and language. Still, the brain appears nearly symmetrical across its midline. The symmetry suggests that corresponding sites on opposite sides can do similar or related things. It is particularly likely that they do related things since they are directly connected together by the neurons whose axons comprise the corpus callosum.

Considering the facts just mentioned, the left hemisphere most likely processes and stores symbolic representations while the right hemisphere most likely processes and stores spatial and affect representations. Representations stored on the left side include symbolic tokens and the verbal thoughts which are brought to mind during events. Representations stored on the right side include visual icons, auditory representations of sounds, affect patterns, and sensory representations of events. If these observations are correct, then the corpus callosum must tie these representations together and associate symbolic, sensory, and affect information from the same experiences. Figure 17.4 illustrates this general principle, and recent research by Damasio (1985) and Damasio, Damasio, and Van Hoesen (1982) provide some supporting evidence.

Reminding is the automatic bringing to mind of one representation when an entirely different representation is processed. Seeing or hearing something can remind us of a prior event in exactly the same way that a verbal description can

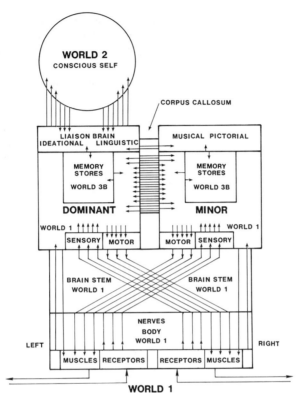

Figure 17.4. The left-brain right-brain dichotomy. (Reproduced, with permission, from K. R. Popper & J. C. Eccles (1977). *The Self and its Brain*. Copyright © 1977 by Springer-Verlag.)

create an emotional experience. Cross-modality reminding, something unrelated just coming to mind, may be one consequence of the asymmetry between the types of information stored on each side of the brain and the functional connections that tie them together.

Evidence presented in the previous chapter suggested that the similarity signals generated by the spatial system initiate recall of corresponding information stored by the symbolic system, and vice versa. In particular, the verbal description of an event, which would be stored on the left side of the brain, automatically elicits recall of the sensory (affect, visual, auditory) representation of the same event, which would be stored on the right side, and vice versa. This is consistent with the observations of anatomy just mentioned and the suggestion that corresponding sites on opposite sides of the brain store related information.

The permanent storage systems are distributed across the cerebral cortex. Although their exact locations are not known and may even differ among individuals, clinical and anatomical evidence suggests certain general principles. Stores which accept inputs from several modalities are located in areas where inputs from those modalities overlap. Thus, within the left hemisphere, the naming stores for visual information are near both the visual and auditory projection areas of the cortex. Consistent with this principle is the fact that naming appears to be one of the important functions of the association area of the cortex of the left hemisphere, that area which lies between the visual and auditory projection areas. We likewise expect the naming stores for sounds (the clanging of a bell or the rustling of leaves) to be located near the auditory cortex while we expect the naming stores for the body parts (identifying a hand or foot when it is touched) to be located near the sensory-motor cortex. As yet there is little clinical evidence either supporting or contradicting this expectation.

The temporal lobes appear to comprise the memory stores of experience although they may serve other functions as well, and the hippocampi either produced the "store now" commands or relayed them to the memory stores. This was described at length in Chapter 6. The hippocampi also process spatial information. Experiments performed by a number of researchers are summarized by O'Keefe and Nadel (1978). Researchers showed that the firing rates of specific cells in the hippocampus of the rat correlate directly with the spatial orientation of the animal during exploration of its surroundings. Although the same experiments have not been performed on humans, nonetheless they suggest that the hippocampus may comprise part of the system which assigns spatial coordinates to experiences. Since spatial coordinates are a part of every stored experience, inputs from the hippocampi may, in addition to producing or relaying the "store now" commands, supply them with the spatial coordinates of the experience being stored. The specific roles of the hippocampi are just now beginning to be understood.

Among the stores of the cerebral cortex are premotor stores that translate symbolic tokens into premotor patterns. The stores that translate them into prevocalization patterns are located near the motor areas which control the vocal apparatus, and the stores that translate them into spatial patterns which control writing or typing are located near the motor areas which control hand movements. Damage to those areas interferes with speech production and writing without disrupting symbolic thought. Thus clinical evidence directly supports the hypothesis that mixed modality memory stores translate between the various types of representations.

The frontal lobes appear to comprise the permanent stores for the programs of thought—the global control stores. For normal individuals, thinking is a learned process. We not only learn how to look at the environment and how to control movements, we learn how to manipulate mental images, how to think with tokens, how to speak, how to listen, how to feel, and how to act. Thus the majority of the control programs for an adult are learned. They must therefore be stored in a storage system. There is considerable evidence that the frontal lobes comprise that storage system. Damage to the frontal lobes does not affect sensory processing, memory, or the control of movements or posture. It does not affect spatial or rhythmic operations. It does not affect speech, either phonetic or morphological. It does not affect writing, although a patient with frontal lesions tires easily. Damage does affect complex abilities such as planning and using verbal thoughts to regulate movements. Syndromes caused by frontal lobe lesions include degradation of voluntary action and an inability to switch from one program of thought to another. Damage also modifies cortical activity in other parts of the brain. These facts are consistent with the suggestion that the frontal lobes hold the control patterns which regulate complex mental processes. These are the control patterns I have called mental procedures, or programs of thought. Although the deeper brain centers are the primary control centers for mental and physical activities, learned control patterns, those which automatically control complex activities, are stored in the frontal lobes. Damage therefore degrades performance of learned activities just as damage to the naming stores degrades natural language performance and damage to the sensory-motor stores impairs movements.

Neural structures lying deep within the brain are the control centers for the brain and body. The brain is organized so that the majority of cells comprising the sensory pathways terminate in nuclei deep within the brain[4] where the axons of secondary cells project to the cerebral cortex.

Only about 20% of the efferent cells which originate at the motor cortex terminate on motor neurons; the majority terminate on relay cells within the brain stem or spinal cord. The remaining efferent cells which regulate the muscles originate in centers within the brain stem. In summary, the final decisions as to what arrives at the sensory projection areas or how the motor neurons will respond to efferent signals are made by centers found deep within the brain, not by the cerebral cortex.

The affect centers, which are also found deep within the brain, evaluate the physical state of the brain and body and mental state of the mind and generate affect patterns which are used by the various control systems to bias decisions, establish goals, and control behaviors. Finally, the control centers which regulate mental activity are also found deep within the brain. The reticular activating system, for example, which is located within the brain stem, controls sleep and wakefulness. These control centers regulate cortical activity and make essential inputs to the purposive system.

The general picture that emerges is that the cortex generates, stores,

---

[4]In the visual system, the optic nerve terminates in the lateral geniculate nucleus. In the auditory system, the cochlear nerve terminates in the cochlear nucleus. Moreover, the auditory pathway, which conveys high-level auditory encodings from the cochlear nuclei, terminates at the medial geniculate nucleus. It is the lateral and medial geniculate nuclei which send projections to the projection areas of the cortex for analysis.

recognizes, and recalls storage representations as required by other systems. It also translates between them. Subcortical systems regulate cortical processing but are not concerned with specific details of the information being processed. They also regulate the transmission of information along the various pathways and therefore focus the attention. Whereas the control functions and circuitry are specified genetically, the patterns that are processed, those that remain at the cortical level, depend entirely on an individual's experiences. They are the memories of experience that are unique to each of us, the patterns which govern our learned behaviors, and the programs which determine our physical and mental abilities.

Figure 17.5 presents a cortical localization chart, which indicates some of the functions performed by various cortical areas. One of the earliest localization charts is due to Kleist (1934) and was translated into English in Luria (1973). More recent localization charts appear in Polyak (1957) and Krieg (1966). The shaded areas in Figure 17.5 and their numbers correspond to Broadmann's (1914, 1925) cytoarchitectural areas. The function labels come from Krieg's (1966) localization chart, with the arrow heads indicating the approximate centers of the areas he suggested. Excellent descriptions of the clinical syndromes which gave rise to charts of this type can be found in Luria (1966, 1980) and Kolb & Whishaw (1985).

INNATE CONTROL FUNCTIONS

When life begins, our memory stores are empty. We have no memories of experience, we do not recognize sounds, we do not recognize faces or objects, and except for simple reflex actions, we can't control movements. Thus our first mental and physical activities must be prewired.

An infant is born with some instincts and innate abilities while others develop as his brain matures. Instinctive behaviors such as sucking, swallowing, and crying, occur at birth; directing the gaze toward a moving object develops slightly later, at an age of about 1½ months. Instincts are prewired behaviors which are executed automatically when an appropriate situation is sensed.

Innate abilities are prewired computational functions of the brain. If there were no innate abilities, we could not learn. For example, if we could not store patterns to control our behavior, we could only act instinctively. Since most behaviors are not instinctive, their control patterns must be learned and stored. Innate abilities include the following: The sensory systems accept barrages of unfamiliar sensory signals, automatically direct the receptors toward meaningful stimuli, and generate storage representations where physical objects and their salient features are made explicit. The affect system monitors the mental and physical states of the body, determines which stimuli are harmful and which are beneficial, and encodes these evaluations to bias future behavior and decisions.

The storage systems accept and store both storage representations and affect patterns, make related experiences available for recall, and automatically synthesize affect patterns from related experiences. These synthesized affect patterns predict future affect states and influence behavior.

The affect system of an infant is prewired. It analyzes the state of the body and generates affect patterns which describe that state. Those affect patterns initiate the only behaviors at the child's disposal—the instinctive behaviors. When the affect pattern indicates a negative state, such as discomfort or hunger, crying is initiated. When the affect pattern indicates a positive state such as tender physical contact, the child becomes alert and attends the stimulus (and hence stores its representation). Regardless of the behavior, both sensory representations and affect patterns are automatically stored and become the child's permanent memories of experience.

Although each experience is unique to an individual, the control functions which store and recall memories and the systems which synthesize affect patterns are common to everyone. The sensory systems create canonical storage representations, which are stored together with their affect patterns. Because the child's experiences are very few in number, similar storage representations are created and the child immediately recognizes them. When an experience is recognized, the associated affect pattern is automatically synthesized and sent to the affect system for analysis. This process is unconscious; it is an automatic innate ability.

Stored experiences automatically influence a child's behavior. Suppose a child was treated roughly by her brother. When the child initially saw her brother, memories in the form of canonical storage representations were generated. When she was treated roughly and experienced discomfort, a negative affect pattern representing danger was generated. Memories of the brother, together with the negative affect pattern, combined to form the record of that experience. When the child sees her brother again, the memory location which holds that memory automatically synthesizes the associated negative affect pattern. This innate process is automatic. As a consequence, the affect system is warned of danger—it predicts trouble—and the child immediately reacts in a negative way, for example by crying or avoiding him. The negative affect state is now automatically produced when the child sees her brother. The innate characteristics of the brain, combined with the child's memories, bias her behavior. The brain is prewired to function that way.

Just as the negative experience in the previous example influences a child's behavior, a positive relationship generally develops between the child and its mother. The mother feeds the child and relieves its hunger pains. She burps it and reduces its gas pains. She changes its diapers and eliminates the discomfort they cause when wet or dirty. She holds and caresses it and speaks softly to it which brings it physical pleasure. The child therefore associates affects which represent security and pleasure with its mother.

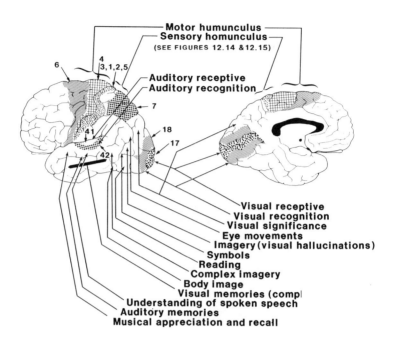

Motor humunculus
Sensory homunculus
(SEE FIGURES 12.14 & 12.15)
4
3,1,2,5
6
Auditory receptive
Auditory recognition
7
41
18
17
42

Visual receptive
Visual recognition
Visual significance
Eye movements
Imagery (visual hallucinations)
Symbols
Reading
Complex imagery
Body image
Visual memories (comp|
Understanding of spoken speech
Auditory memories
Musical appreciation and recall

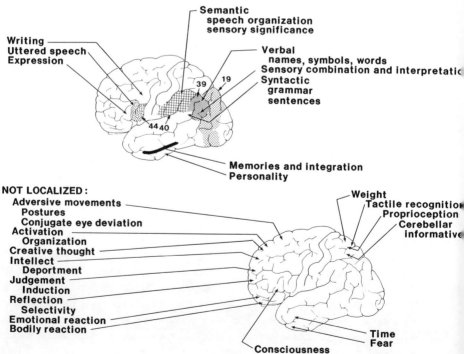

Semantic
speech organization
sensory significance

Writing
Uttered speech
Expression

Verbal
names, symbols, words
Sensory combination and interpretatic
Syntactic
grammar
sentences

39   19

44 40

Memories and integration
Personality

NOT LOCALIZED:
Adversive movements
Postures
Conjugate eye deviation
Activation
Organization
Creative thought
Intellect
Deportment
Judgement
Induction
Reflection
Selectivity
Emotional reaction
Bodily reaction

Weight
Tactile recognition
Proprioception
Cerebellar
informative

Time
Fear

Consciousness

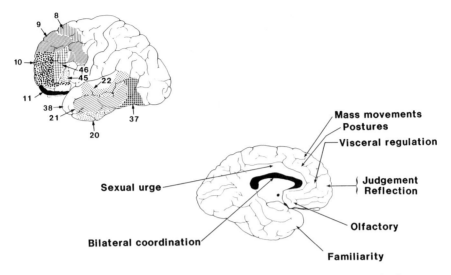

Figure 17.5. Functional organization of various areas of the cerebral cortex.

During the first few weeks of life, a child may become attached to its mother (or person who regularly cares for it) in a special way called **bonding**. Bonding,[5] which appears to be controlled by visual stimulation and initiated by visual recognition, is an attachment which instinctively modifies the child's behavior in very significant ways. Bonding appears to be mediated through a special chemical system in much the same way that arousal from fear is mediated by adrenalin. The role of bonding in the development of the child's personality is a topic of considerable interest at the present time. The underlying biochemical mechanisms are currently unknown.

The child's representations of objects become his or her tokens of thought. Each sensory system has the innate ability to segment its sensory inputs and extract canonical representations of objects for storage and analysis. As a consequence, objects are automatically recognized by the child. Because of the associated affect patterns, objects themselves elicit behaviors in the child. The hunger pains that are relieved when a bottle is placed in the baby's mouth are automatically associated with the bottle, and sight of the bottle triggers the positive affect. Also associated with sight of the bottle and hunger are the

[5]The intense attachment that one adult has for another when he or she is infatuated is probably related to bonding and may even be mediated by the same chemical and affect systems. If you have ever been infatuated, then you already know how your behavior can be influenced, and you understand the intensity of the emotional experience which sight or thought of the other person can bring. If you have never been infatuated, then no amount of explanation can convey those feelings to you.

programs for grabbing and sucking. These programs, initially prewired reflexes, are now stored in the global control stores. When a hungry child sees a bottle, the appropriate program for relieving the pain is triggered. The child immediately stops crying, grabs for the bottle, and starts sucking the nipple. Sight of the bottle, together with the hunger affect, become tokens for programs (behaviors) which when carried out relieve the child's hunger.

Instinctive movements are an essential part of a child's learning to control his or her own actions. (See, for example, Piaget, 1971.) A child initially moves its arms and hands at random because the patterns generated by the motor system are not associated with any sensory patterns. However, the child can see its own hands and arms. The motor store, which has the innate ability to store and associate sensory patterns with motor patterns, stores associations between arm positions (sensory patterns) and motor patterns which propel or hold the arms there. When the child sees a desired object, the object's position becomes the token (premotor pattern) for accessing the motor patterns to grab for the object. It is by this mechanism that stored motor patterns become the primitives of movement control just as the representations of objects become the tokens of symbolic thought.

Controlling movement is not an instinctive behavior for a child because there are no prewired associations between intentions to move and the motor programs which cause the movements. There are also no prewired associations between spatial arrangements of the body and configuration or thrust patterns which achieve them. Locomotion is instinctive in horses, for example, which can stand up and walk immediately after birth. For them, associations between intentions and motor programs exist at birth. They are prewired. A child, however, even after it associates spatial arrangements with configuration and thrust patterns for their attainment, still cannot control its own movements. Before those associations can be used, the child must learn to regulate information transmission along the pathways that route the spatial information to the premotor store where the associations are made, and from the motor store to the muscles where the motor patterns cause the desired movements. Said another way, the child must learn to orchestrate its intentions.

Patterns which route information between different processing systems are control patterns. They are stored in the global control stores, along with the intentions that they implement. For example, if a child intends to grab an object, the child must transmit the spatial position of the object (determined by the spatial system) to the premotor store, where associations between spatial coordinates and configuration or thrust patterns are held. The child must also recall the associated motor pattern and orchestrate it—send it along the spinal pathways to activate the muscles.

The intentions and the control patterns for carrying them out are stored when the child pays attention to what he or she is doing. Paying attention while learning hand-eye coordination is an innate process, which routes spatial coordinates and motor patterns to the premotor stores for storage and control patterns and intentions to the global control store for storage. Once the intentions and their control patterns are available, and once the spatial coordinates and their associated motor patterns are available, the child can finally begin to control its own movements.

When an object is recognized and the child wants it, the desire, an intention, is formed. The desire is formed by the purposive system. How an intention is initially formed is not known, but intentions, once formed, can be associated with affect patterns in the same way that spatial coordinates are associated with motor patterns. The control process for associating intentions with affects is innate. It is done automatically. Once stored, the affect patterns become the triggers for the associated intentions. When a hungry child sees a bottle, for example, the hunger affect and sight of the bottle triggers the intention to grab. The intention is routed to the global control store where the associated control program for grabbing is accessed. The grabbing program comprises the control patterns for routing the coordinates and characteristics of the desired object— the bottle—to the motor store for analysis and for recalling an associated motor pattern from the motor store and orchestrating it. The motor store analyzes the incoming spatial patterns and recalls associated motor patterns. When recalled, the associated motor patterns control the movement. That is, when the motor pattern is orchestrated, the child reaches for the bottle.

STAGES OF LEARNING

A child is able to learn because the brain is endowed with certain prewired control functions and capabilities. However, while some of them are available at birth, others only become available later during the child's normal cognitive development. This section reviews Piaget's developmental stages of cognition and serves as a focus for the remainder of the chapter. My discussion is not intended to assert the correctness of Piaget's theory nor to suggest that other theories are incorrect. My goal is only to relate *general* principles of acquiring knowledge to the computational and storage systems described in this book. A computational theory of human development would require a detailed under-standing of all underlying systems and their control functions; we simply do not have that knowledge at the present time. A computational theory of human cognitive development, in particular, would require a detailed understanding of how specific concepts (physical, numerical, logical) are represented and manipulated. Once again, we simply do not have sufficient knowledge for such a theory.

Piaget studied the development of cognitive capabilities in children and suggested that a child's normal cognitive development can be roughly divided into four stages: (1) sensory-motor (from birth to about 1½ or 2 years of age);

(2) preoperational thought (from about 2 to about 7 years of age); (3) concrete operations (from about 7 to about 11); and (4) formal operations (from about 11 to about 16). The following sections consider those stages of development.

Sensory-Motor Development

During the sensory-motor stage, the child learns to recognize objects and to control his or her hands and body. Hence he or she learns to initiate actions. He or she develops his or her spatial model of the world, begins to understand the concept of time, and begins to develop the ability to create and manipulate mental images. During the preoperational thought stage, the child learns to manipulate internal representations, to classify objects and actions based on perceptual attributes, and to understand local consistency. The child learns to think logically, and is able to follow a train of thought. However, the child is unable to return to a previous step in a thought sequence. The child understands certain physical concepts, such as height and weight, but he or she cannot grasp more complex concepts, such as the conservation of mass.[6] During the concrete operations stage, the child is able to grasp the conservation of mass. He or she learns to manipulate numbers (sequences of symbols), and learns simple abstractions. Finally, during the formal operations stage, the child gains the full, logical capabilities of the adult. Thus he or she learns how to form implications, to form and evaluate mental hypotheses, and to perform complex abstractions.

The development of each of these capabilities demands that the preceding stages in development have already been initiated. They need not be fully developed, however, and once a child begins to use a particular mental capability, he or she can continue to develop it throughout life. On the other hand, if a capability remains unused during a critical period when it first becomes available, the system atrophies and its use appears to be precluded thereafter. For example, a child who does not develop stereo vision by the age of 6 will never develop stereo vision.

Referring now to the networks described in this book, each of the storage networks illustrated in Figures 17.1 and 17.2 become operational at a different stage in a child's development. The sensory buffers, low-level sensory stores, stores of experience, and motor stores are first to develop. They hold low-level representations and associations between low-level sensory patterns and low-level motor patterns. Moreover, because the low-level sensory stores are used to convert low-level representations into high-level representations, the low-level sensory stores *must* acquire stored information before the high-level stores can do so.

---

[6]When water is poured from a narrow, tall glass into a wide, short glass, the height of the water decreases. The child senses that there was more liquid in the tall glass.

Before a low-level store can create a high-level representation, it must store the low-level representations (a similarity pattern) of the objects and their features. (For the auditory system, tokens of sound such as phonemes, words, musical chords, and so forth, are the objects.) Each low-level representation is a template which occupies a particular spatial location in the memory store. Whenever an input pattern arrives at the memory store, it is analyzed. That is, it is matched against every stored pattern—every template—to determine **perceptual** similarity. The resulting pattern of similarity signals is the basis for forming a high-level representation of the current input. A high similarity value in the similarity pattern designates a storage location which contains similar stored information. Thus the high-level pattern describes the input pattern by indicating where similar patterns are stored. It is an **index pattern** for associated low-level information. To create a high-level representation, entries in the correlation pattern are locally combined (for example, averaged) and a subpattern is selected. The high-level representation created by the low-level store consists of the selected subpattern together with the control pattern, which indicates how the selection was made.

Note that if the low-level memory store is empty, all correlation values will be random and the resulting high-level representation will convey no information. It will be meaningless. Also, if the memory store is not empty but does not contain any patterns which are similar to the current input pattern, once again all correlation values will be random and the resulting high-level representation will be meaningless. Thus a high-level representation can only be created if the low-level store contains patterns which match the salient features of objects in the environment—features that the child will automatically select when he or she looks around or listens to sounds.

When a low-level memory store does not produce any high correlation values, the resulting high-level representation is meaningless and the current *novel* input patterns must be stored in the low-level store. The novel input becomes a template for future analysis. The lack of familiarity of the stimulus—its novelty—is exactly what the prewired control system detects when controlling the store. When the surroundings are unfamiliar, the control system stores salient features in the low-level sensory stores, and only when the low-level stores are rich with feature templates can high-level representations be formed. At that time, the low-level store does not store new templates and therefore the low-level features do not enter consciousness. They are not noticed.

Adults as well as children experience unfamiliar situations from time to time and store feature templates as a result. When an individual travels to a foreign country where the facial features of the natives are significantly different from those in his or her own culture, he or she finds it very difficult to distinguish one person from another. They all look the same. Once the facial features have been studied and templates for them have become part of the low-level storage system, then high-level representations can be made and stored. It is then that the people look familiar and can be distinguished from one another. The features, no longer noticed, are processed by the low-level store as it automatically creates the desired high-level representation.

When a person is in a familiar place, the high-level representations generated by his or her sensory systems have many values which indicate similarity. It is then that one no longer needs to pay attention to details, and by not paying attention to details, new low-level representations are not formed. If, for some reason, an unfamiliar object is noticed, its low-level sensory representation is stored and that memory of the experience indicates how it differed from prior experiences. Thus the high-level representation encodes an experience by specifying where the records of similar experiences are stored and how the records of the current experience differs from them. This is how the high-level representation indexes the low-level store.

What is true for one low-level sensory store is also true for another. For example, foreigners speaking in an unfamiliar language sound funny—unrecognizable—as if they were speaking with random noises. The low-level networks do not have the necessary templates to convert the low-level auditory representation into a recognizable (distinguishable) form: Hence the sounds cannot be recognized as meaningful.[7] The stores which hold the low-level representations must contain appropriate templates in order to segment the current incoming sounds and create a storage representation which can be recognized by the high-level stores.

A similar argument pertains to the low-level motor stores,. those which hold the patterns that regulate the muscles. The low-level motor stores hold associations between spatial patterns and motor patterns which achieve them. If those associations are not present, spatial information cannot be used to control the body.

During Piaget's sensory-motor stage of development, the low-level sensory stores consolidate templates for segmenting the sensory inputs while the low-level motor stores consolidate associations between spatial patterns and motor patterns for controlling configurations and changes in configurations. The development of the spatial system and the control programs which utilize it are therefore essential for motor control. Since the spatial system comprises spatial memory, the sensory-motor system, and a major portion of the visual system, learning basic sensory and motor skills parallels the development of the spatial system.

---

[7]In order to understand a language, not only must the words be recognized, which implies the existence of templates for the constituent phonemes, but the words must be associated with their meanings and the sentences must be associated with programs for their meanings as well. The description presented here refers to word recognition only.

Preoperational Thought

Once the low-level sensory stores have incorporated a sufficient number of templates to segment the visual and auditory fields, and once the stores of experience have stored suitably many experiences, the child is ready to access experiences based on external reminders of them. Thus an object or affect may bring to mind an experience. Note that at this stage of development, the control patterns that control reminding are innate and events are brought to mind without conscious intent. Even so, the control patterns are stored in the global control store and associated with affect patterns or other patterns which will enable them to be recalled and orchestrated again at a later time. The associated patterns become the intentions to perform the corresponding mental operation—such as remembering—and the child gains control of his or her own memories and thoughts by this mechanism. That is, the child learns how to control his or her thoughts intentionally: how to recall events and how to manipulate their representations.

At first, representations of concrete objects (for example, visual or auditory representations, or smells) initiate recall which in turn initiates a behavior. In time, as the child learns to manipulate thoughts intentionally, he or she is able to control the associations between representations which relate concepts in the mind. Perceptually similar objects become associated, objects which are used together (e.g., tools in the kitchen) become associated, and objects which occur in the same place (toys, clothes, etc.) become associated. Thus the child learns how to access a variety of representations based only on one of them. In short, the child learns how to classify objects based on perceptual attributes, physical proximity, or temporal contiguity.

As the child manipulates the representations of objects, the representations activate additional representations. Thus the child learns to generate sequences of associations, a preliminary stage in the development of logical thought. (Note that short sequences are stored in individual memory locations as a consequence of the biological structure of memory. This process differs from storing sequences of associations in contiguous memory locations of the memory store so they can be accessed sequentially.)

During preoperational thought, the global control store begins to incorporate the control patterns which regulate the low-level stores and information processing networks. Thus the child learns to perform certain well-defined sequences of mental operations (which may control physical actions as well). The stored control patterns for these sequences are mental procedures or programs of thought and include grabbing objects, crawling toward objects, playing with toys, and so forth. In time, names will be associated with these control patterns (crawling, playing, etc.) and the symbolic system will be able to manipulate them as easily as it does symbolic tokens or icons, but this does not happen at the present stage of development.

Mental procedures are not only associated with the perceptual patterns which initiated them (for example, the sound of the mother telling the child to do something), but they are also associated with the affect patterns which were present before and after they were executed. (Keep in mind the fact that affect patterns are stored with sensory representations as well.) The affect patterns therefore bias the availability of stored mental procedures, as I explained in the previous chapter, and different mental procedures become available, depending on the affect state (e.g., mood) of the child. The other associated patterns become the intentions for performing the corresponding mental procedure.

As the child's mental capabilities develop further, that is, as he or she stores and utilizes more and more mental procedures for controlling the mental apparatus and thoughts, he or she learns to manipulate internal representations instead of performing the corresponding physical actions. In short, the child learns to think logically (although simplistically at this stage) and to follow a train of thought. Still, he or she has not yet developed the ability to interrupt the train of thought and back up to a prior stage from which to progress forward again.

Concrete Operations

Before a child can manipulate symbols instead of objects, he or she must associate the symbols with the objects they represent. Moreover, the child must store appropriate mental procedures to manipulate the representations. For physical objects, the associations are made early and the child, using spatial memory, manipulates icons instead of the objects themselves.

Attributes of objects and processes are much harder to name than the objects themselves, either because the networks that create the representations mature later or because the representations are based on a computational ability which has not yet developed. For example, a child learns to name colors much later than shapes. This suggests that the circuits which extract the representation of a color and focus the attention on it develop later then circuits which store pictorial representations.

Counting is a much more complicated process and therefore develops later in life. In order to count, the child must learn to shift the focus of attention from one object being counted to the next while at the same time access the next token in the sequence "one, two, three, ..." (I am distinguishing counting from naming the number of objects in a collection by pattern matching.) Thus counting requires the child to control his or her focus of attention at the same time he or she controls memory accesses. Both processes must have been previously learned, which makes counting substantially more difficult than either process alone.

Naming spatial relationships is harder than naming shapes and therefore occurs at a later stage in a child's cognitive development. Determining relationships such as "to the left of," "above," and "inside" requires the naming of patterns which control the focus of attention. The patterns which control the focus of attention must therefore be learned before the spatial relationships can be named. For example, determining "to the left of" requires that the control pattern which shifts the visual focus from right to left be recognized by the naming store in a storage location which associates it with the token "left." Since the brain stores and recognizes perceptual representations long before it stores and recognizes control patterns, naming spatial relationships develops later in a child's life than shape recognition.

Controlling spatial memory is necessary for manipulating icons. For example, spatial memory can be used to represent objects which have a constant area, but in order to conserve area when manipulating a mental image, special control patterns must be used. Storing and then learning to manipulate spatial control patterns is an ability which does not develop until a child is 7 or 8 years old. It develops during the concrete operations stage, and hence the young child is incapable of understanding a principle such as the conservation of mass (Inhelder & Piaget, 1964). (The child can memorize a statement for the conservation of mass, but until the principle is associated with control patterns that properly manipulate representations in spatial memory, until the principle becomes operational, it is not understood.)

Formal Operations

A child learns to manipulate the environment at an early age. Thus he or she gains control of the spatial system at an early age. The ability to use the symbolic system is slower to develop. I have already indicated that symbolic operations very often utilize the spatial system, so the spatial system must develop first. In addition, many symbolic operations are sequential. Hence the child must learn to manipulate trains of thought before he or she can process logical implications. Symbolic operations develop very late, precisely because so many low-level systems must develop first in order to have the required mental capacity to process complex logical relationships.

Various fields of study such, as artificial intelligence, are right now addressing questions relating to complex mental activities, such as how the laws of physics are represented, how the imagery system is controlled, and how the spatial and verbal systems interact during ordinary thought processes. There is much yet to be learned, and we are only now beginning to understand the computational structure of complex thought.

ADAPTIVE PROCESSES IN LEARNING

For all practical purposes, the storage systems of the brain have an unlimited capacity for storing new information. Each individual's focus of attention—

those events which he or she chooses to attend—are permanently stored throughout a lifetime. When he or she pays attention to what he or is doing, the motor patterns which control movements are permanently stored. When one scrutinizes unfamiliar symbols on a page of hieroglyphics, those unfamiliar patterns become permanent templates for future visual analysis. When one listens to unfamiliar musical sounds, those symphonic patterns are permanently stored.

If all stored experiences were equally available for recall, if all stored motor programs were equally available for orchestration, if all stored templates were used simultaneously when segmenting the visual field, or if all auditory templates were used when listening to a friend talk, the brain would confront a hopeless computational nightmare of choices for each intended act. But we know this does not generally happen. Only selected memories ever come to mind and when controlling movements, only selected motor programs are available for orchestration. In Chapter 15 I described how the motor system restricted access to selected motor programs.

Each memory store restricts access to its stored patterns—its memories or motor programs—by two fundamental methods. First, in order to access a memory location, it must be activated. It is activated by associations which take place during an appropriate interval of time before the desired access. Controlling this time interval can be used to restrict or limit access to the stored memories. Second, the mechanism for activating storage locations is adaptive. The conditions which are sufficient to activate a storage location at one time may change and no longer be sufficient to activate it at a later time. While learning, the storage access parameters are modified to facilitate or deter access to selected traces. For example, memories which are recalled often become easier and easier to access while those which are rarely recalled are forgotten—they are made difficult to access.

The affect system determines the initial access parameters for each stored item. When we are interested in something or it is important to survival (and hence interesting), the access parameters are set so that the memories are easy to recall. If, on the other hand, we are uninterested, the access parameters are set so that the memories are difficult to recall. I tend to be uninterested in gossip and forget very quickly almost everything told to me. On the other hand, when an item of gossip is repeated, I immediately know I heard it before. The same is true for names, although some stick in my mind forever.

Psychologists have long been studying memory, and there are now hundreds of books on the subject. However, because of the number of storage systems involved, the complexity of their interaction, the complexity of their control systems, and the modifiability of their access parameters, it is often unclear exactly what it is that the psychologist is measuring. In view of our increasing understanding of the computational and storage structures of the human brain, a careful reassessment of much of the memory literature is warranted.

SUMMARY

There are three major computational systems of the brain: the spatial system (which includes most of the sensory and motor subsystems), the symbolic system (which includes the speech apparatus), and the purposive system (which includes the affect system). These systems interact continually in virtually all mental activities and are subservient to the purposive system for planning and controlling decisions.

The cognitive development of the various subsystems generally progresses in an orderly manner. Those systems closest to the external world—the sensory and motor systems—develop first while those which manipulate high-level representations develop later. Whereas some of the control functions for the various systems are prewired, later in life most of the prewired functions can also be learned and stored in the global control stores. Thus instinctive behaviors can be replaced by learned behaviors. Instinctive behaviors only surface during critical situations, and when that happens we say that the individual is "behaving in an irrational way" or he is "acting like a child." When a particular behavior is elicited automatically by a sensory event, it is a reflex, and many reflexes are learned as the cognitive apparatus develops. Mental defense mechanisms, for example, are reflex actions learned at an early age and set into action automatically when triggered by an emotional or stressful situation.

Learning is the modification of behavior caused by four types of changes to the mental apparatus. (1) Storage of new memory traces, (2) modifications to the storage access parameters, (3) storage of new high-level control procedures (programs of thought), and (4) modifications to the memory traces themselves. Because numerous systems and access parameters change, even for the simplest learned activity, little can be said at present to relate the various psychological studies of learning and memory to the computational understanding of the underlying systems described here. In time, a reevaluation of the classical learning literature must be undertaken.

REFERENCES

Broadmann, K. (1914). Physiologie des Gehirns. In Die allgemeine Chirurgie der Gehirnkrankheiten. Neue Deutsche Chirurgie, Vol. 11. Verlag Ferdinand Enke, Stuttgart.

———(1925). Vergleichende Lokalisationslehre der Groshimrinde. Leipzig: Johann Ambrosuis Barth.

Damasio, A. R. (1985). Prosopagnosia. Trends in Neuroscience, 8, 132–135.

Damasio, A. R., Damasio, H., & Van Hoesen, G. W. (1982). Prosopagnosia: anatomic basis and behavioral mechanisms. Neurology, 32, 331–341.

Faught, W. S. (1977). Motivation and intensionality in a computer simulation model. Stanford Artificial Intelligence Memo AIM-305, September 1977, Computer Science Department, Stanford University, Stanford CA.

Inhelder, B., & Piaget, J. (1964). The early growth of logic in the child. Classification and seriation. New York: W. W. Norton.

503

Kleist, K. (1934). *Gehirnpathologie*. Leipzig: Barth.

Kolb, B., & Whishaw, I. Q. (1985). *Fundamentals of human neuropsychology (2d ed.)*. New York: W. H. Freeman.

Krieg, W. J. S. (1966). *Functional neuroanatomy (3d ed.)*. Evanston, IL: Brain Books.

Luria, A. R. (1966). *Higher cortical functions in man*. New York: Basic Books.

―――(1980). *Higher cortical functions in man (2nd ed.), revised and explained*. New York: Basic Books.

―――(1973). *The Working Brain. An Introduction to Neuropsychology*. New York: Basic Books Inc..

O'Keefe, J., & Nadel, L. (1978). *The hippocampus as a cognitive map*. Oxford: Clarendon Press.

Piaget, J. (1971). *Biology and knowledge*. Chicago: University of Chicago Press.

Polyak, S. L. (1957). *The vertebrate visual system*. Chicago, IL: University of Chicago Press.

Popper, K. R., & Eccles, J. C. (1977). *The self and its brain*. New York: Springer International.

Springer, S. P., & Deutsch, G. (1985). *Left brain, right brain*. New York: W. H. Freeman.

POSTSCRIPT

The human brain is a computer, and my goal was to tell you how it processes information. Unfortunately, I only partly succeeded. As you must know by now, we are still a long way from a detailed understanding of the logic of the human brain. Many questions remain unanswered, and my goal here is to ask some of them as a guide to future research and experimentation. What we discover is influenced by what we are looking for, and we are just now learning what to look for.

NEURONS AND NEURAL ACTIVITY

At the present time neurons appear to be the principal computational components of the brain. Still, interactions between neurons and glial cells appear to be crucial to memory function. A considerable effort should be devoted to studying these interactions in hopes of finding the elusive "memory timing mechanism," which converts dynamic patterns into static patterns and vice versa.

The neuron is generally considered to be the smallest computational unit in the brain. Yet, neuroscientists have recently discovered that in some cases parts of neurons, microcircuits, rather than neurons in their entirety enter into computations. If this is so, then the fact that there are roughly one hundred billion neurons may no longer limit our understanding of brain function. In which neural circuits do subneural interactions determine computations? How many computational circuits can distinct neurons entertain? Are the microcircuits of a single cell capable of coordinating different aspects of the same computation or of different computations? Can a single neuron do all the processing of a storage location? Can a single neuron do all the processing of a mathematical computation such as tensor or quaternion multiplication? How does the activity of the neuron that entertains microcircuits affect the computations they perform?

505

From a computational point of view, neurons may be classified according to the function they perform: transforming sensory and control patterns, regulating computations, or initiating biochemical changes (either temporary or permanent). I have called these logical modes of processing transformational, control, and effectual. So far, most laboratory studies have focused on transformational coupling. How does the activity in one set of neurons regulate transmission of information along neural pathways? How does activity in one set of neurons cause temporary or permanent changes in the coupling parameters of other neurons?

The hippocampus has been implicated either as the system that sends the "store now" commands to the stores of experience or as a system along the pathway of control. (This is in addition to other possible functions.) Since the signals it sends initiate consolidation either directly or indirectly, it must either release or cause the release of effectual neurotransmitters. In particular, the target systems of hippocampal outputs are likely to be the systems which permanently store our experiences and the dendritic membranes of the cells that receive the signals are likely to be the sites of the memory traces themselves. Are there, in fact, outputs from the hippocampus whose neurotransmitters differ from other neurotransmitters, and if so, are they effectual neurotransmitters? What are the target cells of hippocampal outputs and what are their synaptic structures? How do their neurotransmitters operate and what part of the target cell is affected?

FAN-IN AND FAN-OUT OF INFORMATION

Distribution or fan-out of information from one neuron to other neurons appears to be unlimited while fan-in appears to be limited to a few thousand inputs in one stage of processing.[1] many times that number of memory locations, and a much higher degree of fan-in (from the memory locations to the output pathway) is therefore essential. Are special types of synaptic contacts (e.g., axo-axonal) used in this regard? If not, how is fan-in implemented? One place to look for special fan-in circuitry is within the layers of myelinated axons in the cerebral cortex. Yet, essentially all studies of the cerebral cortex have focused on its cross section, not sections parallel to its surface. Detailed anatomical studies of the cortex in such planes should therefore be undertaken.

COMPUTATION AND ITS ARCHITECTURE

In some processing systems, computation is combined with structure in an inseparable way. Two examples within the sensory systems are: (1) the analysis of a sound pattern into its frequencies by the cochlea, and (2) the conversion of

---

[1]Fan-in for cerebellar Purkinje cells is estimated to be as high as 200,000 to one, but this is the exception rather than the rule

a retinal image into its complex logarithmic representation by the optic pathways.

What other structural transformations are performed on sensory patterns? For example, what is the nature of the tactile and kinesthetic representations? Are any other transformations performed by the visual system? In particular, the fact that we are able to compensate for perspective when we see a flat surface which is not oriented perpendicular to our line of sight suggests a system which can perform arbitrary perspective or affine transformations on the retinal patterns. What is the anatomy of a network which can perform affine transformations? How are they performed? How are the parameters of the transformation controlled? As a corollary to the above, we are able to recognize symmetries in the visual field even though the retinal projections are not symmetrical. For example, a door appears symmetrical even when seen from an oblique angle. Moreover, when we look at a door, half of it is seen by the left side of the brain and the other half is seen by the right side. Apparently, the corpus callosum plays an essential role in our ability to perceive symmetries and hence determine the parameters of the affine transformations performed prior to visual recognition. What computational architecture allows this type of analysis? Does the fact that each half of the brain processes half of the retinal image play a crucial role in its analysis?

ANALOG VERSUS DIGITAL COMPUTATIONS

Both analog and digital processes are evident in brain function. Neural interactions are for the most part analog. They rely on the stochastic depolarizations caused by diffusion and deactivation of chemical transmitters, movements of sodium and potassium ions, and so forth. On the other hand, bistable circuits allow some neurons to remain either "on" or "off" and to be turned "off" on demand. These bistable circuits might be used to activate memory locations and provide discrete, hence digital, control over particular memories. What are the biological mechanisms which underlie bistable circuits? In what parts of the brain are bistable circuits found? How long do neurons stay "on," and once "on," what turns them "off?" Do their frequencies vary when they are "on," and if so, how?

THE MATHEMATICS OF THE MIND

One of the principal tools for describing the computations of the mind is mathematics, and as you have seen, many different mathematical descriptions are necessary for understanding different aspects of brain function. For example, complex analysis, affine transformations, and Fourier analysis are all important tools for understanding the visual system; matrices, tensors, and quaternions are crucial to our understanding of spatial processing and the control of movement, and statistics and calculus are fundamental for understanding neural interactions. Are other branches of mathematics important? Within the branches of mathematics already considered, are there simplifying assumptions that can make our understanding of human computation clearer? Can an understanding of the underlying computations benefit our understanding of the biological mechanisms which implement them?

INFORMATION

Information has meaning because neural networks are designed to process it in a well-defined way. Static information patterns are spatial arrangements of molecules in neural networks and dynamic information patterns are movements of molecules, hence waves of activity, in neural networks. It is only because neural networks are designed to process patterns in specific ways that they, the arrangements of molecules or the waves of activity, convey meaning. Thus structure—the neural networks and their coupling parameters—and function—the way the networks encode, store, and process patterns—cannot be understood independently.

Static patterns are representations that are encoded at the molecular level in cell membranes, where they determine the coupling parameters, hence computational properties, of the neurons and networks that contain them. How are static patterns encoded by the neurons of the storage networks? How and when do static patterns change? What biochemical mechanisms initiate the changes?

Dynamic patterns transmit and transform information and initiate actions in the systems they are sent to. The initiated actions may be computational, structural, or physical depending on whether the neural networks that receive them are computational networks, storage systems, or muscles. How are dynamic patterns encoded? Are the encodings different for different sensory modalities? Are different representations of the same modality encoded in different ways? Although these are the questions I have addressed throughout this book, nonetheless significant laboratory research is necessary before a detailed understanding will be found.

OBJECTS

An object is an individual, distinguishable entity. We perceive objects. We manipulate them with our hands and we manipulate their representations in our minds. We do not, in general, manipulate pictures of objects. When we perceive a book, a toy, or a pet, we create a mental representation in which the selected object is represented, not the scene, not its background, not a two-dimensional view of it. How are objects represented? How is their three-dimensional structure encoded? What kinds of networks manipulate object representations? What enables us to see them in our minds? How do we integrate their representations with our current world model? How are their physical properties encoded and manipulated? For example, when we imagine dropping a ball on the ground, what we imagine depends on whether the ball is rubber, made of clay, or glass!

We are able to manipulate the representations of several objects at the same time, and we are able to imagine interactions between them just as if the objects themselves were present. In short, we are able to simulate physical interactions in our minds. The mental mechanisms which simulate physical interactions enable us to understand gears and pulleys, chain reactions, and physical causes and effects. Why is there a limit to the number of objects we can imagine at one time? When we mentally manipulate objects, do we manipulate their representations in spatial memory or do we manipulate individual representations in object buffers? How do we project the manipulated representation from an object buffer into spatial memory so the object can be seen in the mind's eye? What part of the brain performs the simulations and what part of the brain controls them? What computations underlie the simulations and what mathematics describes them? Do the same systems simulate interactions between objects that maintain the body posture model? If different systems are used, how do they differ?

MAINTAINING A WORLD MODEL

Each of us maintains an up-to-date internal model of the world, which is updated whenever we move or objects in the world move. As an example, when we drive through unfamiliar territory, we create our own mental model of the territory. Now suppose that some event occurs which requires that we turn around and go back to where we came from. (We might just have passed a gas station and decide to go back and buy gas.) The world remains familiar and things that were selected for the focus of attention remain where we saw them even though they are now seen from a different position and orientation. What is the organization of the temporary memory stores which enables this type of processing? How much information is actually stored and what type is it? Are there differences in the way representations are made and manipulated if the territory is familiar or very familiar—traveled daily? When in unfamiliar territory, what features attract the attention? When in familiar territory, is our scan driven by our experience or do perceptual features attract our attention as they do in unfamiliar territory?

Each of us has a navigational system which maintains the spatial coordinates of the places and objects we have seen. Are the memories used for navigation the same as those of experience? Are navigational memories made only when exploring new territory or are they updated at other times? If at other times, when and why?

PERCEPTUAL AND CONTROL HIERARCHIES

Associative storage networks automatically compare incoming patterns with all previously stored patterns. This means that if a storage network comprises a million memory locations, then a million comparisons are made simultaneously and they are all available in real time. Similarity signals, which indicate the results of the comparisons, may activate memory locations containing similar stored patterns. This makes the stored memories available for recall. At the same time, the resulting similarity pattern represents the input and varies more slowly than it did. In particular, the similarity pattern indicates where related low-level patterns are stored and therefore is an index into the lower-level store for related information. Of what theoretical utility are these index patterns? Sentence patterns are one example, and I have already described how they can be used to access the mental procedures which are stored in conceptual memory. Hence sentence patterns are an index into the mental procedures that are stored there. Are there similar representations at other levels in the hierarchy? For example, the similarity patterns generated by the stores of visual and auditory information may be used to index similar experiences. They can therefore be used to regulate access to related experiences. Are these similarity patterns used in the same way that sentence patterns are used? If so, what is the nature of the information they index? Are there limitations on the way access can be regulated? How does the organization of stored information influence the control structure of the memory store? What do the index patterns of experience correspond to psychologically? Of what significance are the index patterns to the store that holds the index patterns of experience? How does this hierarchy generalize?

The associative storage networks form a hierarchy in which low-level (sensory) patterns are stored at the bottom of the hierarchy while high-level (control) patterns are stored at the top. The temporal characteristics of the representations stored at each level in the hierarchy differ; rapidly varying patterns are stored at low levels while slowly varying patterns are stored at high levels. What is the exact nature of the hierarchy? How many levels are there in the hierarchy? Are there different levels, depending on the modality or system? What representations are stored at each level in the hierarchy? How are the levels determined, and when?

Now consider the hierarchy beginning at the top level and progressing downward. The highest level holds representations of concepts and intentions which vary slowly and last a long time. Mental procedures are an example. High-level representations regulate the lower-level networks by restricting and enabling access to specific memories. The patterns stored at one level in the control hierarchy vary more slowly than the patterns at the next lower level, and they last longer. They are used by the lower level networks to gain access to patterns which are still lower in the hierarchy until, at the lowest level of control, they regulate a computational network, a storage system, or the muscles. How do the control mechanisms used at each level differ? For example, the high-level control patterns initiate activities which last a long time (e.g., a visual search, an intention to type a letter), whereas the low-level control patterns vary rapidly and last a short time (e.g., a ballistic movement). Are different biological mechanisms used at each level, and if so, what are they? How are control patterns from different origins integrated? For example, when we speak our entire breathing apparatus is affected. Thus signals which regulate vocalization and those which regulate blood levels of oxygen and carbon dioxide must be combined in an appropriate way. What are the mechanisms? Which system dominates in the control, and how and when does control switch between the systems?

The psychological correlates of the patterns processed at each level in the hierarchy are well understood. At the bottom of the hierarchy are sensory patterns—the representations of sounds, sights, smells, touch, and affects. These are the direct encodings of sensory experiences. At the next level are canonical storage representation. These representations encode salient features of the items they represent: color and texture, surface orientation, position (with respect to a suitable coordinate system), and movement of objects; pitch, timbre, and location of sound sources; and so forth. Patterns representing words occur at this level as do patterns representing the spatial structures of objects— their connectivity. How is information about spatial structure encoded? How are the storage representations used to guide the visual or tactile analysis of an object? What are the mathematics of the transformations?

At the next higher level are patterns representing concepts. The spatial system retains spatial relationships between objects while the symbolic system maintains organized sequences of symbolic tokens. Sentence patterns are one example at this level in the hierarchy. Notice that each representation varies more slowly than its predecessors. What are the time constants in this hierarchy? How many levels does it have? Do the number of levels differ for different individuals? Do the number of levels differ as a function of intelligence? Moving still higher are patterns representing sequences of relationships—hence relationships between relationships. What are they? Whereas memories of experience are stored at one level in the hierarchy, access patterns which identify related experiences are stored at the next higher level in the hierarchy. This progresses upward until high-level concepts such as intentions are stored.

At the highest level, slowly varying affect patterns are also stored and are used by the purposive system when it selects which intention to carry out. Do the similarity signals at each level in the hierarchy give rise to different sensations of familiarity? Does storage of information at each level of the hierarchy give rise to a different level of consciousness? What are the attention processes at each level in the hierarchy, and how do they differ? What are the access control functions at each level in the hierarchy, and how do they differ? How is information at each level organized? What determines the organization? How does the organization affect intelligence? Performance? Recall ability?

SPECIFYING MENTAL PROCEDURE

Consider now the memories which encode mental procedures. Each mental procedure specifies a sequence of mental (or physical) events which must be performed, and hence each element in the sequence initiates a particular pattern of control. How are mental procedures specified? What types of mental events can be controlled? How do they control particular mental events? How do the control processes differ at each level in the control hierarchy? Under what conditions can mental events be terminated, and how are the conditions specified? How are active mental events terminated? How is control transferred from one element of a mental procedure to the next? How are mental procedures interrupted? Once interrupted, how are they restarted?

The initiation of a mental procedure constitutes a form of discrete control which continues until the lowest level in the control hierarchy where, once again, muscle actions are best understood in terms of forces and tensions, which are analog quantities. It follows that the way we choose to describe the computation depends on the structure of the system, the computation it performs, and the representation it uses. What are the best descriptive mechanisms for understanding mental procedures? Do they differ from level to level in the hierarchy?

PREDICTIONS

Survival depends on how well we predict what is going to happen, both in the immediate future and in the distant future. Predictions take on many forms. Sometimes predictions are in the form of wishful thinking. We create hopes and expectations about the future, and those hopes and expectations guide our behavior. Sometimes predictions are in the form of guesses—both educated guesses and gut feelings. When playing a game like poker, we guess at our opponent's holdings and bet accordingly, based on the statistics of card distributions. When we decide whether or not to trust a stranger we often do so based on our gut feelings about the individual. Sometimes predictions automatically come to mind. When listening to a favorite phonograph record, we often start to hum the next song before it starts to play. We predict what song will play. What mechanisms account for our predictions? How do the mechanisms differ for predictions having different temporal scope—hopes and expectations, guesses, reminding? How do we assign likelihoods to our predictions and how does our behavior differ for different degrees of likelihood?

MEMORY AND LEARNING

I have shown that learning is not the result of simple changes to a single adaptive system, but rather, it is the result of many different types of changes to many independent, yet interrelated, subsystems. Learning includes the storage of new memories, the storage of new mental procedures, and the adaptation of parameters throughout the various participating subsystems. How can the various component changes that take place while learning be distinguished? How can learning experiments be devised so that changes can be restricted to a single subsystem? For example, can we devise experiments where new memory traces are made but access parameters to old traces remain unchanged? Can we devise experiments so that "learning" takes place without the making of new memory traces? Can we devise experiments which depend only on the existence of permanent memories, not on the existence of temporary memories? Can we devise experiments which do not depend on attention processes such as visual or auditory selection?

CLINICAL STUDIES

Numerous studies have been performed by clinicians on patients prior to surgery. These studies have given invaluable insights into the nature of stored experiences. Numerous additional studies should be performed which would give additional evidence both for the organization of the storage systems and the organization of information within them.

Studies of the speech areas have shown that associations exist between sensory representations and symbolic representations. However, these studies have been restricted for the most part to having the patient identify objects when presented visually. (The patient reads written text accompanying the pictures to distinguish between speech arrest produced by the stimulation and aphasia produced by the stimulation.) Similar studies should be performed to investigate naming colors, naming spatial relationships, naming size, naming orientation, naming location, naming relative position, and so forth. Each of these attributes has a different underlying computation and so one would expect the cortical organization to depend on the underlying system and how it supplies inputs to the naming stores. Are memory locations for naming spatial relationships found together with memory locations for naming objects? Colors? Sizes? Are memory stores for identifying faces in one place? Are the naming stores organized by category, pictorial similarity, or what? What about naming sounds—how and where are the naming stores located? What about naming body parts by tactile stimulation?

Similar studies could be performed to determine the locus of higher cognitive functions. For example, the parietal cortex is known to be involved in spatial processing. In what ways would stimulating the parietal cortex degrade spatial abilities? What is the nature of the degradation—conceptual or motor control? Patients having syndromes in which spatial abilities are affected often have difficulties processing logical-grammatical relationships. Can this type of difficulty be induced by cortical stimulation? How localized are the systems which process spatial and logical-grammatical relationships?

Similar questions can also be asked regarding programs of thought. In what way does stimulating the frontal cortex degrade higher cognitive functions? Are mental procedures for spatial processing stored in the same regions of the cortex as mental procedures for symbolic thought? Are they stored in the same hemisphere or in opposite hemispheres?

Researchers have developed several different non-invasive techniques for determining which regions of the brain are active during various mental operations. As the techniques are further refined and better techniques developed, it may be possible to monitor the activity in specific networks. Can similar techniques be developed for stimulating parts of the brain—even individual nerve cells—without invading its integrity? If so, the possibilities for future research are endless!

BRAIN AND MIND

The stance I have taken here is that the brain is responsible for all mental activity—consciousness, thinking, remembering, deciding, feeling. Taken together, these are the processes we call the mind. Without the brain there can be no mind.

Moreover, I have suggested that there are physiological correlates between various computational activities and corresponding mental sensations. As one example, I suggested that consciousness is the sensation correlated with the storage of information (e.g., consolidation) in a storage network. Do sensations depend only on neural activity, or do they depend on nonneural phenomena, such as the presence of specific neurotransmitters, activity of glial cells, or activity such as electrostatic or electromagnetic waves generated by neural potentials but existing throughout the neural tissue? Is consciousness a strictly human process or can a computer be conscious? Can a computer have a mind of its own? Suppose that we program a computer to simulate all human capabilities and we endow it with sensors —eyes, ears, tactile receptors, and so forth— similar to those people are endowed with. Suppose, also, that we give it effectors—hands and voice—so it can freely communicate and interact with us. This computer is so well programmed, in fact, that we cannot distinguish it from a human by simply asking it questions or watching its behavior. The computer is programmed to maintain a complete set of affects, and it is able to describe its emotional state just as you and I might describe our own. It is programmed to learn by experience and to forget (not by losing information but by losing access to information). Would it be conscious? Would it have feelings and emotions? Would it have a mind? At the present time we simply do not know enough about human computations to build or program such a computer. Nonetheless, we can ask the question, can a computer have a mind of its own?

AUTHOR INDEX

SUBJECT INDEX